Community Health Nursing

COMMUNITY HEALTH NURSING

Third Edition

Kathleen M. Leahy, M.S., R.N.
Professor Emeritus of Nursing
University of Washington, Seattle

M. Marguerite Cobb, M.N., R.N.
Associate Professor of Nursing
University of Washington, Seattle

Mary C. Jones, M.S., R.N.
Assistant Professor of Nursing
University of Washington, Seattle

McGraw-Hill Book Company
A Blakiston Publication
New York   St. Louis   San Francisco   Auckland
Bogotá   Düsseldorf   Johannesburg   London   Madrid
Mexico   Montreal   New Delhi   Panama   Paris
São Paulo   Singapore   Sydney   Tokyo   Toronto

Notice

Medicine is an ever-changing science. As new research and clinical experience broaden our knowledge, changes in treatment and drug therapy are required. The editors and the publisher of this work have made every effort to ensure that the drug dosage schedules herein are accurate and in accord with the standards accepted at the time of publication. Readers are advised, however, to check the product information sheet included in the package of each drug they plan to administer to be certain that changes have not been made in the recommended dose or in the contraindications for administration. This recommendation is of particular importance in regard to new or infrequently used drugs.

COMMUNITY HEALTH NURSING

This book was set in Times Roman by Black Dot, Inc. The editors were Sally J. Barhydt and Shelly Levine Langman; the cover was designed by Anne Canevari Green; the production supervisor was Angela Kardovich. The drawings were done by Fine Line Illustrations, Inc. Chapter opening drawings were done by Peggy Woerhle.
R. R. Donnelley & Sons Company was printer and binder.

Library of Congress Cataloging in Publication Data

Leahy, Kathleen M.
    Community health nursing.

    "A Blakiston publication."
    Includes bibliographies and index.
    1. Community health nursing. I. Cobb, M. Marguerite, joint author. II. Jones, Mary C., joint author. III. Title. [DNLM: 1. Community health services. 2. Nursing. WY106 L43c]
RT98.L4   1977   610.73'43   76-26946
ISBN 0-07-036832-5

To
Past, present, and future nursing students,
who by their struggles and creative efforts,
inspire teachers to continue on.

To
Kathleen M. Leahy, the senior author,
who by her past and present commitment,
epitomizes community health nursing as it
has been, as it should be, and as it
endeavors to be.

Contents

Preface

This book was written for nursing students beginning their involvement in the community. This step is not easy and requires an assimilation of many ideas and activities which do not initially make sense to the beginning student. Looking at one's own behavior in addition to the client's and family's behavior can be extremely discomforting and sometimes traumatic at first. Coming into a community which we find familiar in some ways because we too grew up in a community, and which we find strange and complex in other ways because people live and interact so differently and incomprehensibly, requires adaptation and flexibility. Making the transition both physically and intellectually from an institutional setting to an amorphouslike community in which people appear, behave, talk, and act normally is distinctly startling and sometimes perplexing for the student starting out in the role of nurse. Learning to reach out, to initiate, to risk, to consent to new patterns of behavior takes courage, conviction, and determination. However, for those students who are willing to try, to experiment, to accept, the rewards are there—waiting to be discovered and treasured.

For male nursing students, please accept our apologies. We know you are among us and endorse your presence as invaluable to our growth and future development as a profession. Throughout the book, the pronoun for the nursing student is consistently stated as *she,* mainly because of expediency. Please mentally read all pronouns as *she* or *he,* whichever fits your own gender. The terms *nurse* and *community health nurse* are used interchangeably throughout the book and are meant to designate male and female nurses who are practicing community health nursing in communities.

For teachers who elect to use this book as a text, it is not meant to be all-inclusive of the field of community health nursing. Many ideas are introduced that, dependent upon the discretion of the teacher, can be expanded upon in depth by lectures, audiovisual media, experiential assignments, library study, additional references, independent study, and current professional literature, not only in nursing and in public health sciences, but in supporting disciplines, such as sociology, psychology, cultural anthropology, and the humanities. The contents of the book are directed mainly to nursing students entering a community, opening their eyes to concepts and facets that exist, suggesting ways to ease entry, alerting them to phenomena for which to be watchful. The book is meant to be used as one of the tools of the teacher for preparing nursing students to perform community health nursing as it should be practiced.

Sincere appreciation is expressed for the cartoons drawn by Margaret (Peggy) R. Woehrle as a means for illuminating the breadth and depth of community health nursing through humor, analogy, and/or intimation. The cartoons were created to depict special aspects of community health nursing as encountered in the real world and touched on within each chapter. It is hoped that they will provide a link for translating textbook learnings into practical insights for real life situations.

We are grateful for the chapter written by Carrie E. Hall. Her expertise and practical knowledge in the field of Epidemiology contributed to the updating of Chapter 10. She generously consented to write the chapter with limited notice and added inestimably to the usefulness of the book.

Again, we are grateful for the written contributions of former nursing students, who, by sharing their feelings and experiences with their nurse instructors, added the extra dimension of humanistic appeal to the book.

Kathleen M. Leahy
M. Marguerite Cobb
Mary C. Jones

Community Health Nursing

Part One

Chapter 1

Stepping into the Community

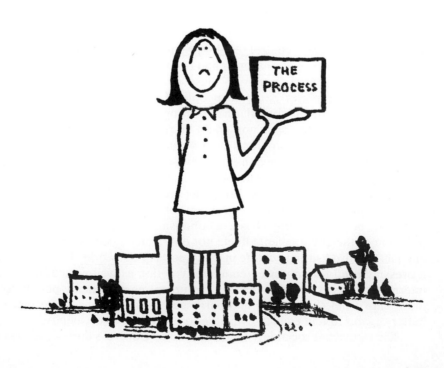

COMMUNITY HEALTH

The promotion and improvement of humankind's total health has a significant bearing on the social revolution now in progress throughout the world (see *The Family of Man*). New thinking and approaches to better health care become mandatory in solving such long-term problems as lack of sanitation, insufficient food and clothing, inadequate housing, and control of communicable diseases and such noncommunicable disease conditions as heart disease, accidents, or disaster. Emerging problems of family pathology, drug abuse and addiction, air and water pollution, polarization of the races, and overpopulation require new methods of solution. Increased scientific knowledge and more imaginative skills and techniques in teaching health care are in order for all community health work.

Community health or public health as a profession had its beginnings about a hundred years ago. Its early responsibility was the control of communicable disease, which was attempted by such measures as control of environment, better sanitation, and strict isolation procedures, particularly for typhoid fever and tuberculosis. As laboratory techniques were developed from increased knowledge of microbiology, earlier diagnoses became possible and medical care became more effective. Other control measures also were developed, such as immunization and the provision of safe water supplies and waste disposal.

Gradually the six basic functions of public health evolved—communicable disease control, environmental sanitation, laboratory services, vital statistics, maternal and child health care, and health education. Public health agencies began to base their programs on these six functions, the emphasis being on people. To carry out these functions effectively school and industrial health programs were developed, since large segments of the population could be reached in this way.

Community health programs built on the six basic functions, including school and industrial health programs, continue to be important, but nearly every nation is experiencing new health hazards that demand fresh approaches to their solutions. Problems stemming from the population explosion include environmental problems of overcrowding, air and water pollution, accidents, drug abuse, alcoholism, and child abuse. Current pollution of the environment affects not only human beings and domestic animals but also fish and wildlife in many parts of the world. This presents a pressing need for concerted community action as well as action on an international basis. Finally, there is the urgent need of many people for more care from the medical and paramedical professions—care that is better organized and equally available to all segments of society.

The significant social legislation passed by Congress during the 1960s and 1970s provided for increased health services and their funding. Examples of this legislation of interest to health workers include:

1 Heart Disease, Cancer, and Stroke Amendments of 1965 (PL 89-239)
2 Health Professions Education Assistance Amendment of 1965 (PL 89-290)
3 The Social Security Amendments Act of 1965 (PL 89-97)
4 The Housing and Urban Development Act of 1965 (PL 89-117)
5 The Comprehensive Health Planning and Public Health Services Amendments of 1966 (PL 89-749) and 1967 (PL 90-174)
6 The Health Planning and Resources Development Act of 1974 (PL 93-641)

Public health appears to be shifting its emphasis to both consumer and environment, accentuating the relationship of the total person to his or her total environment. Underlying this ecologic approach to public health is the vast amount of knowledge that has been accumulated within the past fifty years in the biologic, physical, and social sciences that must be adapted and utilized by the several professions, e.g., medicine, nursing, dentistry, and engineering, in the public health field. The field of public and community health becomes "the meeting ground of all areas of knowledge and professional activity relevant to the health of the public."[1]

COMMUNITY HEALTH NURSING

A description or definition of community health nursing should be based on an understanding and appreciation of the entire spectrum of nursing. Virginia Henderson considers the function of the present-day nurse to be unique. It is, she writes, "to assist the individual, sick or well, in the performance of those activities contributing to health or its recovery (or to peaceful death) that he would perform if he had the necessary strength, will or knowledge. And to do this in such a way as to help him gain independence as rapidly as possible."[2]

Health teaching and counseling and the skilled care of the sick in their homes and other noninstitutionalized centers, by community health nurses from official or voluntary health agencies, is recognized as an essential service in the community's total health program. The nurse functions within the framework of both the nursing and the public health

[1]Hiliary G. Fry, in collaboration with William P. Shepard and Ray H. Elling, Education for Manpower and Community Health, The University of Pittsburgh Press, Pittsburgh, 1967, p. 8.
[2]Virginia Henderson, "The Nature of Nursing," The American Journal of Nursing, 64:64–68, Aug. 1964.

professions, utilizing effectively her knowledge of the content and methods of both professions in her service to the individual, the patient, the family, and the community. There are many definitions of community health nursing, but the most comprehensive definition was established in 1973 by the American Nurses' Association:

> Community Health Nursing is a synthesis of nursing practice and public health practice applied to promoting and preserving the health of populations. The nature of this practice is general and comprehensive. It is not limited to a particular age or diagnostic group. It is continuing, not episodic. The dominant responsibility is to the population as a whole. Therefore, nursing directed to individuals, families, or groups contributes to the health of the total population. Health promotion, health maintenance, health education, coordination and continuity of care are utilized in a holistic approach to the family, group, and community. The nurse's actions acknowledge the need for comprehensive health planning, recognize the influences of social and ecological issues, give attention to populations at risk and utilize the dynamic forces which influence change.[3]

Standards for community health nursing focus on the practice rather than the practitioner and are stated in a systematic approach to nursing practice in areas of assessment, planning, implementation, and evaluation. Based on the above definition, eight standards of community health nursing practice were stated to be:

1   The collection of data about the health status of the consumer is systematic and continuous. The data are accessible, communicated, and recorded.
2   Nursing diagnoses are derived from health status data.
3   Plans for nursing service include goals derived from nursing diagnoses.
4   Plans for nursing service include priorities and nursing approaches or measures to achieve the goals derived from nursing diagnoses.
5   Nursing actions provide for consumer participation in health promotion, maintenance, and restoration.
6   Nursing actions assist consumers to maximize health potential.
7   The consumer's progress toward goal achievement is determined by the consumer and the nurse.
8   Nursing actions involve ongoing reassessment, reordering of priorities, new goal setting, and revision of the nursing plan.[4]

[3]Executive Committee and the Standards Committee of the Division on Community Health Nursing Practice. American Nurses' Association, Kansas City, Mo., 1973.
[4]Ibid.

Philosophy of Community Health Nursing

From the above definition, the philosophy of community health nursing, like that of all nursing, has always been based on the concept of the "worth and dignity of the individual." A hundred years ago, Octavia Hill, a social worker active in slum housing reform, expressed the same idea:

> It is essential to remember that each man has his own view of his life, and must be free to fulfill it; that in many ways he is a far better judge of it than we, as he has lived through and felt what we have only seen. Our work is rather to bring him to the point of considering, and to the spirit of judging rightly, than to consider or judge for him.[5]

Basic to the belief of all nurses is the acceptance that all persons have the capacity and the potential to develop better physical health and improve psychosocial well-being, dependent upon their desires, willingness to change, and adaptability to prescribed therapies. Nursing practice assists individuals and families in adjusting their health needs and wants, resolving health problems in the social, emotional, and physical environments, and facilitating coping abilities to achieve higher levels of wellness.

Family health counseling and primary health-care services appropriate to family and community health nursing practice assist individuals and groups to select, participate in, and evaluate health-related activities. Collaborative liaison actions and appropriate referral to other professionals to maximize patient utilization of health-care services for optimum health underlie all the community health process. As a social activist and consumer advocate, the nurse influences legislation and the legislative process to promote positive individual and collective health.

Each community health nurse develops her own personal philosophy of nursing, tempered by her background, preparation, experience, and personality. Her philosophy will grow and deepen as she acquires experience in working with others—patients, families, communities, and coworkers—and as she adds to her preparation and understanding by continuous study, reading, and thinking. It has been said that "the community health nurse has lots to learn, to teach and to do."

The philosophy that community health nursing is based on "the worth and dignity of the individual" is identified closely with the age-old purpose of nursing, which Marion Sheehan so ably stated to be " . . .caring for, giving comfort and ease, helping persons with health

[5]Octavia Hill, "Through the Ages," *Family Welfare Association of America,* New York, n.d., p. 42.

problems to become healed in body and mind or helping them to live with their infirmities with grace."[6] The nurse who can successfully teach others to "live with their infirmities with grace" has that same ability deep within herself and has achieved a philosophy in accord with that of community health nursing.

Roles and Functions

The community health nurse encounters problems and conditions never imagined by her predecessors. In addition to conditions previously mentioned, the nurse meets such situations as poverty amid affluence, urban sprawl and decay, social injustices, racial strife and tensions, and, in many areas, a decline in the quality and integrity of community life and efforts to improve it. Facing these situations requires marked objectivity on the part of the nursing and public health professions, coupled with the realization that specific knowledge and skills are essential in contributing to the solution.

The family is usually the unit of service for the nurse; therefore the major part of community health nursing is carried on in the home where health care is needed for patients of all ages. In many communities there is an increasing demand for skilled geriatric nursing, largely for the following reasons:

1   The increasing number of elderly people in the population, with many living alone rather than as part of a family group, as in former generations.

2   The growing incidence of chronic diseases usually found in older age groups, e.g., cancer and cardiac vascular conditions.

3   The emphasis as placed today by the medical and nursing professions on commencing rehabilitation of the patient at the onset of the disease or disabling condition or as early as possible.

In her contact with the patient and family, the nurse needs to develop opportunities and plans for teaching health concepts and practices to all members involved. Many parents need help in understanding and appreciating the growth and development—physical, mental, and emotional—of their children at differing age levels, including infancy, preschool, school age, adolescence, and early maturity. Parents sometimes need assistance in guiding their children not only to learn to accept the demands of living within their own group but also to learn to understand, respect, accept, live, and work with people of other races, cultures, mores, religions, and backgrounds.

[6]Marion W. Sheehan, "This I Believe about Nursing." *Nursing Outlook,* 11:641, Sept, 1963.

When entering the home, the nurse is responsible for teaching the patient, or the family member, or other person available for the patient's daily care. This requires a sound knowledge of underlying principles of the physical, biologic, and social sciences, as well as the ability to teach, demonstrate, and use nursing skills, such as the application of sterile dressings to an open, draining wound to minimize the spread of infection and to teach the safe disposal of dressings that have been saturated with drainage. Although a comparatively simple procedure, it requires, if done safely, that the nurse have a knowledge of microbiology, anatomy and physiology, sanitation, and psychology, as well as a deft, sure nursing skill.

The nurse is concerned with the health of the entire family, including those in clinics, schools, industrial plants, and other places of work, as well as those in the home when she visits. She must be aware of extraneous community health hazards, such as poor housing conditions, insufficient and unsafe water supply and waste-disposal facilities, faulty fire protection, and traffic safety. She must be cognizant of possible sources of disease in the community and the routes of spread and methods of their control.

A dimension added to community health nursing is the mental and emotional health services and their integration into the other services the nurse can offer in the home, the school, and places of employment. This integration has been triggered by a wider knowledge and awareness of behavioral sciences, and developing recognition by communities of their responsibilities toward their emotionally disturbed citizens, and a growing understanding of the value of the nurse-patient and nurse-family relationships. Possibly, by the end of the twentieth century, these and other services will have made an impact on the health aspects of people and communities similar to those results brought about by the control of diphtheria, smallpox, poliomyelitis, and insect-borne diseases in the past century. These changing social and health patterns have been the impetus for new and experimental programs and activities in community health services, including nursing.

The need is growing for more nursing services that will provide care and health supervision to patients of all ages and social and economic backgrounds. Nurses are expanding their skills in areas of physical assessment in order that a more complete and definitive nursing diagnosis can be made. There is some increase in nursing services through the provisions for nursing care and supervision in the various health insurance plans, both private and governmental, and programs for continuity of medical and nursing care between hospital and home in urban and rural areas. This increase in service to patients and families widens opportunities for teaching principles and practice of positive health as well as for nursing care of the ill. Group teaching is increasing wherever the nurse can bring like-interest groups together for such classes as prenatal care, child care, nutrition, and home nursing. The nurse should be on the alert for opportunities to develop such classes in housing projects, health centers, or clinics.

Expanded Role

The concept of the *expanded role* for nursing had its beginning in 1964 when Dr. Loretta C. Ford (R.N) and Dr. Henry K. Silver (M.D.) had a demonstration project for community health nurses. Since that time, there has been a proliferation of training and educational programs for family nurse practitioners and for the specialty areas of pediatric nurse practitioners, school nurse practitioners, gerontology, family planning, and diagnostic-disease specialties, to name a few.

The extended or expanded role was based on the premise that more care could be given at a lower cost and that more consumers could be served, especially in the crowded inner cities and rural communities. The Early Periodic Screening Development Test (EPSDT) for ages birth to twenty-one years required more labor to carry out the legislated program, as did the women, infant, children (WIC) program. This necessitated the nurse to acquire skills of physical assessment. Preparation of the nurses took place in a variety of ways from an apprenticeship with a physician, short-term courses, continuing education to formal academic programs.

The utilization of the nurse in the expanded role as a major provider of health care and primary health care is gaining sanction. Nurses practicing in the expanded role are found in institutional and noninstitutional settings, i.e., ambulatory care, clinics, health departments, and individual practice in urban and rural settings.

Because nurse practitioners are able to function with relative independence in clinical settings under the general direction of physicians or a board of health, they are of particular value to health departments. The increasing trend for health departments to become more active in direct health care continues, utilizing the skills of nurses in giving direct health service to people. The expanded functions include some medical diagnosis and treatment which needs more study. The most important fact is that the role remain with nursing for role identity, as too many nurses look at their self-image aligned with medicine rather than with nursing. The reliability of the expanded role is dependent upon the availability of qualified personnel and physician and consumer acceptance. Nursing practice acts have been revised in some states to give special licensure for those nurses meeting the stated qualifications.

Family Nurse Practitioner

The family nurse practitioner, sometimes known as a family nurse clinician or family community nurse practitioner, is given to those community nurses who have had additional educational preparation. The majority of schools preparing nurse practitioners vary in length from one to two years and usually award a master's degree. The curriculum provides expanded knowledge, assessment skills, and therapeutic nursing intervention in providing primary, acute, and chronic or long-term care in ambulatory-care settings. In addition, health promotion, prevention, health counseling, and maintenance of health care are integral components of the curriculum. Systems analysis to maximize social action, capacities within leadership roles, and research are usually identified. Upon completion of an educational program, the nurse is considered a specialist-generalist as in-depth study is given to normal and abnormal findings in the life cycle. The family nurse practitioner has competencies in the ability to:

1 Assess the past and present physical and psycho-social health status of children and adults.

2 Provide health promotion and education, care and referral for acute uncomplicated illness or management of stable conditions with medical collaboration for patients.

3 Provide family health counseling for health maintenance, family planning, child rearing, well-child development, and family relations.

4 Serve in leadership roles in community health services or education settings.

5 Conduct and use research to extend nursing theory and practice to improve the quality of health care and nursing services.[7]

The family nurse practitioner manages the care of upper respiratory infections, urinary tract infections, gastric upsets, gynecological problems, hypertension, diabetes, chronic congestive heart failure, obesity, osteoarthritis, and anxiety or crisis situations in the home.

Family nurse practitioners are found in diverse settings in urban and rural communities. Practice may be in ambulatory clinics in or out of hospitals sponsored by public or private sectors; practice may be with a physician, or independent in an isolated area through collaboration with a physician. The family nurse practitioner is aware of the limits of practice and works closely and interdependently with all health professionals in order to provide the best possible health care to the people served.

[7]*Family Community Health Nurse Practitioner Program*, University of Washington, Seattle, 1975.

Acceptance by consumers, community, physicians, and other nurses is growing. Some hospitals where nurses and physicians collaborate are granting hospital privileges to family nurse practitioners.

Research has increased in the past few years giving evidence of positive results in utilizing nurse practitioners to improve the delivery of health-care services in primary, acute, and chronic or long-term care. Studies in the areas of role, function, setting, preparation, strategies for care, and patient outcome need to continue to further delineate the knowledge base for clinical practice. Like nurses in the expanded role, special licensure is given by state boards of professional licensure to those family nurse practitioners who meet the requirements imposed by the state in which the nurse practices.

School Nursing

The scope of the nurse's activities in the school setting is changing. In 1902, Lillian Wald, the founder of the Henry Street Visiting Nursing Service in New York City, and at that time its director, convinced the city health department of the value of health services for the school child to give first aid and to implement the control of communicable diseases, especially such diseases as scabies, impetigo, scarlet fever, and diphtheria. The immediate success of the program was evident, and schools in other communities soon adopted it. Specialized school nursing continues to function in urban areas, but in some urban and most rural areas, it has become part of the program of county health departments.

The school nurse is a member of the professional educational team employed to aid children in developing their full potential in health and education. Objectives for the school health program are formulated within the philosophy of the school. The nurse organizes and carries out activities according to the standards, policies, and procedures of the specific school. Responsibilities include assessment of the health status of the pupils and school personnel, including health appraisals and screening tests. An important component of the role is the counseling of students, staff, and parents concerning identified needs and being an advocate and liaison between school personnel, medicine, and other disciplines concerned with health care and providing information to or referring the family to appropriate community resources. The nurse provides guidance and health instruction in informal and formal settings, such as in the nurse's office and in the classroom. As a member of the school staff, the nurse is cognizant of and participates in the maintenance of a healthful environment.

An important function is the implementation of emergency care for conditions occurring in the school. Some of the high-risk areas where injuries take place are physical education, industrial arts, and home economics. The nurse identifies students and personnel who are known to have high potential of the need for emergency care in such conditions as diabetes, convulsive disorders, drug or beesting allergies, bleeders, etc.

Record keeping, like in every area of nursing, from kindergarten through grade twelve, is essential. The health history, screening tests, immunizations, illnesses (physical and emotional), referrals to and from health personnel or agencies, conferences, treatments, and home visits should be recorded. The health record generally becomes a part of the student's academic record. Confidentiality must be adhered to at all times.

Home visits are made according to the school policies. Evaluation of the school health program demonstrates the effectiveness of the program and the performance of the nurse. The nurse conducts and/or participates in research of school nursing activities, methods, procedures, and accomplishments for the purpose of changing or upgrading standards.

Certification of school nurses by the state board of education is required by some states and seems to be a growing trend. Since school health programs differ in the fifty states, readers should explore programs and requirements in their own states. There is a potentially high rate of utilization for nurses in the expanded role or nurse practitioners in schools for health education, health screening, and basic diagnosis and treatment.

Occupational Nursing

Specialization as a field of public health nursing began in 1895 with the employment of the first occupational nurse by the Vermont Marble Works, for the care of its employees. The program spread to department stores, factories, and other industrial plants, reaching peaks of development during World War I and World War II.

The occupational nurse has a very important role in the industrial health program. The nurse participates in preemployment, periodic, and special examinations. Because some industries employ part-time physicians or consultants, it is important that the nurse have written policies, standing orders, and protocols. Emergency care is given generally where the emergency occurs such as at the plant, mill, or in the woods, which might be as much as 20 miles from the nurse's office. The nurse may offer classes for training first-aid workers to assist in emergencies. Health counseling and referral for follow-up is an integral part of the nurse's role. In addition, the nurse maintains records and a follow-up system. As a member of the team, the nurse participates in health education programs and encourages research projects to initiate change.

HEALTH SETTINGS

Many members of different social and economic groups in society have a growing awareness of the intrinsic value of health to each individual. There is an increasing recognition that health is no longer a privilege of the few who can pay for it but a right to which every citizen is entitled. There is a definite trend on the part of many communities to accept this belief and to regard adequate health services as one of the responsibilities of government. Communities are realizing, more and more, that not only is a healthful environment essential but also that health services and health supervision are basic to the maintenance of the health of the entire community. This has led to an increase in the number of agencies organized to provide nursing service in homes, health centers, schools, and places of employment.

Community health nursing is practiced in a variety of settings including the official health departments, voluntary agencies, proprietary agencies, ambulatory clinics, schools, industry, free clinics, or special clinics to meet specific ethnic or population needs, such as senior citizen centers and low-cost housing centers. Whatever the setting, the nurse works within the framework set up to carry out certain health-related functions.

The official agencies are those that are tax-supported through federal, state, and local revenue. Examples of the official agencies are the United States Public Health Service, state health departments, and county, district, or city health departments and are generally referred to as *public health agencies.* Voluntary (nonofficial) agencies are private in nature, receiving various sources of support such as gifts, patient fees, United Fund or United Crusade funds, contracts with insurance companies and with medicare and medicaid. Examples of voluntary agencies are visiting nurse associations, the American Heart Association and its components, home health services, and community hospitals. These are generally referred to as *community health agencies.* Proprietary agencies are those in business to make a profit. Examples of this category are many nursing homes and some hospitals.

Local Health Departments

Many counties in the fifty states have county, bicounty, or tricounty health departments or health districts. The idea of a county health department was organized in 1911. The first such departments were in Yakima County, Washington, and Guilford County, North Carolina, and they were set up almost simultaneously. In Yakima County, an organization was needed to control a typhoid fever epidemic, and in Guilford County, health promotion of school children was the immediate objective. All large cities and many smaller ones have municipal health departments, some having functioned since the beginning of the nineteenth century, when their main interest was the control of communicable diseases.

The legal basis for the authority of municipal, county, or district health departments lies in the laws of the several states and in the rules and regulations that define the mandatory activities of local government units relating to health matters. Local ordinances may define additional activities.

Historically, local health departments have come to be charged with responsibilities for (1) developing programs based on the health needs of the community; (2) providing necessary facilities and qualified staff to carry out these programs, and (3) making surveys of community needs and evaluating existing programs as necessary to ensure that these responsibilities are being met. Most local health departments developed their programs around the basic six functions, placing emphasis on the most pressing current problems; for instance, at one time tuberculosis, with its high incidence of death rates, was the most pressing problem in many communities. Health departments in those communities devoted much medical and nursing time to the prevention and control of this disease.

The nucleus of any local health department staff continues to be the health officer (usually a physician), the nurse, the environmental specialist, and the secretary, who is responsible for keeping records and vital statistics. Local programs were and still are instituted and maintained depending on community interest, health needs, budgets, the vision and leadership of the professional staff, and staff availability. As communities come to recognize their health needs and to demand additional professional services, they are more willing to support increased budgets for programs and staff.

With the shift of emphasis from concern for environment to greater concern for consumer, health departments are changing their roles. This results in part from laws recently enacted in the 1960s and 1970s by the United States Congress in relation to social security. Some states followed the federal government and passed similar legislation to meet emerging health problems in their jurisdiction.

This period of transition from the old, accepted "prevention" programs to the wider, more comprehensive, and direct approach to the solutions of health problems with emphasis on the individual and his or her family, raises questions regarding the adequacy of health departments as now organized and administered to meet current problems. Many shifts of practice and emphasis in the health organizations and their administration will become necessary in the near future. There is need also for a careful appraisal of the spending of available financial resources so that the greatest benefit for all people in the community may be obtained, for air pollution and other environmental hazards that directly or indirectly affect the health of people in every part of a community.

This changing concept of community health needs should be implemented by constant study and evaluation of health problems of the individual—such as physical and mental diseases, physical defects, and maternal and child health needs —and of environmental dangers—such as traffic accidents, poor housing, and unsafe dairies and other sources of foods. Following such studies, programs for community protection and safety can be established. The social and economic components of illness must be considered in any assessment and program planning.

Within the metropolitan areas, population shifts have modified the needs for certain health programs and services, and intensified the needs for others. For example, the child population tends to be centered in the suburbs today, thus increasing the needs there for more maternal and child health services; an older age group tends to become centered in cities, necessitating such programs as nursing homes and long-term home nursing services. Furthermore, it is becoming obvious that the child population remaining in the metropolitan areas is to be found, for the most part, in the dependent and low-income groups, who have many health needs.

Many urban, suburban, and rural communities in the past two decades have been experimenting with methods of merging local health departments. The weight of their experiences has shown that essential health services can be maintained with greater efficiency and economy and more effective use of staffs by a combined agency of some type. Various patterns of merged health agencies have been developed by communities, depending on local needs, resources, customs, government, and the interest and participation of the citizens.

Mergers range from a permanent consolidation of two or more agencies into a "combined health district" to the "contract-for-services" type, which allows for an annual contract between two or more health agencies or health departments, stating the specific services to be rendered by one agency to another and the financial obligations and administrative responsibilities involved.

The experiences of agencies that serve wide geographic areas show that communities can be served more efficiently if there is a decentralization to several health districts but with all of them functioning under the same health department policies and practices. Community planning for health programs will continue, but in order to meet new needs and to provide better and more efficient health services, other approaches to health agency reorganization must be developed and tested. The implementation of the Health Planning and Resources Development Act of

1974 (PL93-641) through the designated health services area should improve the health of the residents without increased cost and unnecessary duplication of health resources.

Combination Public Health Nursing Agencies

This type of nursing service has been defined as an agency that is "administered jointly by a voluntary and an official agency, and supported by tax funds, community chests and united funds, earnings and contributions, in which the combined field of service offered by the participating agency is rendered by a single staff of nurses."[8]

During and immediately following World War II, many communities began searching for more effective utilization of the services of the public health nurse. Professional and lay leaders recognized that the duplication of travel and services of both staffs was costly in time and money. Studies relating to the situation revealed that staff nurses from both official and voluntary agencies were visiting the same families, often on the same day.

Combined public health nursing agencies function in approximately one hundred communities in the United States, as a part of both health departments and visiting nurse organizations and in some instances as a part of the schools. The degree to which a combination of merging of nursing services takes place varies with the community. Experimentation with this form of nursing service continues, and new patterns in organization will emerge with study, research, and experience.

State Health Departments

Massachusetts established the first state board of health in 1869. Today, all fifty states have health departments functioning as a recognized part of state government. These departments are charged with the responsibility for assisting local health departments—city, county, district—to promote health in all its phases and provide the safest possible environment for all members of the community.

State health departments are administered in most states by qualified health officers assisted by staff drawn from the many public health disciplines mentioned previously. Other specialists are added depending on the types of industries, health problems, and hazards peculiar to any one state. Each state develops individual programs according to its own needs and resources. Health programs appropriate to Alaska might not meet the needs or be feasible in Kansas or Connecticut.

In the early part of this century, programs were developed to meet pressing community health needs. These programs were built on the six

---

[8]*Nurses in Public Health,* U.S. Department of Health, Education, and Welfare Publication 785, 1964, p. 52.

basic functions mentioned before. Programs were developed around these functions, with nursing participating to some degree in all of them. While it is still important to carry out *these* functions, other functions and programs have become necessary if current community problems are to be attacked. In addition to those previously mentioned, these problems include an increase in recognized mental illness, the need to provide and extend medical care, the toll of accidents with resultant deaths or severe disabling injuries, the increase in drug addiction, alcoholism, and venereal diseases, and the need for family planning and, in some states, abortion counseling.

Some state health departments provide direct services, including community health nursing services to local communities. This may be done for demonstration purposes or, especially in remote areas, from necessity because of a lack of local facilities or scarcity of nursing personnel.

A trend apparent in some states is combination of state departments of welfare and health into one organization. There is insufficient experience at present to determine the feasibility of this move. Students should watch for developments of this and similar trends in their own states.

The Public Health Service

The agency now known as the Public Health Service of the Department of Health, Education, and Welfare was established in 1798. Its main work then was to protect the young nation from disease from without by providing hospitals for ill and injured American and foreign seamen, and to protect the country as a whole from diseases that might spread from one state to another.

Although these original functions are still important, other functions have developed to meet increasing health needs. These include: (1) to carry on research and training in medical and related sciences and community health administration; (2) to aid communities in their planning and development of hospitals, health centers, and related facilities; and (3) to assist states and possessions with finances and trained personnel to apply new knowledge in prevention and control of diseases, maintenance of healthful environments, and development of appropriate community health services.

Medicine, nursing, dentistry, epidemiology, engineering, veterinary science, health education, nutrition, and biostatistics are among the disciplines making specific contributions to the carrying out of these functions. Effective use also is being made of the social sciences. Anthropology, psychology, sociology, political science, and public administration have enabled health workers to gain increased knowledge and understanding of people, aiding them in their work with patients, families, neighborhoods, and the wider community.

Home Health Services

Home health services had their beginning in the early 1880s with the beginning of the Visiting Nurse Association. In the 1960s, with the advent of medicare, other agencies were established to give skilled nursing care in the home, such as a home health agency of a special area or a community home care service of a city or county health department assuming more responsibility for extended care. Most major hospitals today have a home health or home care coordinator program that becomes involved with planning and coordinating care in the home prior to discharge of the patient. The nurse makes referrals to agencies as appropriate, for example, home health services or meals on wheels. Some hospitals and especially health maintenance organizations (HMO) employ community health nurses to provide extended care in the home.

PRECEPTS PRACTICED IN COMMUNITY HEALTH NURSING

As community health nursing developed in large cities and rural areas, changing socioeconomic conditions pinpointed precepts that should be observed to enable the nurse to practice with safety and meet the needs of patient, family, and community. These changing conditions include new findings and practices relating to health, economic, social, and industrial changes, and changes in attitudes of patients, families, and neighborhoods toward health values.

Precept 1 Community health nursing is an established activity, based on recognized needs and functioning within the total health program.

As an activity to meet recognized community health needs, nursing provides supervision and counseling for health promotion, health appraisal, rehabilitation, and prevention of disease and provides care for the sick, toward cure or a peaceful death, in their homes. In addition to the home, nursing services may be carried out in the health center, clinics, schools, and places of employment. Community health nursing is an integral part of the total public health program, coordinating its plans and activities with those of other social and health agencies, and does not function or stand alone in the community.

Nursing services are supported by public and private funds to the degree that the community understands and appreciates its own health needs. The community has the obligation to study and evaluate continuously the nursing services it receives to determine trends of changing family and community needs, to develop new programs as necessary, and to discontinue those no longer pertinent. The decrease in communicable disease incidence resulting from education, immunization, and other control programs, and the increasing need to provide nursing service and rehabilitation for persons in their homes are examples.

Precept 2   The community health nursing agency has clearly defined objectives and purposes for its services.

The multiplicity of social and health agencies in any given community demands that each agency have clearly defined and stated objectives and purposes in order to prevent duplication of certain community services and omission of others. Objectives and purposes vary with the type of agency and the community but should be related to the goals of the agency for nursing service, so that every citizen may be helped to achieve and maintain optimal health.

The philosophy, now in evidence, of the consumer of nursing service having a voice in the development of the objectives and purposes of community nursing is important to implementation of this precept. Such constructive participation by the consumer can result in a more effective nursing service.

The community health nurse works within the administrative framework of her agency, being fully aware of its objectives, purposes, and policies and adhering to them carefully. For the most part, the nurse works alone in the district and frequently is faced with decisions that relate to her work with families and coworkers, such as social workers, school, and industrial personnel. Her complete knowledge and understanding of the agency's objectives, purposes, and policies will help prevent errors that might involve the agency and even community health nursing itself.

Precept 3   An active, organized citizens' group, representative of the community, is an integral part of the community health nursing program.

Community health nursing agencies, public and private, need to share their problems with and seek advice from representative community groups. Nearly every community includes, among its citizens, men and women who have been a part of its past and who will continue to be a part of its future. Their knowledge and experience, shared with the professional workers, can be of inestimable value to the community as a whole and can provide the professional workers with an understanding and awareness of the elements of the complex backgrounds of the community's life, development, and experiences.

An active, organized citizens' group, representing the public, should be invited to participate in the planning and development of health programs that will meet community needs and interests. Such a group can provide continuity for the planning and service of the agency and contribute to the interpretation of community health nursing. It can serve also as a valuable liaison between the agency and the community.

The composition of this group varies according to whether the community is urban, suburban, or rural. Since consideration of community needs is an important function of the group, members should be selected for the contribution they are able to make. Their period of service should be limited, e.g., to three or six years, depending on the needs of the community and its resources. Members may be drawn from such organizations as parent-teacher associations, men's civic and service clubs, women's organizations, church councils, professional groups such as lawyers or physicians, schools, labor and management, and industrial and agricultural groups. Representatives of diverse religious and ethnic groups will aid in the general understanding of community problems, e.g., housing and unemployment.

A citizens' group functions in various ways. Its members may make selected home calls with the nurse so that they can interpret her work with more understanding to other community groups. They can point out to the agency needs for nursing services as they see them in their neighborhoods, districts, or parishes. They can discuss and offer solutions to problem cases presented by the agency. They can assist in the extension and development of nursing services, either geographically or in depth. They can keep the agency informed of trends relating to the economic and social conditions in the community; this is especially valuable when a trend is just beginning. The interest and assistance of this group can also be of great value at budget planning time.

The precept that a citizens' group should be an integral part of the community health nursing program points up that just as the public health nurse should work *with* patient and family, rather than *for* them, community health nursing should plan health programs *with* community members, rather than *for* them.

An advisory committee should meet at regular intervals to be kept informed of the agency's program and to contribute from their personal and community experiences to the solution of problems. They are entitled to share in the successes of the program as well as the failures. Recognition and implementation of this precept is important, as many citizens spend practically their entire life in the community and have much invested in it, and the valuable contributions they can make to the work and success of the public health agency should not be lost.

On occasion, the nurse will find small, informal groups of residents in her district who can be of great help to her in her work, for they can interpret the local needs, cultures, and mores of their neighborhood. Many of these men and women have a potential for leadership and might be considered for membership on communitywide health committees, where their experience and understanding of such neighborhood problems as lack of health centers, child-care centers, and hospital facilities can contribute to the entire community. Recognition and utilization of this resource can add stability and continuity to the agency's program.

Precept 4 Community health nursing services are available to the entire community regardless of origin, culture, or social and economic resources.

Community health nursing is a field of specialization within the broad spectrum of organized public health practice. Its services should be available to all persons according to their health needs, physical and emotional, and regardless of ethnic origin, cultural background, or social and economic resources. Deviation from health of any one member of a family or of the community may affect the health of the entire family or community. The background of the individual or family should not interfere with their receiving the needed services the nurse can provide, e.g., skilled nursing care and health teaching relating to maternal and child care, nutrition, immunizations, and mental and emotional problems. Although community health nursing had its inception in the work of the early church, it is not necessarily a charity and has adapted itself to changes in the social order.

Nonofficial agencies, such as visiting nurse associations, charge for nursing care if the family can arrange to pay. Fees should be within the range of the family's financial resources and should reflect the value placed on the service by the community, the family, and the agency. Fees for visits are charged on a full- or part-pay basis, depending on the ability of the family or patient to pay, especially when the patient is the family's breadwinner. The nurse needs to estimate the period of time care will be needed, as it will be a factor in establishing the fee. Many families who might be able to pay full fees for the nurse's visits for a short-term illness might be unable to do so if faced with a long-term illness, such as cancer. When the family can arrange to pay at least part of the fee, they should be encouraged to do so. Necessary nursing care should not be discontinued because of an inability to pay for it. Part of the nurse's plan is to assist the patient and family in their rehabilitation to attain optimal health so that they may function independently and assume, as soon as possible, their responsibilities for their own health problems. But when for economic reasons a patient has to forego essential nursing care, the goals of the nurse and her agency are lost. In some agencies after the nurse has assessed the situation, arrangements for fee collection are made by the clerical help.

Current policies in most official nursing agencies do not provide bedside nursing care except on a demonstration basis. In some areas this practice is changing; the present trend is for local health department staffs to provide bedside nursing when the community lacks other home nursing facilities. Some states have passed legislation that makes it possible for local official agencies to charge for these nursing visits when feasible.

The precept that community health nursing services are available to everyone is broad in its concept. It permeates all nurse-patient and nurse-family relationships. It contributes to the goals of the overall community health nursing program.

Precept 5   In community health nursing the *family,* rather than the *individual patient,* is recognized as the unit of service.

The community health nurse's work is family-centered, rather than patient-centered, with the home being the usual setting. This is a different approach from that of patient-centered care in the hospital environment. It recognizes the patient or family as the hostess and the nurse as the guest in the situation. The effect of health or illness (physical or emotional) of any one member on the lives of other family members is more obvious in the home than in the hospital, and the nurse is able to observe more closely in the home than in the hospital the effect of suffering, fear, and death on the family.

In studying and trying to understand the home situation, the nurse draws widely on her knowledge and background of the social and behavioral sciences. On the basis of her knowledge of the family composition, its history, resources, and current problems, she employs the epidemiologic approach in meeting family needs. She makes frequent appraisals of the health progress of the family and patient. She recognizes that the family is a segment of the community and of society, and she utilizes the available community resources in her planning. Frequently she functions as a liaison person with other community agencies in securing health and social resources for the family.

The nurse's ultimate goal is to make the entire family independent and knowledgeable regarding health principles and practices. Achieving her goal is facilitated when she plans *with* them rather than *for* them. Her emphasis is primarily on health promotion for all the family through health counseling, emotional support and understanding, teaching, demonstrating, and nursing care; at the same time she provides for the patient's needs.

Precept 6   Health education and counseling for patient, family, and community are integral parts of community health nursing.

Teaching health concepts and practices to the community, family, and patient is interwoven throughout the work of the community health nurse. On a community level she participates with other members of the health team in planning and carrying out community health education concerning immunization programs, safety programs, dependable food and water supplies, reliable waste disposal, or development of mental health programs. Media used to provide community health education include news stories, films, posters, radio and television programs, and talks to individuals and groups. County and state fairs offer excellent opportunities for educating the general public about heart disease, diabetes, and other diseases, and for programs on vision conservation, better nutrition, and accident prevention, among other topics.

In the home the nurse works closely with patient and family in health counseling, focusing on individual needs. She plans with them to meet their goals in health promotion, rehabilitation, and independence in health matters. Teaching the family the importance of immunization and environmental sanitation and teaching prospective parents the care of mothers and babies are examples. As far as possible, the nurse should coordinate her teaching in the home with that of the family physician.

In the schools, the nurse cooperates with principals and teachers in health matters. She acts as a resource for health education, and is available for conferences on health matters with children, parents, teachers, and administrative personnel. In industrial plants, she assists supervisory personnel and others in instituting health and safety programs, and she coordinates her work with other health education activities in the plant and in the community.

The general public is interested in many health matters and fairly well informed regarding them. However, since much of the lay person's information is received from current lay periodicals, the nurse needs to be aware of this source of "health" literature, as it sometimes contains half-truths and needs interpretation. On the other hand, she also needs to keep herself well informed regarding knowledge currently presented in the literature of the medical, nursing, and allied fields.

The nurse's goal in all health teaching and health counseling is to help the individual, the family, and the community to be so well informed regarding sound health principles and practices that they achieve and maintain optimal health by means of their own knowledge and efforts.

Precept 7   The patient and family participate fully in all decision making relating to goals for the attainment of health.

The community health nurse recognizes and respects the right of patient and family to participate in all decision making relating to their health goals. The nurse's function is to help the patient and/or family to recognize the existence of a health need, to assess all aspects of the situation, to consider appropriate activities that will improve the situation, and to arrive at the decision which is deemed most suitable by the patient and family. Implicit in the decision-making process is that the patient and family comprehend fully the meaning of the decision and accept the responsibility for consequential events. An example is the parents' decision to have a rubella immunization for their child after weighing the pros and cons of immunization versus voluntary exposure to a "childhood disease," rubella.

A more involved situation would be the decision a patient and family would have to make regarding open-heart surgery. Although this surgical technique has reached a fairly high degree of safety, there are certain elements of danger in individual cases. The nurse needs to be objective in her teaching, helping the patient and family to make their own decision, and at the same time help them to make a free and responsible choice on their own and to gain independence for future decision making through the experience.

The nurse also observes this precept when working with community groups. Her aim is to involve community members in the planning and provision of health care to the highest possible degree and to help create independent thinking and action on the part of consumers, as well as the ability to live with their decisions. If a community fails to pass a bond issue for necessary money to ensure safe water supplies or a well-equipped fire department, they may have to accept the results of a water-borne epidemic or a heavy loss of life and property following a disastrous fire, but the decision should lie with the community.

Precept 8 Periodic and continuing appraisal and evaluation of the health situation of the community, family, and patient are basic to community health nursing.

Although this precept has been recognized for a long time, its importance has been accentuated in recent years by the rapidly changing patterns in community and family life and by the new discoveries in medicine that shorten recovery and convalescent periods. In some situations, changes in the circumstances of the community, family, or patient may be so subtle that they pass unnoticed unless the nurse and the agency maintain continuous appraisal and are fully aware of their implications. The term *periodic* is a fluid one, and its meaning depends on many factors. In a family, community, or neighborhood experiencing rapid changes, it may mean every month or oftener; in other situations a review or appraisal might not be necessary more than once every six months.

The family health appraisal is a tool for the nurse in helping the family to achieve health independence. Family situations can be dynamic, a birth or death may cause a complete family reorganization, and a severe illness or change in the health status of any one member may have repercussions for every member. Also a change of residence or a change of occupation with resultant change in income may have marked effects on the physical and emotional health situation. At intervals, these changes need to be assessed by family and nurse in the interests of planning for the family health program. By consultation with family and patient and by careful observation and case recording, the nurse can evaluate the family health progress, determine the priorities, and adjust her nursing plans.

An awareness of the progress that is being made and of the degree of independence that the family seems to be achieving helps the nurse to establish her priorities in planning for her daily work in the district and the home calls to be made.

Communities, too, are dynamic and changing constantly for better or worse, some at a quicker rate than others. Periodic study of the neighborhoods in her district enables the nurse to be informed of changes that will affect the lives of the families there. What changes are taking place in relation to population shifts, age groups, business areas, recreational facilities, and housing? Changing transportation facilities, such as an increase or decrease in bus routes, parking lots, arterials, and highways, affect a neighborhood. The need for additional buildings for schools and hospitals, or their abandonment, points up community changes involving growth or decay.

From these periodic appraisals of patient, family, and community, the nurse gains a basis for evaluating the effectiveness of her work and of her own growth and development.

Precept 9   The nurse is prepared professionally to function as a health worker in the community.

A hundred years of experience with community health nursing has proved to society that the nurse must be prepared professionally to serve as health worker in the community and that this preparation should be based on a firm foundation of nursing knowledge and skills, including theory and practice in community health procedures. She needs special competence in adapting learned nursing procedures to the home care and rehabilitation of the patient. Since community health nursing is a family-centered activity rather than a patient-centered one as in the hospital, the nurse also needs a broad background in such social and behavioral sciences as anthropology, sociology, and psychology to meet effectively problems that involve interpersonal relationships, community organization, and social pathology.

The community health nurse brings not only broad preparation and technical skills to her work, but she also must continue to grow and to improve her performance skills in interviewing, teaching, problem solving, group work, and leadership. She needs to keep up with recent knowledge in nutrition, social work, epidemiology, and behavioral sciences as well as in nursing and medical care.

This precept that the nurse be prepared professionally for her work is the cornerstone in the foundation of community nursing, for without previous professional preparation and an awareness of current knowledge in nursing and medical care, as well as in the allied fields, her work could not measure up to the community's needs.

Precept 10   The community health nurse functions as a member of the health team in serving community, family, and patient.

All successful teamwork is based on a common interest of the team members and there should be no division of concern among them. The community health nurse often finds herself functioning on various teams at one time or another. One such team would include members from her own agency or nursing division such as other staff nurses, paranursing personnel, students, the district supervisor, the nursing director, clerks, volunteers, and other nonprofessional personnel, all of whom work together to provide the best possible community nursing service.

The nurse also participates on a community team composed of workers from the allied health fields and interested community members. Although the ultimate goals of this team are the same as those of the nursing team, the emphases may vary. This interdisciplinary team usually includes, besides the nurse, a health officer, family physician, social worker, nutritionist, and environmental specialist. Members of other health disciplines can be added as needed, as well as such interested community members as school personnel, clergymen, volunteer community workers, and in most situations, the patient or the patient's family.

The nurse has several roles on the interdisciplinary team. She acts as an interpreter of nursing in the team's assessment of the patient's physical, mental, and social needs and in planning means to meet these needs, and in turn keeps the nursing team aware of the thinking and action of the community team. She also participates in the team action regarding improvement of environmental resources. The nurse also functions as a leader by influencing the quality of health and nursing care that can be provided to the community by helping it to become aware of the need for health programs.

With the recognition of the value of continuity of nursing care, it is possible that a third team is emerging composed of hospital personnel as the head nurse, staff nurse, resident, intern and/or family physician, and the community health nurse, all of whom would know the patient. This team can coordinate plans for continuity of nursing care, thus providing for fewer interruptions in the care of the patient during the transition from home to hospital to home. The patient and family frequently participate on this team and assist with the making of plans and their implementation.

In making the team effective, each member must recognize the contribution of all other team members in achieving the planned goals and objectives, which are the health, safety, and comfort of patient and community.

Precept 11 The community health nurse provides nursing care for the individual patient as ordered by the patient's physician.

The provision of nursing care for the individual patient as ordered by the patient's physician is basic to all nursing. Every nurse, in her care of the sick, works under the direction of the physician in charge of the patient. Violation of this precept jeopardizes the entire community health nursing program. The nurse receives orders for care from the physician responsible for the medical care and supervision of the patient. In most instances this is the family physician, but it might be a physician from a hospital clinic, a school system, or an industrial plant.

When a family or patient refuses medical care, although it appears necessary to the nurse, she has no recourse but to withdraw from the situation. This has occurred on occasion. It is a difficult step for the nurse to take, especially if the patient is an infant or a child, but this precept must be held inviolate. Before taking such a radical step, however, the nurse should report the situation to her nursing supervisor or her health officer. Except in great emergency, a nurse does not care for a sick patient without medical orders.

Most community health nursing agencies have a policy, approved by the local medical society, that the nurse may make, without medical supervision, two nursing visits to a family with illness for the purpose of providing nursing care. If during the first visit, the nurse believes that the patient should be under medical supervision—and he or she is not—she must advise the family that a physician should be called. Depending on her judgment, she may give nursing care during the visit according to the agency's standing orders, which have been approved by the medical advisory committee of the agency, the county medical society, or the local health officer. At this time also she may counsel the family on health matters such as general nutrition, rest, comfort, and safety of the patient. The next day, the nurse may visit the family to see whether a physician was called and to ascertain the physician's orders for nursing care. If the family has not called a physician and does not plan to do so, the nurse should determine their reasons. If it is a matter of finances she can explain the community resources for free medical care. If the family does not wish to have medical care for other reasons, the nurse cannot continue to provide nursing care.

As in the hospital, the nurse in the public health field reports regularly to the physician in charge, regarding the patient's condition, and secures additional orders as necessary. When the nurse visits the home for health teaching and counseling, she keeps the family physician informed, in writing or by telephone, so that they may work together in assisting the family to achieve independence and self-sufficiency in health matters.

Precept 12 The community health nurse makes full use of family and other service records.

The maintenance of accurate records and their use are important to both family and agency. The family record is indispensable to the nurse in her daily work and is an important element in making continuity of nursing care possible. Good recording covers all nurse-family, as well as nurse-patient contacts and interaction. The nurse uses patient and family records in planning for home visits and for other means of serving the patient. Her visit plans will be based on the accomplishments of previous visits that she and other nurses, if any, have made to the family or patient and on the current situation of the patient or family. Records are invaluable to the nurse assuming care of the patient for the first time. A review of the records prior to her first visit will save both her time and that of the family. The nurse's knowledge and understanding of situations will reduce family stress at the time of a first visit by a new nurse.

The quality of the agency's services to the community is reflected in its records. A periodic critical study of them helps the agency to evaluate its program in relation to its current objectives, and assists in determining its long-term objectives. The records are a source of statistical information and are valuable in determining costs, in ascertaining needs for additional staff members, and in planning budgets. They provide a guide in making staff assignments to the different nursing districts.

Community health nursing agencies have legal authorization to operate, their records are legal documents and as such are subject to subpoena by the courts, but in all other situations they are strictly confidential. Within the policies of the agency, a report of the contents of the record is shared with the family physician or with a professional staff member of another agency, such as a social worker, when requested.

The staff nurse is responsible for maintaining her records so that they are current, accurate, complete, and legible. The information should be recorded objectively, the nurse being aware at all times of the many uses the agency will make of the record.

Precept 13 The community health nurse does not provide material relief but directs the patient or family to appropriate community resources for necessary financial and social assistance.

The community health nurse does not provide material relief, since there are community agencies organized for this purpose. The nurse's concern is for the patient's immediate health needs and for the promotion of health, physical and emotional, and prevention of disease. By providing material relief, even transportation to the clinic or health center, except on the request and approval of the cooperating agency, the nurse might be jeopardizing the long-range planning of other community workers. The nurse is responsible for knowing the programs and functions available from social agencies and for cooperating with them, utilizing their services, and referring patients and families to them.

The timing for the referral and the family's readiness to accept it needs careful consideration. The family should participate in the planning for the referral, which should never be made against their will but only with their understanding and acceptance.

It is basic to this precept that when a nurse provides material relief, no matter how little, she tends to nullify her teaching. Unconsciously she is buying patient and family cooperation in health matters, for instead of incorporating her teaching into their thinking and making it their own practice and action, they are waiting to be paid for it.

Precept 14   Nursing supervision of the staff nurse is provided by qualified nursing personnel.

Supervision is an educational and advisory relationship between supervisor and staff nurse. Its aim is to develop the abilities and skills of the nurse so that she can meet her professional responsibilities with an increasing productivity and effectiveness.

Supervision in community health agencies by qualified nurses is essential for continuous improvement of the nursing service to patient and family, for the overall planning of the staff nurses' work, and for coordination of their activities within the agency. It is also a stimulus and guide for the staff nurse in her health teaching, family counseling, and nursing service, and for her own growth and development.

Methods of supervision vary with agencies, but the methods most frequently employed include planned and continuing staff orientation, joint study and review of family case records by supervisor and nurse, supervised home calls or clinic experiences, and individual and group conferences relating to the nurse's work and to the continuing development of the agency's program. Staff members need to be aware at all times of the agency's planning and work if a balanced development is to be maintained. An adequate and satisfactory program of supervision will assist not only in the growth and development of each staff member but also in the continued improvement of the quality of nursing service that the agency provides the community.

Precept 15 The community health nursing agency provides a continuing staff education program.

Such a staff education program is essential to maintain sound nursing practice in hospitals and community health agencies. Planning for in-service education takes into account the professional needs and interests of the staff nurses. Consideration is given also to the special skills and knowledge required by the agency. The staff must be kept informed of new situations and conditions arising in the community, such as a sudden increase in the incidence of a communicable disease, a change in the health and welfare resources in the community, e.g., the formation of a local council for alcoholism, and new federal, state, and local regulations relating to health matters.

Periodic, planned staff meetings for sharing experiences and information with other members of the health team in the community also provide an opportunity for widening professional knowledge and skills, not only in nursing but also in other phases of the community health program. Many agencies send one or more staff members to conferences, institutes, summer schools, or professional meetings in other parts of the state or country on the premise that the entire staff will share in the reports of these educational experiences.

A sound in-service program is based on the dynamics of medical and nursing care and an appreciation of the ever-increasing body of knowledge with which the nurse must be familiar and the additional skills she must acquire for use in her daily practice with patients and families and in her contacts with coworkers.

Precept 16 The nurse assumes responsibility for her own continuing professional development.

The responsibility of the nurse for her own continuing professional development is a precept basic to all nursing; it is the other side of the coin of the precept just stated relating to the agency's recognized responsibility and obligation for providing in-service and staff development programs. The staff nurse is equally responsible for her own continuing professional growth and education. It has been said that the ultimate goal of an education program is to shift to the student the burden of pursuing his or her own education. Continuing education is considered by many leaders in all fields to be the greatest single challenge to professional personnel.

Each nurse needs to establish her own immediate and long-term goals in order to continue building and developing her education, both professional and general. She can do this by various methods, such as reading professional journals and periodicals on nursing and allied subjects, attending and participating in the meetings of her professional organizations, and not neglecting books, journals, and lectures in the humanities and the arts. For the most part, the nurse will find libraries, art galleries, concert and lecture series available in either her own community or an adjacent one. As a professional person, the nurse should plan to invest some of her own time and money in her growth and development through attendance at summer sessions in colleges and universities, and by working toward higher degrees whenever possible.

SUMMARY

The precepts of community health nursing relate to the *organization* of community health nursing, to the *work* of the individual nurse, and to the *nurse* herself. They are guidelines only and are to be followed in any situation with sound judgment and common sense. The majority of these precepts pertain to nursing in general, not to community health nursing alone. Their implications for all nursing will tend to increase as the philosophy and practice of continuous care of the patient from home to hospital to home becomes accepted by patient, family, and community, as well as by the nursing, medical, and allied professions. Students of nursing have become aware of many of these precepts from their experience in clinical situations in the hospitals. They are stated here, however, within the framework of community nursing.

The responsibilities of today's community health nurses are succinctly summarized by Cline and Howell as "to help individuals, families and communities to develop and utilize their potential for healthful living through cultivation and use of their own and external resources, and to provide nursing care for the sick and disabled in their homes."[9]

The means by which the nurse carries out these responsibilities include visits to patient and family; work with neighborhood groups, such as parents' classes and prenatal classes; health supervision in places of employment; and assistance to teachers of children of all age groups. Community health nursing must be based on an understanding and appreciation of the needs, social relationships, and cultural mores of the patient, family, or group.

[9]Nora Cline and Roger W. Howell, "Public Health Nursing and Mental Health," in Stephen E. Goldston (ed.), *Mental Health Considerations in Public Health,* U.S. Department of Health, Education, and Welfare, Public Health Services and Mental Health Administration, National Institute of Mental Health, Chevy Chase, Maryland, 1969, p. 146.

SUGGESTED READING

Archer, Sarah Ellen, and Ruth Fleshman: "Community Health Nursing: A Typology of Practice," *Nursing Outlook,* **23:**358–364, June 1975.

Bergeson, Paul, M.D., and Nancy Melvin, R.N.: "Granting Hospital Privileges to Nurse Practitioners," *Journal of the American Hospital Association,* **49:**99–101, August 6, 1975.

Blum, Henrik L.: *Health Planning,* Human Sciences Press, New York, 1974.

Bryan, Doris: *School Health in Transition,* The C. V. Mosby Company, St. Louis, 1973.

Draye, Mary Ann, and Lorric Anderson Stetson: "The Nurse Practitioner as an Economic Reality," *The Nurse Practitioner,* **1:**60–63, November–December 1975.

Dunn, H. L.: *High Level Wellness,* R. W. Beatty Co., Arlington, 1961.

Farrand, Linda L., and Marguerite Cobb: "Perceptions of Activities Performed in Ambulatory Care Settings," *The Nurse Practitioner,* **1:**69–72, November–December 1975.

Guidelines for the School Nurses in School Health Program. American School Health Association, Kent, Washington, 1974.

Hanlon, John Jr.: *Public Health Administration and Practice,* 6th ed., The C. V. Mosby Company, St. Louis, 1974.

Igoe, Judith Bellaire: "The School Nurse Practitioner," *Nursing Outlook,* **23:**381–384, June 1975.

"An Interview with Dr. Loretta Ford," *The Nurse Practitioner,* **1:**9–12, September–October 1975 (editorial).

Milio, Nancy: *9226 Kercheval: The Store Front that Did Not Burn,* The University of Michigan Press, Ann Arbor, 1971.

McNeil, Jo, R.N., M. N. Bergner, and Lawrence Bergner, M.D., M.P.H: "Use of Mobile Units to Provide Health Care for Preschoolers in Rural King County, Washington," *Public Health Reports,* **90:**344–348, July–August 1975.

Oda, Dorothy S: "Increasing Role Effectiveness of School Nurses," *American Journal of Public Health,* **64:**591–595, June 1974.

Skrovan, Clarence, Elizabeth T. Andrews, and Janet Gottschalk: "Community Nurse Practitioner," *American Journal of Public Health,* **64:**847–852, September 1974.

Splane, Verna Huffman, R.N. (guest ed.), "Community Health Nursing in Canada." *The Nursing Clinics of North America,* W. B. Saunders Company, Philadelphia, December 1975.

Tinkham, Catherine V., and Eleanor F. Voorheis: *Community Health Nursing and Process,* Appleton-Century-Crofts, New York, 1974.

U.S. Department of Health, Education and Welfare, Secretary's Committee to Study Extended Roles for Nurses: "Extending the Scope of Nursing Practice." *American Journal of Nursing,* **71:**2346–2351, December 1971.

Williams, Carolyn A.: "Nurse Practitioners Research: Some Neglected Issues," *Nursing Outlook,* **23:** 172–177, March 1975.

CHAPTER 2

Conceptualizing a Frame
of Reference

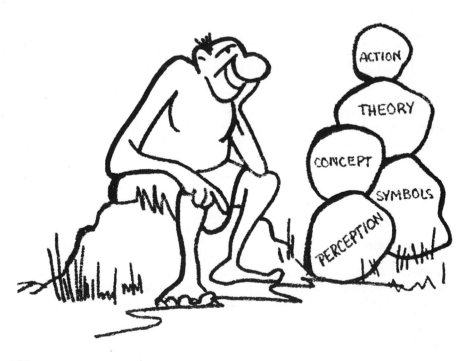

Theory has been described as a game with words. Words are symbols of one's view of the world.[1] If the words have meaning and are descriptive of interrelated concepts which are observable and familiar to nurses, then a basis for studying phenomena in the real world is established.

As we grow and develop, each of us perceives the world from our own perspective, based on life experiences. We develop our own concepts (mental images) by directly perceiving a thing, object, person, or event. Our concepts serve to provide symbolic representations of the world and describe characteristics and attributes of objects and events. For nurses in particular, concepts can be thought of as word symbols or abstract ideas which give meaning to sense perceptions, permit generalizations, bring order to disconnected observations, and provide a means for communicating and exploring interrelationships of observable phenomena.[2]

PURPOSE OF A CONCEPTUAL FRAME OF REFERENCE

Theories are intellectual tools and form the basis for applying concepts and direction to nurses who seek knowledge, understanding, and prescriptions for effective actions. Theories provide guidelines for successful actions. By applying a conscious use of a selected theory while studying a family, the community health nursing student is enabled to synthesize classroom theory with actual practice. In so doing, she learns that theory has practical value, that new and useful data are elicited because of the requirements of the theory, that family members learn and understand new ways of behaving when the theory is completely explained, and that they become aware of positive results as a consequence of their experimental change of behavior.

The conceptual frame of reference advocated for community health nurses is presented in a simplistic fashion so as to provide a beginning foundation for using known and familiar theories with clientele in communities. It is based on a model in which optimal health is viewed as a total life process and is attained differentially by each individual. The process of seeking and maintaining optimal health evolves from birth and proceeds in the direction of three growth patterns—developmental, learning, and socialization. Every person develops, learns, and socializes; passes through phases in which the tasks and goals are identified, according to a chronological age norm; experiences life events; and progresses individually toward the final task, death. Whether a life is seen as successful, tragic, indifferent, or accomplished depends on the person evaluating the life. All life evolves regardless of an evaluation. The task of

[1]Imogene M. King, *Toward a Theory for Nursing,* John Wiley and Sons, Inc., New York, 1971, p. 13.
[2]Ibid., p. 12.

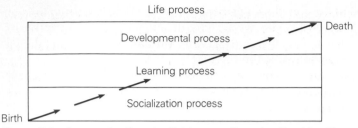

Figure 2-1 Arrows signify potential for growth and optimal health.

community health nurses is to assist each individual who is ready to grow and develop in the direction of achievable optimal health according to his or her individual capability and readiness. The nurse is a "helping" person, who by synthesizing her scientific and behavioral knowledge into effective individualized activities, assists her client to move in a constructive growth-potential direction.

The visual representation of the conceptual frame of reference is pictured in Fig. 2-1.

The life process for each individual evolves from birth to death. The three growth patterns—developmental, learning, and socialization processes—are subconcepts of the life process concept. The three growth patterns are experienced by every living individual and progress at different rates congruent with cultural background, life-style, values, and psychophysiologic capacities. The arrows are purposely placed in an upward forward movement from birth to death—signifying the potential of progressive growth, realization of new potential, and attainment of optimal health for each person. Even though death may not be viewed as an ultimate goal, it is a final destination for each person. The arrows also represent the need of every individual to grow and maximize potential whether it be from life experiences, books, schools, trial and error, or relationships with helping persons such as parents, teachers, peers, mates, or nurses. When the nurse recognizes a developmental, learning, or socialization need, it is a signal for helping the prospective client to grow and move toward the goal of greater optimal health and self-actualization, provided the client can be convinced as to the desirability of redirecting a particular life-style.

DEFINITION OF CONCEPTS

Health is viewed as a total life process and/or a dynamic state in the life cycle of an individual, which implies continuous adaptation to stresses in the internal and external environment through optimum use of one's resources to achieve maximum potential for daily living.[3] In other words, life is a continuous growth process during which situations, events, or developments that happen must be seen as opportunities for increasing wellness if optimal health is the desired goal of the individual. Health encompasses the whole man and relates to the way in which the individual deals with the stresses of growth and development while functioning within the cultural pattern in which he was born and to which he attempts to conform.[4]

Life process is the continuing orderly evolvement of an individual which is characterized by dynamic changes that occur naturally and situationally from birth to death. It is a continuous state of "becoming."

Developmental process is the evolutional change which every individual experiences physically, biologically, and psychologically as he or she matures naturally and situationally. This change becomes increasingly complex as it progresses.

Learning process is the change in behavior that is acquired by each individual as a result of practice and can be repeated when the need is aroused.[5] The change of behavior may or may not be directly observable.[6] It is a process in which new sensory and cognitive meanings are gained by the learner.

Socialization process refers to the use of communicative language as a means of social effectiveness. In the process of interacting with others, the individual transmits meanings verbally and nonverbally, which reveal—as well as camouflage—feelings, thinking, and actions.

APPLICATION OF THE CONCEPTUAL FRAME OF REFERENCE

When a nursing student first meets a client or family, it is necessary to assess if the health problems or needs are of a nature that a helping person can assist in the resolution of the problems or potentiate growth in family members toward more optimal health. If the student decides that the client or family can be helped, it is necessary to negotiate an agreement with them to work toward a mutually acceptable goal. Ideally, the mutually acceptable goal (or contract) is written on paper and signed by the clients and nurse. The student begins to visit the family on a regular basis, develops a person-oriented relationship with family members, and

[3]Ibid., p. 72.
[4]Ibid., p. 67.
[5]Em Olivia Bevis, *Curriculum Building in Nursing,* The C. V. Mosby Company, Saint Louis, 1973, p. 40.
[6]Ibid., p. 41.

experiences the realistic task of trying to persuade clients to modify identified health activities. By selecting a theory which seems appropriate for use with the family, the student often facilitates constructive changes in the family's behavior. The theory frequently serves as a mechanism for understanding family behavior, provides specific guidelines for actions, teaches family members about new and useful ideas. In using theories, students often seek out reference books to become completely familiarized with all the elements of the theory. When they observe the successful implementation of a given theory, they gain respect and appreciation for the theoretical approach as well as recognition of their own learning. When the family understands the basis for the theoretical approach and likes the accomplishments gained through the use of the theory, they are armed to deal with future situations with intelligence and predictable success.

Suggestions for theories which can be used effectively with families have been categorized under the subconcepts for the life process as shown in the following section. The aim of categorization is mainly to assist students in the selection of theories which are geared to help clients with specific behaviors, changes, or processes. New, familiar, and unfamiliar theories can be categorized under any of the three subconcepts representing the life process concept. The listed theories represent only a segment of possible theories that can be applied with families. Any particular categorization can be challenged, dependent on the viewpoint and perception of the nursing student.

Examples of some theories that can be used with families for promoting growth are categorized in Table 2-1.

A CASE STUDY, USING OTTO'S STRENGTHENING THEORY

An example of a case study written by a senior nursing student is cited to reveal how the use of a specific planned theory with a client works.

> Cindy is eleven years old with a diagnosis of meningomyelocele and has had a problem with stool incontinence at home and school. She had not taken the initiative on her own to clean herself up until I started working with her. This had led to increasing problems of social isolation at school and much frustration and embarrassment for the family. Since her family thinks Cindy is very apathetic and could care less when it comes to being clean, I decided to try Otto's strengthening theory.
>
> I hypothesized that if Cindy had a good self-concept, she would be more motivated to carry out her own self-care and hygiene. In saying this, I am proposing that she has a poor concept of herself and needs motivational tools which will assist her to improve in her hygiene.

Table 2-1

Theory	Reference source
***Developmental process* (evolutional change of individuals)**	
Stages of man in development of personality	Erik Erikson, *Childhood and Society*
Individual and family developmental tasks	Evelyn Duvall, *Family Development*
Hierarchy of needs	Abraham Maslow, *Motivation and Personality*
Crisis intervention	Donna Aguilera, Janice Messick, Marlene Farrell, *Crisis Intervention, Theory and Methodology*
Stages of adaptation	Elisabeth Kubler-Ross, *On Death and Dying*
***Learning process* (change of behavior acquired by individuals)**	
Behavior modification or social learning	Gerald Patterson, M. Elizabeth Gullion, *Living with Children*
Potentiality or strengthening	Herbert Otto, *Guide to Developing Your Potential*
Life events or stress	Thomas Holmes, *Journal of Psychosomatic Research,* 1967
Territoriality	Cornelis Bakker, Marianne Bakker-Rabdau, *No Trespassing*
Cognitive dissonance	Leon Festinger, *Scientific American,* 1962
***Socialization process* (use of communicative language)**	
Communication patterns	Virginia Satir, *Peoplemaking*
Active listening	Thomas Gordon, *Parent Effectiveness Training*
Transactional analysis	Thomas Harris, *I'm OK—You're OK*
Self-disclosure and authenticity	Sidney Jourard, *The Transparent Self*
Law of interpersonal relationships	Carl Rogers, *On Becoming a Person*

Since Cindy is a child, I wracked my brain to think of a way to present this theory to an eleven-year-old. Cindy loves to play games, so a game it became. She would name ten things she liked about herself or was good at, and I would name ten things I liked about her. We would share them together and then tie them in a bright pink ribbon. This would be her nice list. Then on mutual agreement we would draw up a work list, and this would be things she needs to work on or would like to change.

On my next home visit, the minute I got in the door, she could not wait to tell me that her bowel program was working. She had not been incontinent since the day it was started, and she was pleased. Cindy lives on a farm, so I asked her to show me the animals. We chased the cows, petted the pigs, and held and petted the chickens, with her dog, Smokey, accompanying us. Then we sat down on a huge rock which she explained to me was her favorite, because she spends a lot of time sitting there.

We talked about the animals, and when she started talking about games that she liked to play, I told her that I had brought a game for us to play. She was all ears. After explaining my game to her, she said, "but I do not like anything about myself." She stated that she could write a list of things she did not like about herself. She felt that people are always finding things wrong with her now. However, she said, after a time, that she might be able to name some good things about herself but not her personality, because she did not like it at all. We went for a short walk, then went into the house to play the game.

It took her quite some time to think of five items, but after she had done those, she wanted five more to complete. I filled out my cards at the same time. Then we shared them with one another, alternating as if playing a card game. Table 2-2 gives each of our lists.

I found it surprising that she mentioned only parts of her body. She was amazed at the things I said about her, and said, "You know I do like those things! I love to eat and be with people." We took the nice list and tied a hot pink ribbon around it.

Table 2-2

Mine	Cindy's
Fun to be with	Nose
Pretty smile	Nails
Likes to play games	Feet
Tries hard at things she wants to do	Toes
Cheerful	Fingers
Likes to be with people	Ears
Likes to eat	Arms
Has a family	Legs
Pretty eyes	Eyes
Pretty, thick hair	Hair

We then composed a short list of things which she would like to change. These were that her bowels would be regular, that she would wash herself to decrease her odor, and that people would spend more time with her. It was agreed that we would share this list with her mother. Cindy wanted to call this her bad list, but I explained that these things were not bad because they were part of her. They only needed to be worked on, if she wanted them to change. At this time, she expressed the fact that she did wish that people would tell her good things about herself once in a while.

I have not worked with children for quite some time. I had forgotten how intense their own feelings can be. It really hurt when Cindy came right out and said, "I really do not like anything about myself, and especially my personality." I was sort of taken aback at that moment. I realize how very important it is to take the time to really listen to a child, for so much can be learned from them. I never considered it before, but self-esteem is really important to develop as one grows. If we do not feel good about ourselves, what will motivate us to achievement?

Otto's strengthening theory was used purposefully with the client, Cindy. In playing the game, the student gained concrete data which revealed Cindy's limited view about her own assets. By sharing the lists, Cindy was made aware that she had strengths with which she could agree, and the process of building self-esteem was started. In using Otto's theory, the student hoped to provide Cindy with a belief in her own potentiality and a basis for increasing self-confidence in doing the things she desired to do. The game was a modification of Otto's personality inventory method and was devised to catch the interest of the client. The use of the theory was effective in revealing to the student the status of Cindy's self-concept and in revealing the client's need for constant reinforcement of her strengths as a means for motivating greater desire to explore the extent of her capabilities in giving self-care, making friends, and feeling good about herself.

SUMMARY

A conceptual frame of reference based on the use of theories for providing guidelines for successful actions with individuals and families was outlined. Health was described as a total life process which is attained differentially by each individual. Within each life process are three growth patterns—developmental, learning, and socialization. The identification and utilization of theories, categorized according to the three growth patterns, was suggested as a useful frame of reference for community health nurses to utilize as a basis for analyzing the application of the nursing process with individuals and families.

SUGGESTED READING

Aguilera, Donna C., Janice M. Messick, and Marlene S. Farrell: *Crisis Intervention, Theory and Methodology*, The C. V. Mosby Company, St. Louis, 1970.

Bakker, Cornelis B., and Marianne K. Bakker-Rabdau: *No Trespassing!* Chandler & Sharp Publishers, Inc., San Francisco, 1973.

Bevis, Em Olivia: *Curriculum Building in Nursing*, The C. V. Mosby Company, St. Louis, 1973.

Duffey, Margery, and Ann F. Muhlenkamp: "A Framework for Theory Analysis," *Nursing Outlook*, 22(9):570–574, September 1974.

Duvall, Evelyn Millis: *Family Development*, J. B. Lippincott Company, Philadelphia, 1962.

Erikson, Erik H.: *Childhood and Society*, W. W. Norton & Company, Inc., New York, 1950.

Festinger, Leon: "Cognitive Dissonance." *Scientific American*, October 1962.

Glasser, William: *Reality Therapy*, Harper & Row, Publishers Incorporated, New York, 1965.

Gordon, Dr. Thomas: *Parent Effectiveness Training*, Peter H. Wyden, Inc., Publisher, New York, 1970.

Harris, Thomas A.: *I'm OK—You're OK*, Harper & Row, Publishers, Incorporated, New York, 1969.

Holmes, Thomas H.: "The Social Readjustment Rating Scale," *Journal of Psychosomatic Research*, 11:213–218, 1967.

Jourard, Sidney M.: *The Transparent Self*, D. Van Nostrand Company, Inc., Princeton, N.J., 1964.

King, Imogene M.: *Toward a Theory for Nursing*, John Wiley & Sons, Inc., New York, 1971.

Kubler-Ross, Elisabeth: *On Death and Dying*, The Macmillan Company, New York, 1969.

Maslow, Abraham H.: *Motivation and Personality*, Harper & Brothers, New York, 1954.

Miller, Jean: "Cognitive Dissonance in Modifying Families' Perceptions." *American Journal of Nursing*, 74(8):1468–1470, August 1974.

Otto, Herbert A.: *Guide to Developing Your Potential*, Charles Scribner's Sons, New York, 1967.

Patterson, Gerald R., and M. Elizabeth Gullion: *Living with Children*, Research Press, Champaign, Ill., 1968.

Rogers, Carl R.: *On Becoming a Person*, Houghton Mifflin Company, Boston, 1961.

Roy, Sister Callista: "Adaptation: A Conceptual Framework for Nursing," *Nursing Outlook*, 18(3):42–45, March 1970.

Satir, Virginia: *Conjoint Family Therapy*, Science and Behavior Books, Inc., Palo Alto, Calif., 1967.

———: *Peoplemaking*, Science & Behavior Books, Inc., Palo Alto, Calif., 1972.

Zimbardo, Philip, and Ebbe B. Ebbesen: *Influencing Attitudes and Changing Behavior*, Addison-Wesley Publishing Company, Inc., Reading, Mass., 1969.

Chapter 3

Relating and Communicating

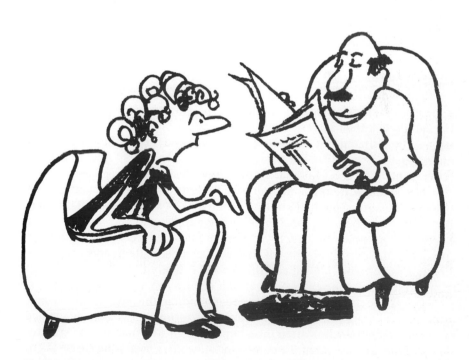

"And in about two minutes . . . this hostile, overaggressive female who doesn't express her feelings appropriately is going to have to slug you one!"

For the nurse beginning to practice community health nursing, the necessity for relating effectively and productively with others is known to be a crucial determinant for her subsequent practice. Because of inner awareness of this knowledge, many nurses often approach the first families with high anxiety and attempt to practice the role of the community health nurse according to accurate or inaccurate preconceived ideas, past experiences with community health nurses, and expectations of proper professional nurse behavior. What happens thereafter is dependent upon the innate skills of the nurse and the behavior of the family receiving the visit.

The nurse must know *why* she is knocking on the door and meeting the family, and she must be able to convey the purpose for her visit in words that the family can understand and accept and with behavior that is congruent with her words. She must be open, honest, and genuine. With an approach like this, the family is inclined to reciprocate with similar behavior. Because it is important to work *with* families, understand reciprocal verbal and nonverbal communications, and work toward goals which are agreed upon together, it is vital that the nurse initiate the relationship process in a way that the family member can accept and support.

USE OF SELF WITH OTHERS

Many books have described the advisability of knowing oneself and have explored ways of increasing self-knowledge, but few have interpreted the difficulty of knowing oneself both as a person and as a nurse. Nurses frequently ask themselves, "Can I be me and a nurse too?" In encouraging a senior nursing student to be genuine with the family she was visiting, an instructor was told, "For three years I have been told how to behave professionally. I don't know if I know how to be me!"

In a book written for the purpose of getting better acquainted with oneself, the author pointed out that we all make two wishes in life. One is for success in our relationship to other people and the second is for success in our undertakings. If we were to make a third wish, it should be to understand ourselves, since if that wish can be made to come true, the first is certain to be fulfilled and the second is likely to be. The initial step in understanding the self is observation of how we act in the world.[1]

In all the fields of nursing, understanding the self is important; however, in the setting of the community, the observation and cognizance of the behavior of self is often thrust upon one like an unexpected stiletto. The action and reaction of the consumer of health services has to be taken

---

[1] Jo Coudert, *Advice from a Failure*, Dell Publishing Co., Inc., New York, 1965, p. 245.

into account and given careful consideration, and subsequent behavior of the nurse intervener must be modified in accordance with the purpose of the encounter. The nurse frequently represents the middle-class setting and culture and consequently interacts with people from a middle-class point of view, which involves an expectation of others to have values and beliefs similar to her own. Meeting consumers from settings and cultures different from her own requires acute observation skills, sensitivity to verbal and nonverbal cues, ability to be adaptable and flexible, and an intuitive sixth sense, which is sometimes needed to guide her toward appropriate behavior. An early sufficient grasp of the characteristics of lower-class families in poverty and the cultures of minority families such as blacks, Chicanos, Indians, and Asians must be known so that the establishment of a beginning relationship can be facilitated.

Consumers who live in poverty tend to distrust helping persons on first acquaintance, particularly if the nurse or health representative epitomizes characteristics that they lack. The distrust is based on several factors, some of which are (1) despondency regarding their own potential for achievement; (2) disbelief that their life and environment can be changed; and (3) negative previous experiences with professional people who tried to help but lacked understanding of vital essentialities inherent in their culture or life-style. In preparation for working with consumers who are different, it is imperative for the nurse to be accepting of all differences, no matter how great or small, and to be cognizant of the effect she induces in others.

To start with, the nurse should be aware of her personality style as a person and as a nurse. Is she friendly, charming, talkative, serious, reserved, or quiet? Jourard stated that many nurses acquire a fixed way of behaving in the presence of patients. He called it their bedside manner or character armor. Use of the bedside manner stifles spontaneity in the person using it and protects the nurse from possible hurt coming from the outside. Character armor serves effectively to hide a person's real self, both from himself and from others.[2] If a person avoids a bedside manner or a "charming front," how can a nurse "sell" her purpose for visiting the consumer? By being herself and believing deeply that she can assist the consumer toward greater health. An inescapable nurse is one who is open to her own experience, who genuinely cares about people and about herself. She knows it is important to care about herself. She is a person who is always in the process of maturing and growing. She can look into her own memory, background, and experience and find that she has suffered, thought, felt, wished, and enjoyed just about everything human beings anywhere under the sun have experienced. This openness to herself makes it possible for her to establish empathic contact with families.[3]

Talking and Listening

When the nurse is a spontaneously talkative person, she must be aware of the effect of her verbosity on the consumer. If the constant output of words is repelling or elicits few responses from the patient, the purpose of the encounter may be nullified. The gabby nurse needs to be able to control her talk, be sensitive when her words dominate the dialogue, and maintain a discipline of self-articulation. On the other hand, the quiet nurse who finds it difficult to verbalize extensively generally is able to elicit responses from patients fairly easily because she is often a good listener. Her difficulty arises when she meets another quiet person and the conversation is filled with frequent uncomfortable silences. The quiet nurse needs to be particularly prepared before a home visit with specific information to which the consumer may be responsive and be able to force herself to talk when the conversation takes a lull and needs direction. If she practices role playing or rehearsal of information she wishes to give with another person before making the home visit, this may make her feel more at ease during the actual visit. Learning to talk effectively is facilitated when the nurse is accepting of herself, honest, and spontaneously open to her experiences, and does not hide behind the mask of being a quiet person.

Intelligent and effective listening takes conscious effort and is the key on which a successful interview is based. Listening to a patient takes skill, which is best accomplished in a competent, professional, and friendly way. It denotes a voluntary effort to comprehend meanings and can be used in several ways. It can mean that (1) the nurse acts as a sounding board against which the patient can ventilate and recognize what he or she feels; (2) the nurse elaborates and expands the words the patient has used and gives him or her a sense of prestige and importance in exerting greater effort to clarify or crystallize meanings; (3) the nurse provides psychological support by listening to the patient's feelings in relation to the problem, and the burden is lessened because the problem is shared; (4) the nurse creates an environment in which the patient is comfortable in expressing thoughts; and (5) the nurse is willing to expend energy toward gaining greater understanding and empathy with the patient.

A patient's willingness to verbalize is highly dependent upon the nurse's response to what is said, and if she listens with sensitivity she plays a major role in facilitating her own recognition of the patient's

[3]Ibid., pp. 136–137.

expressed needs. Wilson stated that it is desirable for nurses to do reflective listening and described it as a process that involves the listener's conscious or unconscious assessment and selection of clues from the auditory influx of data, his interweaving and interconnecting of this data with his own existing psychic organization, and his resultant behavioral responses.[4] Reflective listening implies an integral *relation* between verbalization, listening, and response and promotes a creative, progressive relationship between nurse and patient that is dependent on their mutual listening abilities. When both nurse and patient experience feelings of satisfaction about their interactions, this implies cooperation and responsibility regarding the purpose of their exchange and provides impetus to strive toward accomplishment of their mutually set goals.

Friendliness and Professionalism

Many nurses feel a deep concern about their manifestation of professionalism. They wish to be open, honest, and genuine, but these attributes seem to conflict with their concept of professionalism. Nursing students report that they receive ambivalent messages from experienced nurses about the characteristics of professionalism. Can a professional nurse be a friendly nurse? Can she reveal herself as a personable being?

Not many years ago the professional nurse image purported to be organized, orderly, clean, courteous, and knowledgeable and her manner was one of crisp efficiency. She was called "Miss Doe" and never revealed any personal characteristics that would betray the fact that she had human weaknesses. This imagery tends to persist even though behavioral scientists currently encourage more openness, genuineness, and warmth.

To be involved in a helping relationship, Carl Rogers has set some penetrating questions upon which to reflect. They are:

1 Can I *be* in some way which will be perceived by the other person as trustworthy, as dependable or consistent in some deep sense?

2 Can I be expressive enough as a person that what I am will be communicated unambiguously?

3 Can I let myself experience positive attitudes toward this other person—attitudes of warmth, caring, liking, interest, respect?

4 Can I be strong enough as a person to be separate from the other?

5 Am I secure enough within myself to permit him his separateness?

6 Can I let myself enter fully into the world of his feelings and personal meanings and see these as he does?

[4]Lucille M. Wilson, "Listening," in Carolyn E. Carlson (ed.), *Behavioral Concepts and Nursing Intervention*, J. B. Lippincott Company, Philadelphia, 1970, pp. 153–168.

7 Can I receive him as he is? Or can I only receive him conditionally, acceptant of some aspects of his feelings and silently or openly disapproving of other aspects?

8 Can I act with sufficient sensitivity in the relationship that my behavior will not be perceived as a threat?

9 Can I free him from the threat of external evaluation?

10 Can I meet this other individual as a person who is in process of *becoming,* or will I be bound by his past and by my past?[5]

If the nurse internalizes these questions and uses them as a guide for her behavior with the patient, she is less apt to hide behind a mask of "professional" helpfulness and is more inclined to be genuine and honest with the person to whom she is relating. She is comfortable about revealing significant personal thoughts and feelings and sharing past experiences when a disclosure seems purposeful and has potential meaning for the patient.

In a nutshell, the friendly nurse also can be the professional nurse. The friendly nurse is preferred by most consumers. The difference between a purely friendly and a professional relationship is that the professional is purposeful and goal-directed in her behavior with the patient, whereas the friend responds to interactions spontaneously and with no particular intent to change behavior.

Well and Sick Patients

Since most nurses are perceived as persons who work mainly with sick patients, an initial difficulty for some beginning community health nurses is to relate with "well" persons as the focus of their attention. They may be accustomed to working with patients who are sick enough to be bedridden or who are in the process of being rehabilitated to activities of daily living. Such patients have the advantage of a diagnosis and a prognosis, and the nurse feels comfortable in her role as caretaker. However, many of the consumers of health services in community nursing are well persons who are coping in their own way with the conditions of their world. The community health nurse is an intervener who becomes acquainted and offers her services in an effort to improve their health status. They may recognize a need for improved health but are not always cognizant of the role that a community health nurse can play in assisting them. This fact requires the nurse to interpret and communicate to the consumer her special ability to relate, to give services purposefully and in a nonthreatening manner, and in so doing, to imply that the coping measures of the consumer will be greatly enhanced by her

[5]Carl R. Rogers, *On Becoming a Person,* Houghton Mifflin Company, Boston, 1961, pp. 50–55.

intervention and will be more effectively adaptable to ever-changing daily tasks.

To elaborate, all human beings experience some degree of tension daily and have individual ways of coping with stress, which they regard as perfectly normal or as their own idiosyncrasies. In an effort to maintain balance or order in their lives, they make use of coping measures which have been satisfying to them in the past, such as chewing gum, cursing, taking a long walk, and other common activities which help to release excess energy. However, when equilibrium is not achieved at a particular time and tensions seem to mount, as evidenced by exaggerated or irritated reactions to minor daily events, coping devices inevitably become more pronounced and are less effective in alleviating stress, and a state of emergency or crisis ensues. It is at this strategic time that the nurse intervener can most effectively initiate a helping relationship. Jones cited the case history of a woman who was pregnant, had marital problems, an alcoholic husband, and little money. The patient was coping with her problems by feeling discouraged, eating quantities of bread and jam, and constantly criticizing her husband. The nurse on early acquaintance was responsive to the patient's concerns, listened to the description of her worries with sensitivity, and by means of discussion, encouraged ideas or activities that the patient could try that she had not considered or attempted previously. As a result of the progressively supportive nature of the relationship between the patient and nurse, changes occurred within the family because the patient voluntarily started to try new methods of coping, such as dieting and attempting to praise her husband instead of nagging him. As the patient noticed subtle, perceptible improvements within her household, her self-confidence gradually returned and her eagerness to try more and more measures to alleviate trying conditions within the home was accentuated. She reported her accomplishments to the nurse with satisfaction and pleasure.[6]

Salesmanship of Self

In community health nursing the nurse sometimes recognizes that she may be mistakenly received as a salesperson at the door. To counteract such an impression she immediately introduces herself, the agency she represents, and her purpose for visiting. At the same time, if the visit is her first one to the family, she presents herself as favorably and convincingly as she is able in order to gain entrance into the home. Because of the initial need to "sell" herself and her services, the nurse must be conscious of her personality style, her approach, her strengths,

[6]Mary C. Jones, "An Analysis of a Family Folder," *Nursing Outlook,* **16**:48–51, December 1968.

and her limitations. She must also be aware of her behavior on an initial visit if she is anxious and uncomfortable, so that accurate evaluations of nurse-patient interactions later can be studied by her or with the help of a consultant or supervisor. She can increase awareness of her style by attempting to objectively view herself as a third party by writing process recordings of her interaction, by listening to herself and the patient on a tape recorder, or by use of videotapes if they are available. Preceding a home visit she can role-play an anticipated situation with other nurses or with her supervisor, or following a home visit, a description of an actual situation can be enacted with the nurse playing herself or the role of the patient. New insights are often gained through role playing or psychodrama because the enactment of a role not only causes words to be spoken but actual physical sensations to be felt that are autonomous to the situation. Another effective method of increasing self-understanding is to role-play yourself in a given situation with another person, followed by a reversal of roles. Observing another person playing your role according to their perception of your behavior can be illuminating and clarifying.

In a study of community health nurses interacting with patients, Mayers found that each nurse had a basic, generally unchanging, interactional style. In other words, if the nurse was inclined to be a nondirective listener, that style was used in every client situation. If the nurse was directive, she was consistently so. Of importance about this finding is the fact that each nurse has an individualistic consistent style.[7] However, how many nurses have an accurate perception of their own interaction style? Many tend to avoid conscious appraisal of themselves as an act of humbleness or avoidance of knowing. Many intellectually explain how they come across to others, based on their *intended* messages. However, most individuals dislike hearing their own voice on a tape recorder when they first listen or seeing their body language by means of videotape. Consequently, their interactional style can be quite different from what they believe it to be. Learning about your own interactional style *accurately* and objectively is sometimes jolting and difficult; however, it must be done, and each nurse must learn to accept herself as she sounds, appears, and behaves. Accurate feedback is gained from tape recordings, videotapes, and honest feedback from others.

Another important finding from Mayers study was the high correlation of patient-focused interactions with positive client response. In other words, nurses who were client-focused communicated a sense of concern and caring, followed up on patient cues, and consequently had more successful interactions—regardless of their individualistic style. Nurses who were nurse-focused were more inclined to react to patient's cues

---

[7]Marlene Mayers, "Home Visit—Ritual or Therapy?" *Nursing Outlook,* 21:328–331, May 1973.

from their own perspective, act upon their own idea of solutions without consulting the patient, and seemed less involved with the patient's situation.[8]

It is possible for all nurses to be client-focused and learn to interact therapeutically, even though individual styles vary. To be client-focused requires the desire to be so, the ability to listen and observe sensitively and accurately, and the initiative to follow up on verbal and nonverbal cues coming from the client.

WORKING WITH INDIVIDUALS

A wide variety of people are encountered in community health nursing, representing the basic fabric of which the community is composed. The nurse must be aware that she interacts with differentiation, dependent upon her degree of comfort, to representative members of the community whether they are members of lower, middle, or upper classes; minority and cultural groups; youth, middle-aged, and geriatric groups; or those with special disease classifications. Her encounter with a specified patient will be based on her experiences, observations, understanding, and acceptance of the different characteristics of which the individual is representative. For example, a young, middle-class nurse who has never entered a poverty-stricken home might initially relate differently to a representative of the lower-economic classes, particularly if the home is filthy according to her standards and the consumer is apathetic and unresponsive to her suggestions, than she would to a representative of the upper class whose home is beautifully furnished and whose manner is pleasantly courteous. The manner in which a nurse responds to a given situation is often dependent upon her expectations, past experiences, values, prejudices, and adaptability to unfamiliar stimuli.

Because she must deal with all types of persons, the nurse is best prepared to function effectively when she feels a deep interest and curiosity about others. By consciously transferring her thoughts to the identified patient or family member, she helps herself to communicate clearly, to be responsive to the other's reactions, and to judge if the encounter has meaning. Her interactional skill also is enhanced by reading references about the characteristics of the group of which the patient is a member because clues and guidelines given in readings aid in observation and verification of existing or nonexisting patterns of behavior. By being attentive to the patient and accepting the patient as he or she is, the nurse communicates a respect for that person's autonomy and a sense of "caring" for the patient as a distinctive individual. In Chap. 5 characteristics of a variety of representatives of a community are discussed. By

[8]Ibid., p. 331.

delving deeply into additional books and periodicals, the nurse can prepare herself effectively to be cognizant of the many physical, economic, environmental, social, and psychological factors which are affecting the consumer's life-style.

INTERPERSONAL APPROACHES

Since consumers of health services are individuals and families representative of widely different backgrounds and experiences, the interpersonal approach of the nurse must be sensitive to the responsive patient behavior. Professional books and periodicals representing nursing, social work, medicine, and psychology have described a variety of known approaches that can be implemented. In addition, new methods of interacting with patients and families are reported with increasing frequency. This fact emphasizes the importance of continuing self-education and maintaining familiarity with up-to-date literature and references. The selection of a given approach or mixture of components can be adopted for use and attention given to the responses of the patient to determine if the selected approach is effective in securing the patient's attention and implementing the desired change of behavior. At the same time the nurse must be aware of her interviewing skills and constantly practice to improve her ways of relating so that the patient is helped to feel at ease in talking to a professional person. Some of the known therapeutic and nontherapeutic interpersonal statements or responses have been described in detail by Hays and Larson. They claim that every comment the nurse makes to the patient (or within his hearing) can be evaluated as having therapeutic or nontherapeutic value; i.e., it either contributes to his emotional growth or it reinforces his illness.[9] When a nurse consciously practices the described therapeutic techniques, she finds that they do facilitate commentary from patients, and that with practice her interactional therapeutic skills become more spontaneous and natural.

Some therapeutic questions or statements that are helpful in eliciting information or commentary from the patient are "How have you been managing the past few days?"; "Is there some way I can be of service to you?"; "You appear worried about something"; "How have things been going lately?"; or "It sometimes helps to talk about your concerns with someone who is not a member of the family." At the same time that the nurse verbalizes these questions or statements, her nonverbal behavior should be one of interested concern and intent listening. By making brief comments or asking pertinent, open-ended questions, which are used to

[9]Joyce Samhammer Hays and Kenneth Larson, *Interacting with Patients*, The Macmillan Company, New York, 1964, p. 2.

encourage the patient to continue talking, the nurse gains an impression of the patient's perspective or the way the patient views personal concerns. By eliciting the patient's perception of his or her immediate health problems *first,* the nurse then has a base from which to operate. She is made aware of the patient's attitude, and his or her method of handling current problems, and consequently she is able to devise a plan of implementation that is feasible for the patient's situation.

Some approaches which have been used successfully with consumers and which recognize them as necessary participants in the interactional process include the mutual, strengthening, inquiry, and goal oriented approaches.

Mutual Approach

This approach makes use of the patient and the nurse as equal participants in any interchange that involves determining the purpose for visits, planning for implementation of goals, evaluating outcomes, and clarifying feelings and/or behavior.

When the purpose for visits on a continuing basis is the focus of attention, a discussion takes place whereby the patient is encouraged to pinpoint a health concern with which the patient would like assistance or a difficulty in daily life with which the patient is dissatisfied, and the nurse then interprets skills, resources, and materials to which she has access that may be of assistance to the patient. As a consequence of this interchange of information, a *mutual agreement* or *contract* is made by the patient and nurse to work toward the stated, agreed upon goal, and plans are made for continued contact. At the same time, it is desirable that each participant know what constitutes the work he or she must do to prepare for the next visit, so that movement toward the stated goal will be achieved in progressive steps and at a pace that is reasonable for both the patient and the nurse.

For clarification of feelings and/or behavior, the nurse is generally the one who initiates the discussion to take this focus. The following example was recorded in a family record by a student nurse:

> Sue appeared uncomfortable and did not know what to say. I then told her how I felt about our nonexistent relationship and that I too was uncomfortable. Sue then told me a little about herself. It is hard for her to talk with strangers and she doesn't talk much anyway. After this, she talked more freely.

By recognizing the patient's nonverbal behavior and revealing her own feelings, the nurse communicated a discomfort with the one-way conversation, requested the patient to share her feelings, and facilitated a much more satisfactory interchange.

Strengthening Approach

During the educational period when a student is learning to become a nurse, she is encouraged to look for deviances from the norm. She is alerted to symptoms that are indicative of a pathology and patterns of behavior that are not accepted as healthy behavior. For example, symptoms can be identified that are descriptive or indicative of specific biologic diseases, emotional dysfunctions, or unacceptable social conditions. Because of the identifiable nature of the symptoms, the student learns to look for those signs which represent pathology and often anticipates manifestations of progressive disease. Concurrent with learning to identify and anticipate pathology, the nurse also experiences performance evaluations of her work with ill patients. When her nursing performance is evaluated, she seems to be conditioned to expect critical statements rather than positive reinforcing statements regarding her skills. Otto stated that in our problem-centered culture most people's perception of their own personality strengths and resources is very limited. Research has shown that the average healthy, well-functioning person with one or more years of college training, on being asked to list his strengths, writes down only five or six items. If asked to list his weaknesses, he can usually fill one or two pages.[10]

It is generally accepted that all persons have unrealized potential and frequently live a life within self-imposed boundaries or limitations inflicted by others. One way for assisting these persons, including patients and/or nurses, to recognize their strengths and disclose thoughts about potential is to do a personality inventory of strengths. This method is new to many persons, and the results of such an inventory can be strengthening to individuals as their self-image and self-confidence soar to a new level of acceptability. Sometimes a false idea of humbleness blocks their receptivity to the idea of personality strengths. Yet if these persons believe in themselves and their innate skills, they must recognize those strengths that exist and realize that a deepening and broadening of their positive capabilities can yield results beneficial to themselves and to those around them.

Nurses themselves and patients are enriched mentally and emotionally from a personality inventory of strengths. It is a procedure that a person can do alone or one in which two persons can share identification of strengths for each other. Herbert Otto prepared a list of headings under which strengths could be identified.

Sports and outdoor activities
Hobbies and crafts

[10]Herbert A. Otto, *Guide to Developing Your Potential,* Charles Scribner's Sons, New York, 1967, pp. 171–172.

Expressive arts
Health
Education, training, and related areas
Work, vocation, job, or position
Special aptitudes or resources
Strengths through family and others
Intellectual strengths
Aesthetic strengths
Organizational strengths
Imaginative and creative strengths
Relationship strengths
Spiritual strengths
Emotional strengths
Other strengths such as a sense of humor[11]

In the practice of writing down assets, additional related strengths often come to a person's mind and should be added to the list. When two people are using the inventory method, they inspire each other with many additional ideas. It must be remembered that the process of taking inventory of strengths is strengthening in itself to all participants.

Nurses who have used the strengthening approach with patients have received a variety of reactions, mainly positive. Patients are initially surprised to have strengths pointed out to them but respond with pleasure, and if the approach is a consistent one, they increasingly show evidence of an improved self-image and confidence in decision making. One situation in which the strengthening approach was conducive in moving the patient toward an increase in self-respect involved a nurse's weekly visits to a young mother for emotional and practical support; the nurse decided to try the method, explained the process to the patient, and asked her to write down her own strengths in preparation for the next visit. The nurse assured the patient that she too would write down the patient's strengths as she had observed them. On the subsequent visit the patient read her list of strengths first. They were mainly positive statements regarding her relationship with her husband and child. None made a direct reference to herself. When the nurse read the list of strengths that she had observed in the patient's behavior and life-style, the young mother perceptibly straightened up in her chair, responded with a radiant glow, and exclaimed, "Do you really see that in me?" In this case, by accepting the positive opinion of the nurse, the young mother was started on the road toward development of greater self-respect, which involved the recognition and internalization of *her* strengths. This she needed, the nurse believed, in order to cope more effectively with her daily life.

[11]Ibid., pp. 236–239.

Inquiry or Problem-Solving Approach

The inquiry approach is based on the idea of encouraging the patient or family member to think his or her way through to new understandings by himself or herself. The nurse serves as a facilitator in introducing this process and making use of questions that stimulate thought, expression, and divulgence of new insights. It is known that thoughts are often fuzzy when the mind is mulling all aspects of a given problem, and the act of verbalizing one's thoughts tends to clarify and crystallize ideas which have been previously vague and disjointed. Language influences thought and the putting together of an idea verbally helps to organize and clarify the problem. When the individual attentively figures out a personal problem with the assistance of a facilitator and considers possible methods for solution, he or she attains greater depth of understanding of the issues involved, is more apt to follow through with devised solutions, and feels satisfaction with the conclusions and self-directed learning.

The role of the nurse in facilitating an inquiry approach is to elicit those problems that are of concern to the patient. As the concerns of the patient unfold, by being responsive to the patient, the nurse can pose questions that enable the patient to delve investigatively and sometimes with discovery into all aspects of the problem. If there are omissions or patterns of information given, the nurse can assist in looking for the gaps by asking the patient pertinent questions or recognize the patterning by making comparative analogies or checking her perception of the information she has heard from the patient. The nurse's goal in the inquiry approach is to stimulate the patient to think by creating an environment responsive to the patient and enabling the patient to verbalize concerns in a self-investigative, creative way. Rather than giving direct suggestions or advice, the nurse elicits the knowledge the patient has about his or her problems, the possible solutions and resources with which he or she is acquainted, and the possibility of implementing activities which the patient believes to be feasible. Through this approach the patient is an active participant in his or her own learning, is enabled to find answers to his or her own questions, discovers the joys of doing his or her own problem solving, and consequently feels a boost of self-esteem. The nurse may have known the best answer to the problem and given the needed advice early in the interview, but by engaging the patient into doing his or her own problem solving, the probability that the patient will carry through with the "discovered" solution is greatly enhanced. At the same time the sharing of information and wrestling with a problem between nurse and patient produces a supportive relationship that is satisfying to both. There are times when the patient is unaware of the role the nurse plays when she facilitates inquiry, and the patient thinks he or she has done all the problem solving unassisted. At these times the nurse may express pleasure that the patient is so adept at problem solving or she may recap the sequence of the interview as it progressed.

The following example illustrates the facilitating role of the nurse as she talked to a mother who was concerned about her fourteen-year-old boy, who had been known to steal but on the day of the interview was playing hooky from school. The nurse makes use of the inquiry approach and she also takes advantage of the teachable moment when it occurs.

Nurse: Now, why do you think Mike played hooky today? He hasn't been in any real trouble for quite awhile, although he has been stealing by picking things up.

Mother: (then recounted his habit of "lifting things" and told about her husband's sister, who is married and has a habit of "lifting things") I don't intend to excuse myself, but really, there has been no stealing on my side of the family. I've thought about it very carefully. My husband and his sister and her twin brother do "lift things," but the sister does it more than any of the others.

Nurse: (getting back to Mike) You asked me why Mike stole and why I think he may have played hooky. Shall we look at this together?

Mother: Well, I sure would like to understand why he does things like this.

Nurse: There are several theories or ideas why children steal. We can look at these and think about it. One idea is that the child is looking for love and affection and he steals because he is trying to grab on to love. Another idea is that stealing is attention-getting. It is one way to be a "big man" around one's friends, to be important. Another idea is that stealing and behaving badly is a way of getting back at your parents or authority figures. It will get your parents in trouble. Because he has not stolen this time, but played hooky, and you and Mike have been fighting about the dishes this week, I would tend to subscribe to an underlying dynamic that he is hitting back at *you.* Here is one way that will really hurt you, and get you into trouble.

Mother: I hadn't thought about that. I really would like to understand him better. (Said with sincerity.)

Nurse: He knows you have been angry with him. Have you said any kind things to him at all this week?

Mother: (looked at the table for awhile in thought. Then she raised her head and said) No, I don't think I have.

Nurse: Well, no matter how badly the children have behaved, they need praise. You may have to look hard sometimes to find something to praise them about that is real, but look, and look hard and give praise and appreciation to the children, especially those who misbehave the most. At the same time you need to stand firm—as you are doing—on your expectations for them.

Mother: I wonder what I should do to him.

Nurse: What do you plan to do?

Mother: I'm really going to lay into him when he comes home. I'm really going to tell him what I think about him and his friend (a pause). But I've done that before and it doesn't work.

Nurse: I offer this as a thought. Why not tell him you know he is angry with you about this past week and you realize he's trying to get back at you and hurt you. Tell him he has succeeded. Let him know he really has hurt you, and ask him how he feels now and if hurting you has done him any good.

Mother: I never thought of that. Do you suppose it would help?

Nurse: I really don't know, but it is an honest approach, isn't it?

Mother: Yes, it is. I've never approached him in that manner. I suppose I might as well try it. Nothing I have done has worked.

Nurse: There is one thing about discipline; you must fit it into the framework of *your* family and the values *you* hold. Consistency is the key, and teenagers in the rebellion of seeking the independence of adulthood still want the security of limit setting. This is how you tell them you love them, that you care what happens to them.

Goal-oriented Approach

The goal-oriented approach makes use of the fact that any person will actively strive to attain a goal that he or she truly desires when it is believed to be within reach. The optimal time to set a goal or goals is when the individual feels dissatisfied with a specific condition or aspect of life. Upon reflection and considerable thought, a person can be encouraged to decide what he or she wants, then set definite, desired goals. Goals must be known and desired, must be clearly stated and preferably written, must have a deadline for achievement, and in reality, must have the possibility for attainment.

Life is a continuous process of development and maturation from birth to death. Developmental tasks are dealt with as the person progresses in age. Tasks such as learning to walk and talk, to relate effectively with others, preparing for marriage, adjusting to physical changes of middle age, and adjusting to retirement often are taken for granted and managed as the particular stage of development and age are reached. However, life at any stage also has periods of obstacles and challenges which each individual can view as opportunities if one wishes to realize potential for growth and make optimal use of any situation. One method of coping with life's problems is to set goals. Goals help to focus attention on coping mechanisms, facilitate movement or progression toward a desired end, help in motivation, give a sense of inner, compelling urge, and often expand the individual's view of existing opportunities. When goals are reached, the reward of achievement develops increased self-esteem and confidence.

The role of the nurse in utilizing the goal-oriented approach is to introduce it as a method for the patient, explain the purpose and desired ends of goal setting, and offer encouragement and support as the patient needs it when obstacles are encountered. When the nurse makes use of goal setting in her own life, she can serve as an excellent model and proponent of the efficacy of the method. She can offer examples of benefits and pitfalls from her own experience. She can stress the importance of *clearly stated goals, written goals,* and *time limits* for achievement. She can discuss the difference between goals and wishes as one of commitment. A wish is a desire that a person may dream about and truly want. It can be changed from a wish and become a goal when one is committed to achieving it by writing the culmination of the desire in clearly stated terms, setting a target date for achievement, and persisting in the belief that the goal can be and will be attained, regardless of the obstacles that may appear.

The nurse can utilize the goal-oriented approach in planning her own work for and with the patient. This is shown in the nursing care plan written specifically for the patient. The nurse can also introduce the patient to goals by advocating the use of the goal-oriented approach. She can assist the patient in writing a clearly stated goal that is conceivably attainable within a specified time limit. Together they can work toward achieving the stated goal. By involving the patient in goal setting and demonstrating success in achievement, the nurse serves as a teacher in opening up new avenues for the use of goal setting. For example, the patient may be encouraged to write his or her own personal goals which will benefit his or her life. Personal goals do not necessarily need to be shared with others; sometimes a personal goal is best attained when the individual writes it privately and works toward it alone. At other times the individual needs the reinforcement of a helping person such as a husband, wife, friend, or nurse. This person's role is to give positive encouragement as it is needed to overcome motivational obstacles and periods of discouragement and to reinforce the individual's belief in his or her ability to attain desired goals.

An example of a goal-oriented approach utilized by one nurse with a patient was demonstrated when the nurse visited a young woman who stated the desire to lose weight. A discussion ensued about the variety of crash diets which the patient had utilized in the past, the successes and failures that had been experienced, and the pitfalls that often occurred. The nurse asked the patient what weight she wished to attain and tried to determine if the patient were truly in earnest about wishing to lose weight. When the nurse sensed that the patient's motivation was purposeful, she suggested the goal-oriented approach. Together the nurse and patient wrote down the desired loss in weight and the target date for achievement. In this instance, the patient weighed 135 pounds and wished to lose

15 pounds. A target date for achievement was set for two months hence. The weekly goal of weight loss was determined to be a minimum of 2 pounds. A chart for notation of weekly weights and specified target dates was devised. The nurse advised the young woman to set up the chart where it would be seen constantly and remind the patient of her resolve to lose weight. The nurse also encouraged the patient to cut out pictures that would image her goal and put them where she would see them frequently. In this case the patient chose a photograph of herself when she had weighed 120 pounds. She put the chart with blank spaces for weekly weights and target dates and the photograph of herself on the door of her refrigerator. In addition, she pasted a statement in large lettering which read, "I weigh 120 pounds and it looks *good.*" Together the nurse and patient worked out a low-calorie diet that the patient felt she would be able to follow and that would enable her to lose the 2 pounds needed per week. On every subsequent visit the nurse requested the patient's account of how things were going. When success was achieved in losing the 2 pounds weekly, the nurse gave praise and reinforced the patient's self-discipline. When pitfalls were encountered, the nurse encouraged the patient to recall the events preceding the period when the diet was forgotten. Together the nurse and patient looked at the stresses which the patient had experienced and talked about ways in which the patient might respond differently if a similar event or temptation occurred. The nurse maintained a constant belief in the patient's ability to lose and communicated this belief to the patient verbally and nonverbally. When the patient attained her goal of 15 pounds weight loss ahead of her target date of two months, she felt elated and proud of her accomplishment and emanated a new sense of self-confidence in her demeanor.

THERAPEUTIC RELATIONSHIP SKILLS

When the nurse meets a family for the first time, a relationship is initiated which has the possibility for moving in any number of directions. If the nurse is offering her skills to help the family with a health problem, she desires the relationship to become a therapeutic one. Initially, as two people interact, they work out together what type of communicative behavior will take place in their relationship. From all the possible messages given to each other, they select which messages are acceptable or unacceptable. The cues for acceptability or unacceptability are given verbally or by nonverbal behavior. In this way they reach a mutual definition of the relationship. For example, on making a home visit and meeting a mother with a young baby for the first time, the nurse may enter the living room of the home and say. "That is a beautiful flower arrangement. Did you do it?" The mother may respond with pleasure and the conversation will focus on flowers temporarily. Later in the interview, the family cat may choose to jump on the nurse's lap, whereupon the nurse reacts with horror and pushes the cat away. The look of displeasure on the mother's face will be a cue to the nurse that her behavior was unacceptable. By being observant of all cues and initiating different subjects for discussion, the nurse and patient consciously and indirectly agree on limits within which the relationship can be developed.

In order for any relationship to be successful, Truax and Carkhuff state that three characteristics are essential for the therapist to possess. These are accurate empathy, nonpossessive warmth, and genuineness.[12] To be facilitative toward another human being requires that the therapist be deeply sensitive to the other's moment-to-moment experience, grasping both the core meaning and significance and the content of his experiences and feelings. To understand empathically means that the therapist must have some warmth and respect for the other person. This is best expressed by being "real" or truly genuine with the other person. To be genuine means to be honest and open, to meet the other person without defensiveness or without playing a role that is "phony." Nonpossessive warmth is of central importance to any trusting relationship. The warm person has a sense of liking people and practices a friendly interest and acceptance of the other, regardless of differences or appearances. The quality of being nonjudgmental is of vital importance and has to be constantly exercised before it becomes a natural aptitude. To have a truly empathic understanding of another person, warmth, respect, trust, and even love for that person must be mutually communicated.[13] It is caring deeply about what is happening and what might happen to that person. It is at this point that a therapeutic relationship is established and the growth of the patient begins to take place. The development of a therapeutic relationship takes time and several contacts, not happening immediately.

Rapport and Therapeutic Relationship

Rapport can happen immediately between two persons, but not necessarily between all persons. Rapport is a process, a happening, an experience undergone simultaneously by the nurse and patient. It is composed of a cluster of interrelated thoughts and feelings which are transmitted and communicated to each other. The nurse and patient remain separate and

[12]Charles B. Truax and Robert R. Carkhuff, *Toward Effective Counseling and Psychotherapy*, Aldine Publishing Company, 1967, p. 25.
[13]Ibid., p. 32.

distinct human beings who share a series of mutually significant experiences together.[14] Both are involved. They perceive each other and relate as human being to human being, instead of as nurse to patient. For example, when two people's eyes meet and something "clicks," it often means a good rapport in which meanings of words are understood, enthusiasm is transmitted, and a mutual warmth of liking for each other occurs. Humor is shared and all behavior is accepted at face value. However, if two people meet, are courteous to each other, listen attentively and politely to all words spoken, but nothing is communicated when the eyes meet, this represents a pleasant acceptance but not necessarily a rapport. Because there are individuals in the community who have had little opportunity to experience moments of relatedness, it is particularly vital for the community health nurse, if possible, to facilitate the vivid awakening of a meaningful human-to-human encounter with specified patients. Rapport is a dynamic process and is developed with consecutive contacts and interactions, which lead eventually to a therapeutic relationship.

The therapeutic relationship may be developed slowly or rapidly, depending on the circumstances of the nurse-patient situation. The nurse facilitates the development of trust by being warm, open, honest, genuine, and flexible. She creates an atmosphere in which the patient feels free to express his or her feelings, whether positive or negative. She actively tries to understand why the patient feels as he or she does and assists in developing personal understanding. She listens keenly, sensitively, and with complete attention. She communicates that she genuinely "cares." The patient responds to the relationship by feeling secure and comfortable. Any initial anxiety is reduced and a reassuring sense of worthiness and respect develops. The patient feels that perhaps help can be obtained and becomes ready to change any views or behavior if it seems expedient. All interactions are directed purposefully toward a mutually agreed goal of health. During the early stages of the relationship, there are periods of progression and regression. It is the nurse's task to be sensitive to the moments of regression and identify possible reasons for the patient's behavior. She may need assistance from special consultants to define the weakened link in the process and to be able to intervene subsequently in a helpful manner with the patient.

In conclusion, the therapeutic relationship is a connection or bond between nurse and patient that connotes mutual trust, respect, caring, sharing, and understanding. By its nature, it facilitates the growth of the patient toward a goal of health which the patient desires and is made possible through the purposeful intervention of the assisting nurse.

[14]Joyce Travelbee, *Interpersonal Aspects of Nursing*, F. A. Davis Company, Philadelphia, 1966, pp. 155–156.

COMMUNICATING

The effectiveness of much of the community health nurse's work is dependent on her communication skills, not only those of speaking and writing, but also those of observation and listening—not just hearing, but *listening* with an open mind even if she is not in agreement with what is being said. In simple terms, *communication* means "effective transmission of information." The key word is "effective." Communication is a two-way process, including both the giving and receiving of knowledge, ideas, information, attitudes, and opinions.

A ready command of language, which was invented to facilitate communication, is requisite for developing communication skills. A discriminating knowledge of words and their specific meanings, plus the ability to use them with accuracy are essential in successfully presenting thoughts and ideas to patients and families, community members, and professional coworkers, either by writing or by speech. The importance of accuracy in spelling and in meaning can scarcely be overrated. An example is the two words "discreet" and "discrete," pronounced the same but with a difference in spelling and meaning, yet at times used interchangeably by persons who do not understand the meanings. It has been said that linguistic differences are a perpetual source of international misunderstanding. This is equally true on a person-to-person basis. The nurse must be certain that words have the same meaning for her patients as they do for her. A classic example is the nurse who asked a pregnant mother to save a twenty-four-hour urine specimen. The mother withheld her urine for twenty-four hours at a cost of much discomfort and some pain.

Four specific skills are employed in communications, namely, reading, writing, listening, and speaking. "These four skills are unevenly distributed in human beings. Some of us are good writers; some are good talkers; some, good listeners; some, avid readers. All of these skills can be improved immeasurably if we want to improve them.[15]

Inherent in the use of communication skills is the social responsibility to strive for clarity, accuracy, and truth. In speech, it is a choice of words, use of voice tones and inflections; in writing, a choice of words, correct spelling, punctuation, sentence construction, and paragraphing. The listener and the reader have the responsibility for making an honest effort to grasp the meaning of the speaker or writer.

Successful communication may be carried on by nonverbal means also. The tone of voice, a smile (Lillian Wald said a nurse could smile in twenty-seven different languages), a gesture (such as a shrug of the

[15]C. M. Siggins, "A Professor of English Looks at Communication Skills," *Nursing Outlook,* **9:**666–668, November 1961.

shoulders), silence or inaction when action is indicated, all can communicate in an expressive way and merit attention. Children have long been recognized as masters of nonverbal communication.

Frequently problems arise from unconscious nonverbal communication, partly because persons are not aware of their nonverbal behavior and partly because they are unaware that it is evident. The nurse must watch for her own nonverbal communication when talking to the patient and family. It could either strengthen or weaken her teaching. Those watching her might misinterpret a facial expression or a shrug of the shoulders as impatience with them, not herself, or they might think it was a lack of interest in them on the nurse's part. The nurse who will listen calmly and with poise to the patient's or family's difficulties and problems without revealing her own inner feelings or attitudes will be more helpful than the nurse who shows her impatience and frustration with the general situation by her facial expressions or gestures. The nurse needs to listen for unexpressed hopes and fears. Listen to the young woman expecting her first baby. What is she really saying? What are her hopes? What are her fears? People may communicate what they are thinking or feeling by body posture, movements, and facial expressions, so that the nurse needs to watch, listen for, and learn to recognize the significance of these nonverbally expressed feelings with a comprehending silence. What is *not* said with words may be as important as what *is* said.

While working with patients and families, and with coworkers, too, the nurse will note clues to unspoken feelings and ideas. Sometimes an unexplained pause or hesitancy in speech or a sudden change of subject may be a person's way of saying that he or she does not wish to continue with the conversation. On the other hand, the hesitancy or pause may indicate that the person is thinking and searching for the exact word or phrase to express his or her thought. The nurse should consider this and allow time as necessary. Many older persons and those for whom English is a second language are not always facile with words and need adequate time in which to phrase their thoughts and ideas. Sometimes this may apply to children as well. It is important, therefore, to be understanding and patient and not to misinterpret a sudden pause or change of topic. The nurse's skill in interpreting this comes with thoughtfulness, observation, practice, experience, and understanding. Occasionally, the patient or family will tell the nurse what they assume she wants to hear, and then her hope of being effective lies in listening carefully and searching for the nuances. During a visit, the nurse may gain insight into the family situation by close observation of surroundings. A painful neatness or an extreme untidiness may communicate the patient's or family's reaction to an unhappy situation. Such feelings may be expressed in other ways as well. This requires the nurse to be alert and understanding at all times.

THE NURSE AS A ROLE MODEL

The nurse must be cognizant of the fact that she is seen as a role model by her clients, positively or negatively, consciously or unconsciously. For this reason, she must be aware at all times of the way she influences others. Her actions, behavior, appearance, and manner of speaking should be purposeful and designed to create the impression for which she is striving. She should take note of her dress and grooming since her appearance has an impact on clients. She needs to consciously recognize and include all family members as she interacts with them, since this does not go unnoticed by family members. Her manner of asking questions, making inquiries, stating information, giving verbal reinforcement for positive acts, being courteous and considerate—all are absorbed in some fashion by clients as they observe and listen to the nurse. Individuals often mimic other significant persons, particularly if they admire a characteristic or behavior. They tend not to realize their mimicry. When nurses are aware of clients or children copying a hair style, a way of dressing, a behavior, a manner of speaking, a phraseology, they should not be surprised but complimented that the client was attentive and impressionable. Even though all nurses may not want to be role models, they must recognize the client's potential of copying behavior and perform as they would like to be remembered.

TEACHING AND LEARNING

Objectives and Goals

If you don't know where you are going, you will end up somewhere else.

L. Peter[16]
Teaching and learning are interlocked. In teaching, the nurse's underlying objective is to help the patient and family to learn to meet and solve their own health problems. In addition to establishing her objectives for teaching, the nurse also helps the patient and family to determine *their* objectives and expectations for learning.

Objectives are defined as being the goals or outcomes sought.[17] Or, put in another way, an objective is a description of what things will be like when a goal has been achieved. It is a statement identifying the intended conditions for the conclusion of an activity. An objective is a destination.[18] Behavioral objectives are explicitly written to describe specific

[16]Laurence J. Peter, *The Peter Prescription,* William Morrow & Company, Inc., 1972, p. 141.

[17]Vivian C. Wolf, "Educational Objectives," *Journal of American Association Nurse Anesthetists,* December 1972, p. 436.

[18]Peter, op. cit., p. 141.

types of behavior that individuals and families are expected to demonstrate as an outcome of their learning experiences. For example, if the goal of the nurse is for an individual to take a medication for hypertension every day without fail, she will write objectives which anticipate the outcome behavior she is expecting of the patient. Some sample objectives are as follows:

1 Relates correct understanding of the importance of taking hypertension medication
2 Describes in detail the individual's daily procedure of taking hypertension medication
3 Distinguishes the difference between the hypertension medication and other medications that are taken concurrently
4 Selects a daily schedule which aids in remembering the correct time of day to administer the medication

It will be noted that each objective is written from the perspective of the client's learning, begins with a verb that specifies observable or measureable behavior, describes the terminal performance that is anticipated as an outcome, states one learning outcome rather than a combination of ideas, and is written at a level that can be attained realistically by the client.[19] For accomplishment of client objectives, it is important to involve the client in determining what he is able to do, and what he agrees to do. When others participate in the setting of an objective, understanding and acceptance will result.[20]

Nurses must get into the habit of writing objectives for activities or programs in which they are engaged. The writing of objectives clarifies the purpose of the activity or program, sets boundaries of expectations regarding outcomes, provides consistency of direction toward the goal, acts as guidelines for anticipated performances. The actual composition and writing of useful behavioral objectives is difficult initially, but the process becomes easier with practice. Questions to think about while writing objectives that are designed for clients are:

1 Are learning outcomes appropriate for this client?
2 Are all possible learning outcomes remembered?
3 Are the objectives attainable for the client?
4 Are the objectives in harmony with the basic principles of learning?
   a Is the client *ready* to proceed successfully with the objective?

---

[19]Norman E. Gronlund, *Stating Behavioral Objectives for Classroom Instruction,* The Macmillan Company, New York, 1970, p. 11.
[20]Peter, op. cit., p. 146.

b   Is the client *motivated* or does the client want to work toward the attainment of the objective?

c   Is the client apt to *retain* the terminal behavior as something he or she will continue to use?

d   Is the client apt to *apply* the terminal behavior in other new situations?[21]

e   Does the client understand and accept the intent of the objective?

Before the nurse can teach effectively, she must know the learner. What are his or her goals and objectives in relation to health? or does he or she have any? Those who live close to the poverty line and move from one family crisis to another frequently have no objectives. The nurse will sense the lack of motivation toward optimal health in many low-income families, where there is the constant threat and fear of unemployment with resulting inability to pay the rent or buy sufficient food and clothing. The lack of independence engendered by welfare may be another reason for low motivation. These families are more concerned with their critical situations than with long-range problems of health. A practical approach is usually the wisest one in teaching low-income groups.

Behavioral objectives which show tangible movement toward desired outcomes, are readily attainable, are written at a level understandable and achievable, and are acceptable to the family will be successful, particularly if the nurse has taken the initiative to elicit the interests and desires of the family before writing and interpreting the meaning of the objectives to them.

Health Teaching

Teaching employs many forms of communication, verbal and nonverbal. In planned teaching, the nurse applies, in one way or another, the four specific communication skills mentioned earlier: reading, writing, listening, and speaking. She may implement these with demonstrations and other types of visual aids: care of the patient, equipment, charts, pictures, slides, films, and television. At the same time, she communicates or teaches, often unconsciously, by other means such as her own standards, attitudes, feelings, and interests, or by her appearance, manner, mode of dress, tone of voice, and acceptance of others.

Teaching sound health practices to patient and family was recognized early in its history as basic to all community health nursing. That it was an accepted part of the early public health nursing programs in the United States is shown in a daily report of a pioneer district nurse in Boston, when she wrote, "Almost every day I find some former patient carrying

[21]Gronlund, op. cit., pp. 29–30.

out many of the simple directions that have been given during some former sickness."[22]

In thinking of the family, the nurse must give realistic consideration to what a family is. Any definition would have to consider not only the so-called "normal family," but also the "broken family" or the "solo parent," families of varying racial, educational, and cultural backgrounds and families on all economic levels. The nurse encounters all these types in her work, and the needs, expectations, and health and medical goals will vary from family to family.

The teaching done by the nurse takes place in various locales, the home, health center, school, industrial plant, and at community gatherings, such as meetings of the parent-teacher associations and neighborhood clubs. Some junior and senior high schools depend on the nurse to teach one or more classes of a planned course in the curriculum in health education or the home nursing course in the home economics curriculum. If the nurse accepts such a responsibility, she should determine the subject matter that she will be expected to cover, the objectives for the entire course, and those which are to be met in her particular presentation.

At times the nurse is asked to speak at meetings of the parent-teacher association on health matters relating to school children, such as drug abuse, nutrition, safety measures, or communicable disease control. At the beginning of the school year, and at other times also, the nurse may be asked to attend a teachers' meeting to present some phase of her program and to discuss some of the health problems current in the school and community which the teachers will encounter, such as the possibility of an influenza outbreak, or problems that relate to an influx of a new population in the community.

The teacher-nurse conference in the school can be a planned teaching and learning experience for both teacher and nurse. By sharing their knowledge of the health problems of the children under their care and direction, they can work together with children and parents toward the solution of many of these problems. Because of unexpected needs of a patient or family, some teaching has to be done without prior planning in order to meet a specific situation. The nurse must be alert to take advantage of these opportunities.

Time is always a factor in the nurse's teaching, for there is seldom enough, especially on a home call. This is frequently true also in a scheduled contact at the clinic or even in a formal class presentation. This lack of time enhances the need for the nurse to make a thorough preparation for her teaching.

[22]Isabel A. Hampton et al., *Nursing of the Sick, 1893,* McGraw-Hill Book Company, New York, 1949, p. 123.

In working toward her goals to help patient and family learn to meet and solve their health problems, the nurse may encounter some resistance to change, and this is normal. Change is unsettling to some people, particularly the elderly. It is difficult for most of us to give up established behaviors in which we are comfortable and in which we feel we have certain skills for something unfamiliar. When a patient or family does not fully understand the new situation or if they think they would be more uncomfortable than under present conditions, they will resist.

An example is that of a young man who unexpectedly learns he has diabetes, which will involve a new way of living for him such as learning self-administration of insulin, eating a different diet, and accepting a degree of control of certain activities, including athletics, camping, and travel. In such instances the nurse will encounter resistance that must be met with understanding and appreciation of the feelings of the young man and his family, recognizing that these changes will cause uncertainty, discomfort, and anxiety until he finds usefulness and satisfaction in his new way of living.

The nurse must watch for both the readiness and resistance factors involved in change. The best teaching may be done by careful, intelligent listening, allowing patient and family opportunities to think through the situation for themselves by talking it over and gaining a perspective. A situation such as that which faced the young diabetic is difficult to accept and the nurse must not let herself become so involved emotionally that she is not free to think objectively.

There are several components of success in teaching. Perhaps the three most important are: (1) The teacher's mastery of the subject. This entails continuous study for the nurse, in order not only to add to her general knowledge but also to add to her knowledge and understanding of nursing and of the natural and social sciences. The importance of this point has been emphasized by the "knowledge explosion" in many fields, particularly medicine, with the new drugs, new laboratory findings, and new approaches to long-established treatments. (2) The teacher's appreciation and enjoyment of her subject. Her enthusiasm for it and her interest in sharing her knowledge will help to stimulate learning on the part of the patient and family. (3) The teacher's genuine liking for people—all people of varying cultures, creeds, and backgrounds—and in particular the patient, the family, or the community group she is trying to teach.

Continuous evaluation of the achievement of the objectives—her own as well as those of patient and family—will enable the nurse to make her teaching a learning experience for herself as well as for others. It will help her to assess her ability and skills to bring about behavioral changes for better health practices by patients and families under her care.

The true measure of success in health teaching is not so much what people *know* as what they *do.* The community health nurse meets expectant mothers from many walks of life who still have not seen a physician at the end of their seventh month of pregnancy; they tell the nurse, "I know better, but I just haven't gotten around to seeing my doctor yet." Was their behavior due to fear? to ignorance? to habit? or to apathy?

Learning

Closely allied with teaching is learning. It covers a wide range of activities, from the acquisition of manual skills to the mental processes of problem solving. Learning is one of our principal activities, but how it actually takes place is not known. There is comparatively little information regarding the mechanism of the transfer of knowledge from instructor to student, an instructor being any one of a number of things—a book, a picture, an observation, or a person. There is general agreement, however, that learning is evidenced by a change of behavior. These behavioral changes involve not only the individual's overt actions, but covert actions as well in ways of thinking and feeling. Learning may be thought of also as a learner's development of ways of satisfying motives or attaining goals.

The individual has not really learned unless the changes in behavior persist. If learning is to become relatively permanent, it must be used either in mental activity or in physical practice. Many people in low-income groups tend to be action-oriented rather than word-oriented and find learning easier when the demonstration and return demonstration of teaching or of role-playing is used. This becomes an important way of teaching for the nurse in the home and the health center. Teaching a mother how to examine her baby is one example. Another example would be by a role-playing situation in which the mother would play the role of her preschool child who says "No," with the nurse playing the role of the mother as she perceives that role.

Curiosity is a vital factor in the psychology of learning of any age group. It should be stimulated but at the same time given direction. A child's effort to learn why and how a match makes a flame can be disastrous without supervision and guidance.

Principles of learning   Many principles of learning have been formulated by various schools of psychology. Some that apply to the work of the nurse are included here.

1   Learning takes place more effectively when an individual is ready, both physically and mentally, to learn.
2   Individual differences must be considered if effective learning is to take place.

3   Motivation, either from within or without the individual, is essential for learning.

4   What the individual learns in any given situation depends on his or her perception of the situation.

5   An individual learns what he or she actually uses or what has relevance for him or her.

6   Learning takes place more effectively when the individual has a sense of satisfaction and when he or she feels the learning is personal.

7   Evaluation by learner and teacher is essential in determining whether desirable changes in behavior are taking place.

These principles bear consideration as the nurse plans and conducts her teaching and develops accompanying learning experiences. None of these principles functions alone, but they are interdependent and interact with each other. A consideration of these principles follows.

Learning takes place more effectively when an individual is ready to learn   This principle of the readiness element in learning points out that what is to be taught must not only be relevant to the individual but must also meet one's needs and interests and be within the range of mastery and achievement. This principle is basic to all teaching of patients. For example, most pregnant women are interested in and ready to learn about the anatomy and physiology of pregnancy and of the birth process. Many mothers seek information about good nutrition for their school-age children, and ask for assistance with emotional problems of their teenagers.

Much of the success in teaching the patient and family depends on utilizing their interests and expressed needs. In the situation of an unwanted baby, the nurse may encounter an emotional block on the part of the mother or the family to learning about the baby's needs and care. When the readiness to learn is not present, what can the nurse do to stimulate it? A great deal depends on her initiative and insight. She can determine some interests of the patient and family and try to capitalize on them. The well-planned use of visual aids will help. In addition to the birth atlas, there is available literature prepared by government agencies, insurance companies, commercial companies such as milk and baby food companies, and the voluntary agencies such as the American Heart Association or the American Cancer Society.

Timing is a factor in readiness to learn. A mother's interest in learning may lag if she is more concerned with putting her washing on the line or preparing dinner than with the information the nurse has to offer. Readiness to learn may be inhibited also by the presence of neighbors or children, and there is always the chance that the mother frankly may not be interested at the time. The nurse must be sensitive to these and other hidden causes that may underlie the lack of readiness, and she must evaluate the situation carefully. Often it is wiser, under the circumstances, to plan for a return call under more fortunate circumstances, and close the visit.

Individual differences must be considered if effective learning is to take place In her work, the community health nurse observes wide variations in the cultural, ethnic, religious, economic, and educational backgrounds of the families assigned to her. She also notes differences in the life experiences, ages, and interests of these families. The pregnant woman who lost her previous baby has certain needs and fears that are different from those of her young neighbor, a primipara. These individual differences occur among families living in the same neighborhood, and sometimes the nurse sees marked differences between members of one family. Alertness in the nurse and consideration of the background differences of individuals, families, and neighborhoods will enhance both teaching and learning.

Motivation, either from within or without the individual, is essential for learning Motivation is difficult to ascertain. It is related to readiness, and without it, whether from within or from without, little learning by the patient and his or her family with resultant changes in behavior can take place. To gain an idea about the client's or family's concerns, the nurse must elicit and identify *crucial* issues with which the individuals are involved. What is important at that moment in time? What do they *care* about?

In a situation of a hydrocephalic, grossly obese twenty-year-old female who was not yet bladder- and bowel-trained, the nursing student, on a first visit, received the urgent message that the family was *most* concerned with clearing up the existence of two tiny bedsores on the buttocks. The family's motivation to attain the following behavioral objectives was at an optimum level: (1) treat the bedsores with soap and water following every elimination and (2) provide light treatment for a period of thirty minutes to bedsores three times every day.

By being attentive to the family's first and foremost area of interest, the nurse was completely accepted, and suggestions and assignments were heard. At a later time, the nurse hoped to determine other areas of interest about which the family was interested and for which she felt an inner concern, such as the obesity and the need for bladder and bowel training.

Many patients and families are motivated on their own to learn because they appreciate that what the nurse has to teach will promote their comfort, safety, and security. In addition, many recognize the long-term values of health instruction and what it can mean to their permanent health, e.g., the nurse's instruction regarding dental health and hygiene. On occasion, the nurse needs to challenge and to motivate the patient and family to learn. Praising and showing appreciation for what has been learned and put into use constitutes one way. The nurse's effort to make the family independent of her in meeting their health needs can motivate them to learn more. Sometimes she may motivate them unconsciously by her enthusiasm for teaching, her evident knowledge of health matters, and her interest in the patient and family as persons.

Motivation by fear or threat leads to negative teaching and should be avoided. However, the teaching the nurse has done regarding immunization, without apparent effect at the time, may result in a marked change of behavior by a family or a community that is galvanized into action by the report of the health department that cases of communicable diseases, such as smallpox or poliomyelitis, are occurring in the community.

Motivation may come also from satisfactions gained in the use of previous learning, with a resultant desire to learn more in order to gain further satisfaction. Many young mothers, as they gain skills and competencies in the care of their new babies, are motivated to learn more about child care as their babies grow older. Sound interpersonal relationships between nurse and family will be a positive element in stimulating motivation and determining behavior—social, emotional, and intellectual—which develops from the learning situations.

What individuals learn in any given situation depends on their perception of the situation Patients and families frequently will see things differently from the nurse because of their backgrounds and life experiences. What individuals see, hear, understand, and know affects their learning. In community health nursing, language difficulties and cultural and religious customs may interfere with the learning of the patients and their families. Furthermore, misinterpretation can occur easily if members of the family think they understand what the nurse is saying and doing, when actually they do not. Periodic repetition of important points in the discussion by the nurse, and the use of pertinent questions from time to time on the material covered, will give her an idea of how much or how little has been understood. In certain instances, the nurse may need to change her approach in teaching and try other means in order to help patients and their families increase their perception and learning.

Individuals learn what they actually use or what has relevance for them The effect of this principle is recognized by students in many fields. How easy it is to forget a foreign language when there is no opportunity to use it, either by speaking or reading. This principle emphasizes the value to the learner of the return demonstration in the demonstration method of teaching. When a technique such as the administration of insulin has been taught by the demonstration method to patients or family members in the hospital, health center, or home, the nurse should observe a return demonstration as soon as possible, to assure herself that the basic principles of the procedure have been comprehended and are being applied with an appreciation of their importance.

Learning takes place more effectively when individuals have a sense of satisfaction and when they feel the learning is theirs This principle is related to the principle of readiness to learn, and it depends on the goals and interest of the individual learner. The wise selection of the learning experiences by instructor and student will bear on the implementation of this principle. The experiences must be within the range of accomplishment by the learner, not too difficult, but not too easy if satisfaction is to be derived in carrying them out. In any plan for teaching, the instructor needs to consider how to incorporate this principle. Basically it is the goal of all teaching, and can provide satisfactions for both student and instructor.

Evaluation by learner and teacher is essential in determining whether desirable changes in behavior are taking place Evaluation may be carried out in a variety of ways and is helpful to both the learner and the teacher. For example, the nurse may discuss with the mother the learning experiences she had that were associated with the care of her previous baby. Is she able to utilize the knowledge and carry out the skills she acquired in the care of that baby when caring for her new baby? What additional skills and knowledge does the mother feel she needs? What additional skills and knowledge does the mother appear to the nurse to need? Can a family meet new health needs and problems as they arise in daily living and solve them satisfactorily on the basis of their previous learning experiences? Both nurse and family need to ask themselves these and similar questions from time to time. The nurse applies this principle to her own work when she evaluates the progress made by family and patient in learning to meet their own health problems. Have they made sufficient progress in meeting their own needs so that she can close or discharge the case until such time as a new health crisis arises for which help is needed? In evaluating the learning that has taken place, the nurse should take the long view. Results of change in behavior leading to better health practices by patient, family, or community need time to be identified; the process may even take years.

The principles of learning selected for discussion here are guidelines or suggestions to help the nurse to attain a measure of success in an important part of her work, health teaching. As the nurse gains experience in her teaching and continues her observations, evaluation, and study, other principles which she can utilize will become apparent to her.

Concomitant Learnings

In addition to the primary learnings that are the principal objectives of planned learning activities, there are concomitant learnings that also concern the instructor. These learnings include such intangibles as attitudes, ideals, appreciation, pride in accomplishment, and habits of conduct. They may have positive or negative values and will occur simultaneously with the primary learnings. Both types of learning may be derived from the same activities.

When the nurse carefully demonstrates formula making in the home, observing principles of cleanliness and accuracy, maintaining neatness of the work area, and making skillful use of the equipment, the mother will gain an appreciation of the importance of these factors, as well as of the actual techniques of formula making. If, on the other hand, the demonstration is conducted in a careless, slovenly, and haphazard manner, the converse may be true.

In all her work, the nurse should not lose sight of the concomitant learnings that are constantly taking place, sometimes without her thought or knowledge. In evaluating her teaching of patient and family, the nurse should look for evidences of concomitant learning and should be objective in recognizing both the positive and negative aspects.

TECHNIQUES OF TEACHING

The community health nurse will always have a responsibility for teaching patients and their families in the home. However, the demand for group teaching is increasing as communities become more aware of and interested in health matters. Group teaching is more economical in time and effort than individual teaching, but it requires methods and approaches that differ from those used with the individual patient or family in their own environment.

Teaching Plan

Preparation of a teaching plan, whether for a group or individual, is the first step in organized teaching. The instructor begins such a plan with a statement of goals and objectives for both the learner and herself, for teaching should be defined in terms not of content to be covered or techniques to be used but of goals and objectives of both instructor and learner in the ends to be achieved. For example, a mother might request the nurse to bring her information regarding means of birth control on her next visit. On that planned visit, the nurse's objective as teacher would be to acquaint the mother, by use of the family-planning kit, with the variety of existing birth control devices. On the other hand, the mother's objective as learner would be to determine for herself the most feasible means of birth control for her own use.

The nurse should not impose her own health standards or values on the learner without first studying or investigating the existing situation.

She should determine, with the help of the learner, what needs are being met satisfactorily for those concerned and what needs are unmet to the degree that achievement of optimal health is seriously affected by the current situation. From there, she works out ways of filling the unmet needs. The means of implementing desired change should be explored with the learner.

In addition to setting objectives that can reasonably be attained by a group, the instructor needs some information about the class. For instance, is it an expectant parents' class? The nurse should have some pertinent information about their community or neighborhood, its health facilities, and health needs. What behavioral changes or learning are desired *by* and *for* this group? What content would facilitate achievement of the aims?

A story is told of the women in a certain North African village during World War II whose cooperation was required during the African invasion. They were alerted to the situation but requested to keep it secret, which they carefully did. Their cooperation contributed markedly to the success of the Allied Forces. The commanding officer wished to repay them for their loyalty. On learning that all water used in the homes had to be carried from the village well, he ordered water to be piped to each house. When this was done, the women were outraged. Going for the water each morning was a social activity in the village. At the well the women met their friends and neighbors and learned the local news, births, marriages, and deaths. When there was no reason for gathering at the well each morning, the local mores were disturbed and the need for human contact was no longer being met.

The teaching plan is a blueprint, a suggested guide. It should be so flexible that it can be adapted easily to the needs of patient, family, or community group. The teaching method best suited to the subject and circumstances should be selected. It might be a lecture, formal talk, discussion, demonstration, or any combination of these methods, or it might be the problem-solving approach. Visual aids to accompany the teaching plan should be selected carefully. They might include any of the following: demonstration of equipment and techniques, charts, posters, maps, graphs, books, slides, films, health literature, and reports. Aids to be used, and when and where, should be noted on the margin of the teaching plan. Not only visual aids but verbal illustrations may also be listed in the margin. A question or two is helpful if the instructor sees that interest is waning in some members of the class.

The nurse outlines the content of the lesson, keeping the stated goals for that lesson and the principles of learning clearly in mind. Clarity is essential. It has been said that if you cannot phrase your ideas in simple terms, you do not understand them fully yourself. Terminology should be used with discrimination; such words as "carcinoma" or "nephrectomy" should be avoided, as they carry little or no meaning for the laity. Finally, a lesson plan should provide space in which to record an evaluation of the class session. Noting questions that were raised during or at the end of the class is helpful in making the evaluation.

Lecture Method

The lecture is usually selected if formal teaching seems appropriate to the situation, as in a large, organized class or a community gathering, a situation in which it is desirable to present certain information to many people. The real value of the lecture method lies in arousing the listener's curiosity so that he or she will develop an interest in seeking further information and knowledge. Therefore, thorough preparation is mandatory.

A careful but not detailed outline is required, based on current and accurate information. If statistics are to be used, they must be the most recent available and must be clearly interpreted. The outline is only a guide. No more than three main ideas should be developed, as an instructor cannot do justice to more in the forty-five- to fifty-minute period usually allotted. In general, the lecture has three divisions, an introduction that establishes the framework of what is to follow, the development of the theme, and the conclusion or summary, to which nothing new is added. There should be only enough facts and figures to illustrate the three ideas; more could be confusing. The instructor should have enthusiasm and interest for the subject, be knowledgeable, and be responsive to the group interest.

If visual aids, such as slides or films, are to be used, it is essential to check the equipment, e.g., the projector, before it leaves the office and again at the meeting place before the group assembles. Do all the electric connections work? In selecting visual aids the instructor should verify that they contain the desired information to support the theme of the lecture. Before visual aids are presented, the audience should be briefed on their content; at the conclusion of the showing, this content should be related to the overall subject of the meeting.

If the audience is not too large and if there is enough time, a discussion may follow. It provides the instructor with an opportunity to clarify any necessary points. In the discussion, the nurse should be on guard against those members of the group who want to do all the talking, describing their personal experiences, often irrelevant, and preventing general discussion.

Demonstration Method

The demonstration method is effective when teaching such nursing activities in the home as body exercises, body positioning, dressing a wound, or making a formula. It is difficult to learn to carry out a procedure by listening to a description of it. An anonymous patient once wrote:

I can soon learn to do it
    If you can let me see it done,
I can watch your hands in action
    But your tongue too fast will run.

In planning the demonstration, the equipment used should be the same as that found in the home, the same as that the patient or family will be using. In other words, not the shining chrome sterilizer in the health center, but an ordinary saucepan found in any home kitchen should be used in teaching the sterilization of equipment.

The demonstration lesson plan should note where and when each step will occur. Even though she is familiar with the procedure, the nurse should review each step prior to performing it in the teaching or class situation. Before commencing the demonstration, it is important to check that everyone in the group is able to see the demonstration and to hear the instructor.

It is expedient to demonstrate only one method of carrying out a procedure; otherwise the learner may be confused. However, the instructor may mention that there is more than one method but that only one method is being demonstrated at this time. It is helpful to have a few questions ready in case attention appears to be waning and the group needs a little thought stimulation. Neatness of the work area, organization of equipment and materials, and the nurse's manual dexterity in carrying out the procedure will be observed closely by the class. Because she sets standards for accomplishment by the group, her skills are important. Consciously or unconsciously, they will try to emulate her. The nurse must be aware of the opportunities for concomitant learnings and must consider them in planning her demonstration. She must never be guilty of implying, "Do as I say, not as I do."

The demonstration method is expensive timewise and should therefore be used on a group basis whenever and wherever possible, e.g., for mothers waiting in a clinic or for a class in a housing project. There are times, however, when an individual demonstration in the home or clinic is necessary to meet a specific need or situation. Demonstration is especially helpful when there is a language barrier. In such a situation, extreme care should be taken to avoid errors and to proceed slowly and carefully, checking each step with the learner.

As stated previously, a return demonstration is an integral part of this method. It enables the nurse to see how well the underlying principles of the procedure were grasped, understood, and incorporated into the learner's thinking. It also permits the nurse to check on her teaching and to determine what concomitant learning, positive and negative, has taken place. The demonstration method, even though it is time-consuming, probably is used more frequently than any other type of teaching by most community health nurses. The nurse must constantly evaluate her skills in its use and the results obtained. She must continually ask herself how she can improve her skills.

Problem Solving

Problem solving is an important technique in all public health work, including community health nursing. Epidemiology, a part of a nurse's daily work, is problem solving. The nurse uses the epidemiologic approach in relation to much of her work in homes, in schools, and in the community. From whom did the little two-year-old boy contract his tuberculous infection? How can a beginning outbreak of mumps in the third grade be controlled? What might be the source of the food poisoning that occurred following a school picnic?

Problem solving has been defined as a planned attack upon a difficulty or an obstacle for the purpose of finding a satisfactory solution. Clarity in the statement of the problem and critical thinking are essential in this method. It can be used as a teaching technique with patients, families, and community groups. One important goal in community health nursing is to teach the patient, family, and community to become independent of the nurse in meeting and solving their own health problems.

This is illustrated by Nancy Milio in her book *9226 Kercheval: The Storefront that Did Not Burn.* She points out that eventually she realized she could withdraw from the health center and its direction because those concerned no longer needed her help and guidance; furthermore, she came to see that they could only grow strong and secure without her.

Following the recognition that a problem exists, five steps are taken toward its solution: (1) Define and limit the problem. Until it has been clearly defined, and its limitations have been recognized, little can be done toward the next step. (2) Analyze the problem. This step involves a consideration of the factors present and their relationships. Every nurse has observed a physician in the problem-solving process of analyzing such data as x-rays, laboratory reports, physical examinations, and the outcome of interviews with the patient before arriving at a diagnosis. (3) Determine possible solutions to the problem, on the basis of a discriminating review of the problem and the facts involved. (4) Select the most likely solutions to the problem and test them. (5) Put the solution or plan into effect and evaluate the results.

When using the problem-solving approach with a patient and family, the nurse may find that the steps are not always so clearly defined as they are presented here, and that they may not occur always in exactly the same sequence. However, there must be an understanding and definition of the problem, some critical thinking relating to possible solutions, and a plan for effecting the solutions and testing them.

Group Discussion

As a method of facilitating teaching and learning, group discussion can be used by the nurse to arouse interest and provide information in health matters. The nurse prepares as carefully for this type of teaching as for any other. She reviews the subject selected for discussion and prepares herself to be the resource person. This method is more successful when members have a fairly common background or a similar interest, such as a group of parents with the common problem of drug abuse among their teenaged children. These parents would face many similar problems, emotional, social, health, and economic. A satisfactory size for such a group is from about five to not more than fifteen members. Having fewer than five or more than fifteen members inhibits purposeful discussion within the group. With fewer than five, an insufficient number of viewpoints may be presented, and with more than fifteen, it is not possible to secure an expression of opinion from each group member and there is less opportunity to raise pertinent questions.

The physical setting for the group discussion is important, such as ventilation, adequate space, lighting, and elimination of outside noises as far as possible. Members should be able to see and hear each other at all times. Usually chairs are placed in a circle or around a table. The nurse is included in the group but does not have a position of authority, as in a formal classroom. Members are introduced and an effort is made to pronounce their names carefully and correctly. Usually the group selects its leader and recorder and the nurse acts as the resource person and facilitator.

The leader's role is important, for he is responsible for helping the group to feel as comfortable and at ease as possible and for following the discussion carefully to see that it is kept within the limits of the subject matter. From time to time the leader asks the recorder to report on what has been said or accomplished. The leader tries to secure the viewpoint of every member, tactfully preventing any one person from dominating the discussion and encouraging the shy members to contribute their ideas. On occasion, if a crisis arises in the discussion, the nurse may suggest that role playing be tried in order to clarify the situation. A summary by the leader or recorder concludes the meeting. Usually a subject that lends itself to group discussion extends over several meetings, since not a great deal can be accomplished in one meeting alone. Until a sense of unity and cohesion has developed among group members, little progress in learning can take place.

At the end of each session, the nurse makes an evaluation for her use. Did all the members participate? If not, why? What important points of the subject were not covered? How might they be covered at the next session? Did she, the resource person and facilitator, talk too much? Was she prepared with the information needed by the group?

One nurse tried this method successfully in a suburban area with a group of parents of mentally retarded children. They represented a wide segment of the local community which had this one problem in common. The group included the custodian of the local grade school, a chemistry professor from a nearby college, a clergyman, several businessmen and women, and some housewives, about twelve in all. The custodian was selected to be the leader. As she observed the group interaction, the nurse realized how many facets of the problem they presented and discussed that would have been difficult for her to do on an individual, one-to-one basis; she also saw that these parents were coming to realize that they were not alone with their problem but were able to share it with others who had appreciation and understanding.

Interviewing

Purpose distinguishes an interview from a casual conversation. The following account reveals the purposefulness with which a nursing student interacted with a client:

> I initiated my interview with Lola by asking her, "How are things going?" This gave her the opportunity to take the lead in the conversation, and focus on the issue of most concern to her at the moment. By doing this first, I felt the client would be better able to concentrate on subjects I had planned for teaching in relation to the problems which were mutually identified during our last visit. In addition, the client would feel you care about her as an individual with her own life and unique problems, not just as "another case."
>
> I always greet the dog, Tramp, at the beginning of the visit, pet him, and ask how he has been feeling. To Lola, this is giving recognition to her personal possession and loved one. Tramp is the most worthwhile thing she feels that she has. She states that she could never leave him. She gives him medicine when he is ill, and shares her food with him. By accepting Tramp, I show that I accept Lola and her way of life.

In its simplest form, interviewing is a method of securing information, such as facts, opinions, or personal histories. When used on a professional level, interviewing, according to Abramovitz, involves "a process of interaction and communication between people. Through this process individuals can mutually clarify feelings, attitudes, and meaning-ful information. In this way professional people can gain increased understanding of the behavior and personal reactions of individuals they serve."[23] Abramovitz points out further that the interview process can help individuals come to recognize and understand their own problems.

Meanings are transferred from one person to another during an interview. For the individual transmitting a message to another, the meaning is what he believes is so. For the person receiving the message, the meaning is as he perceives the message. However, it cannot be assumed that the meaning to the second person is identical to that of the first person. Each person lives in his own world of reality, and reality is *not what is,* but what each person *believes it to be.*[24] Consequently, communicating clear messages from one person to another is much more complex than the average individual assumes. People behave in terms of their personalized perceptions of discovered meanings, and they view the world from a perspective of attitudes and values which have been learned from experience and which provide a frame of reference for subsequent meanings. Because people have internalized attitudes and values which constitute their own world of reality, the helping person must attempt to understand meanings and behavior as individualized by the client.

An *attitude,* as defined by Rokeach, is a relatively enduring organiza-tion of beliefs around an object or situation predisposing one to respond in some preferential manner. A *value* is a type of belief, centrally located within one's total belief system, about how one ought or ought not to behave, or about some end-state of existence worth or not worth attaining. Values are abstract ideals, positive or negative, representing a person's beliefs about ideal modes of conduct and ideal terminal goals. Once a value is internalized it becomes, consciously or unconsciously, a standard or criterion for guiding action, for developing and maintaining attitudes toward relevant objects and situations, for justifying one's own and others' actions and attitudes, for morally judging self and others, and for comparing self with others. Within each person is a value system which has a heirarchical organization or a rank ordering of ideals or values in terms of importance. To one person truth, beauty, and freedom may be at the top of the list, and thrift, order, and cleanliness at the bottom. To another person, the order may be reversed. Many individuals have inconsistent values within themselves and are not conscious of their contradictory beliefs. For example, a person may be asked to rank a set of values in order of importance and find that he ranked freedom first and

    [23]Abraham B. Abramovitz (ed.), *Emotional Factors in Public Health Nursing,* University of Wisconsin Press, Madison, 1961, p. 72.
    [24]Arthur W. Combs, Donald L. Avila, William W. Purkey, *Helping Relationships,* Allyn and Bacon, Inc., Boston, 1971, p. 82.

equality last, or salvation first and a comfortable life second, or making money first and health sixth. When the discrepancy of the ranking is pointed out to the respondent, awareness of the dissonance may lead to a cognitive reorganization of values and possibly a change of behavior. Values clarification is a method by which clients are helped to consider whether their stated beliefs and values match their behavior and actions.[25] If not, the individual must decide how to handle his apparent dissonance or contradictory behavior. Any decision made is a reflection of what we value.[26] Nurses who use the values clarification method concentrate on making responses which encourage clients to cogitate about their life and ideas. For example, for the client who rates making money first and health sixth, the nurse can point out, with realism and drama, how maintenance of health is essential and desirable while in the process of making money and enjoying its benefits. The purpose of values clarification is to stimulate the problem-solving capabilities, self-direction, and responsible behavior of clients.

Essentials for a successful interview of any type include a satisfactory environment, privacy, and the assurance of confidentiality. The home is a suitable place for the community health nurse's interview, especially if the interview is her first contact with the family. As the host, the patient (or family) will feel more secure and relaxed in their own environment. For the nurse, the intrafamily relationships and the atmosphere of the home will be more apparent and will provide clues on which to base her interview. Furthermore, the photographs, framed certificates of birth, confirmation, and marriage seen in many homes, and also the books, musical instruments, and arrangements of household living will provide silent answers to some of the nurse's questions and cues for others.

Settings other than the home can be used for the interview, such as the office, a clinic, a health center, a place of business. When interviews take place in settings other than the home, the nurse is the hostess and the patient or family are guests. In her role as hostess, the nurse must take this into consideration, recognizing that they may not be as comfortable as in their own home. During an interview the patient and family need ample time to develop their point of view. It is as valuable for the nurse to listen as it is for her to talk, and knowing *when* to do each is a skill in itself. The nurse should determine how she herself is reacting to the expectations of the interviewee.

In her eagerness to help, the nurse should be careful not to impose on others her own attitudes and standards in such matters as cleanliness,

---

[25]Milton Rokeach, *Beliefs, Attitudes, and Values,* Jossey-Bass Inc., Publishers, San Francisco, 1970, pp. 112–160.

[26]Nena O'Neill and George O'Neill, *Shifting Gears,* M. Evans and Company, Inc., New York, 1974, p. 157.

mode of dress, food, medical care, or social behavior. An understanding tolerance is important here. It has been said that the true meaning of tolerance is to be found in the Sioux Indians' definition: "If you wish for tolerance you must ask the Great Spirit to help you never to judge another until you have walked for two miles in his moccasins." This is especially true when patient and family are trying to meet their problems not only in the light of their own traditions, culture, and religious customs but also within the general patterns of American culture. The nurse must try to recognize what the patient and family really want, need, and are ready to accept from the professional services she has to offer.

The nurse needs to look for and consider causative factors in the patient's background that may be operating in his or her behavior. Her expressed appreciation for what the patient has accomplished and the difficulties he or she has encountered will help to establish rapport. A judicious use of sympathy and empathy enters the relationship. There will be times when the patient or interviewee needs help in differentiating between reality and confusion created by his or her own defenses. Setting limits to prevent the patient from wandering too far from problems under discussion will help.

In planning for the interview, the nurse considers and selects those questions that will elicit the information needed, questions that are concise, clear, and pertinent to the situation. These questions need to be phrased carefully, with no evidence of disapproval by the nurse of her personal value judgments. Weissman has listed some concerns that community health nurses and other public health workers have expressed in relation to their skills and techniques in the interviewing process. Following are some of these concerns:

1   How can the interviewer ask questions that will elicit meaningful responses?
2   How can the interviewer secure information and understanding about some of the underlying emotional aspects of problem situations?
3   How does the interviewer deal with her own anxieties and tensions during an interview?
4   How can the interviewer comfortably meet silences on the part of the interviewee?
5   Can a silence be constructive?
6   How can the interviewee be encouraged to break the silence?
7   How can the patient's or the family's anger or unwillingness to talk be handled?
8   What does it mean to be supportive, and how is it done?[27]

[27]Isabel G. Weissman, "Make Interviewing a Creative Process," *California's Health*, **22**(22):201–203, May 15, 1965.

Questions which have been found to be helpful in eliciting desired responses are:

When did it start?
How did it happen?
How often does it happen?
Where did it happen?
In what way do you let other people know how you feel?
What would you like different in this situation?
What have you done about this situation so far?

A question to avoid is "Why?" In most instances, a "why" question elicits a defensive response. As an experiment, the nurse can ask a series of "why" questions of a friend and observe the friend's progressive self-protective responses. Questions that may be answered with a "Yes" or "No," e.g., "Does May eat the right kind of breakfast?" are usually of little help to the nurse. Such a question elicits little information about May's eating patterns. A more specific question, such as, "What did May eat for her breakfast this morning?" would provide a more helpful answer.

It is advisable also to think twice before giving advice! Human behavior seems to dictate that each person will do as he or she wants to do or as he or she perceives what must be done. When this person asks advice, he or she often is weighing possible alternatives, is curious what the nurse will advise, is "playing an acceptable game," or is waiting to hear a solution he or she will *not* use. The clairvoyant nurse will avoid giving advice, and instead, will elicit the possible solutions the client has been considering in an effort to encourage self-direction and responsibility.

It is important to remember not to ask two questions during one verbalization. The client is forced to decide which question takes top priority for answering and, consequently, the direction of the discussion can be changed.

When a relationship of trust exists between nurse and client, direct appropriate questions can be asked which will elicit direct honest responses. Some nurses tend to seek information via the circuitous indirect route rather than being open, honest, and direct about the questions for which they want answers. When clients trust the nurse, they feel comfortable about responding honestly, directly, and without embarrassment.

"I" messages are an effective means of verbalizing language which states meanings the interviewer is thinking about. The client, upon hearing the "I" message of the interviewer, can affirm or deny the meaning of the statement and not feel overtly attacked. For example, the nurse interviewer can say, "I sense, at times, that your baby's crying is more than you can stand." Or, "I am uncertain if you are taking the medications as regularly as you say." In these instances, the nurse is conveying a message she wants the client to hear, and the client can accept or deny the implications of the message. The relationship between the nurse and client is not necessarily disrupted, and clarification of concerns may be facilitated. An "I" message can be initiated by the nurse when she feels uncomfortable during the interview. For example, she can say, "I am uncomfortable with this silence. I am uncertain if it is because I cannot tolerate silences or if you are waiting for me to say something?" Again, if the nurse perceives the client to be angry, she can say, "I feel you are angry and am not certain if it is due to something I said or did?"

When the nurse engages in *active listening,* she utilizes several techniques which assist in clarifying the concerns of clients, including emotional aspects of problem situations. *Paraphrasing* is repeating a message back to the client, but putting the thought together with the client's words or with new words to convey what was heard. *Perception checking* is closely related to paraphrasing but deals more overtly with the meaning of the message as heard by the nurse. The content of the message is repeated to the client and concluded with, "Is this what you mean?" or, "Is this how you see it?" *Behavior description* is very effective in giving objective feedback to clients. It consists of reporting your observations of specific behaviors or actions without interpretation of a good or bad value. For example, the nurse can say, "You are telling me how troubled you are with all your problems, yet you are smiling." Or, "I notice you clench your fist every time you talk about your son." For beginning nurses, practice of these interviewing interventions is recommended so that utilization of them becomes natural and spontaneous. Frequently, important information is gained through the use of these techniques—information that was not anticipated but turns out to be valuable.

There are several components of the communication process which must be understood as underlying all messages and meanings which are transmitted from one person to another. They also contribute to the way in which the listener interprets the message. The *content* of the message is the cognitive level which most adults listen for and deal with. The *vocal process* of the speaker transmits meanings that the listener interprets according to his perception of tone quality, style of speech, and method of delivery. *Body talk* reveals nonverbal behavior descriptive of the emotional status of the speaker. Use of the *metaphor* (a figure of speech in which one thing is likened to another) assumes the understanding of the listener according to the perspective meant by the speaker. The *life theme* or script of the speaker is apparent to all the senses of the listener as he receives and interprets the message from his frame of reference. Upon examination of the components of the communication process, it must be realized that most adults deal mainly with the content of messages, and because they miss cues revealed by the remaining components, they misinterpret or misunderstand messages. The remaining components of the communication process are understood much more readily by children as they are attentive to the speaker, but not necessarily to his words.[28] The effective nurse must use all her senses to the best of her ability when she interacts with a client in a therapeutic relationship and interprets meanings as intended by clients. Abramovitz points out that skillful interviewing is a medium in which "an integrated understanding of people is combined with the knowledge of one's own professional field in order to enable the patient to help himself."[29]

The interview should close with a summary of the positive things that have been accomplished, some of the things yet to be done, and suggested plans for another conference or interview at a later date. However, the interview is not complete until the salient points have been recorded and placed in the folder of the family or patient. The planned date for the next interview and what is hoped to be accomplished at that time should be a part of the record.

One type of interview, that with the venereal disease patient, is on the increase because of the rapid rise in the nationwide incidence of syphilis and gonorrhea. Such interviews may take place in the home, the health center or clinic, the school, or place of employment. Because of the implications and the attitudes toward these diseases, this type of interview requires special skills in establishing confidence and developing rapport with the patient in order to gain his or her cooperation in undertaking a program of treatment promptly, which is not only important to the patient's health but is of equal importance also to his or her family, to future children, and to the community's health and protection.

There should be an appreciation on the part of the nurse that this type of interview may be uncomfortable, embarrassing, or even painful for some patients. Others may be receptive to the health information the nurse offers and be more cooperative. As in all interviews, the nurse should be sensitive to behavioral cues, be objective, understanding, nonjudgmental, and help the patient to take the long view of his or her situation. Her goals are to help the patient and to protect the community.

[28]Peter J. Hansen, *Family Counseling: A Workshop for Nurses,* Notes taken during workshop, October 1975.
[29]Abramovitz, loc. cit.

As the nurse records an interview, she has an opportunity to evaluate it. Skills in interviewing do not come easily but require constant practice and evaluation, so she should ask herself the following questions:

1   Were the purposes and objectives of the interview met?
2   Did the interviewee have adequate time to participate in the interview and express his or her point of view?
3   Was the interview, as far as possible, kept with an "open end" and not too structured?
4   Was the interviewee permitted to talk freely and without interruption unless he or she rambled or became too repetitious?
5   Did she maintain a critical, objective, and impartial attitude while listening and talking?

By evaluating her interviews, the nurse gains an awareness of her progress in developing the necessary skills and techniques, for interviewing is a professional skill that can, for the most part, be developed only by constant study, practice, and self-evaluation.

SUMMARY

The emphasis on and importance of attainment of relationship skills for community health nurses was stressed as having *high* priority if successful practices with individuals, families, or groups are desired. To be a truly helping person who will be accepted and often appreciated by the consumer, the nurse must possess three characteristics: accurate empathy, nonpossessive warmth, and genuineness. When consumers are asked to describe the kind of nurse they would like to have serving them, they invariably bring out their desire for a nurse with warmth, humor, friendliness, and a special liking for them.

Community health nurses use a variety of different approaches when they work with individuals and families. Descriptions and examples were given of some specific approaches which can be successfully implemented dependent upon the individualized responses of individuals and families.

When the nurse communicates and/or teaches, behavioral objectives are essential to describe the anticipated desired outcomes for individuals and families. Learning may take time to produce results, i.e., a change of behavior. There must be motivation from within and from without. The nurse needs to begin where the learner is, and by determining what is already known and accepted, proceed from the known to the unknown, developing relationships between the two. The content of her teaching must fit the needs of the learner with appropriate learning activities. Planned time for review, reconsideration, and evaluation at spaced intervals is necessary, depending on the ability of the individuals and families to learn and put into practice what they have gained from the nurse's teaching.

SUGGESTED READING

Bakker, Cornelis B., and Marianne K. Bakker-Rabdau: *No Trespassing!* Chandler & Sharp Publishers, Inc., San Francisco, 1973.

Beier, Ernest G.: *The Silent Language of Psychotherapy,* Aldine Publishing Company, Chicago, 1966.

Brammer, Lawrence M ⋅ *The Helping Relationship: Process and Skills,* Prentice-Hall, Inc., Englewood Cliffs, N.J., 1973.

Branden, Nathaniel: *The Disowned Self,* Bantam Books, Inc., New York, 1971.

Caplan, Gerald: *Principles of Preventive Psychiatry,* Basic Books, Inc., Publishers, New York, 1964.

Carkhuff, Robert R.: *Helping and Human Relations: Volume I,* Holt, Rinehart and Winston, Inc., New York, 1969.

⎯⎯: *Helping and Human Relations: Volume II,* Holt, Rinehart and Winston, Inc., New York, 1969.

Carlson, Carolyn E. (ed.): *Behavioral Concepts and Nursing Intervention,* J. B. Lippincott Company, Philadelphia, 1970.

Combs, Arthur W., Donald L. Avila, and William W. Purkey: *Helping Relationships,* Allyn and Bacon, Inc., Boston, 1971.

Cumming, John, and Elaine Cumming: *Ego & Milieu,* Aldine-Atherton, Inc., Chicago, 1962.

Dunn, Halbert L.: *High-Level Wellness,* R. W. Beatty Co., Arlington, Va., 1961.

Frankl, Viktor E.: *Man's Search for Meaning,* Washington Square Press, a division of Simon & Schuster, Inc., New York, 1963.

Gronlund, Norman E.: *Stating Behavioral Objectives for Classroom Instruction,* The Macmillan Company, New York, 1970.

Haley, Jay: *Strategies of Psychotherapy,* Grune & Stratton, Inc., New York, 1963.

Jourard, Sidney M.: *The Transparent Self,* D. Van Nostrand Company, Inc., Princeton, N.J., 1964.

Mager, Robert F.: *Preparing Instructional Objectives,* Fearon Publishers Inc., Palo Alto, Calif., 1962.

Mayeroff, Milton: *On Caring,* Harper & Row, Publishers, Incorporated, New York, 1972.

Mayers, Marlene, "Home Visit—Ritual or Therapy?" *Nursing Outlook,* 21(5):328–331, May 1973.

Moustakas, Clark: *Personal Growth,* Howard A. Doyle Publishing Company, Cambridge, Mass., 1969.

O'Neill, Nena, and George O'Neill: *Shifting Gears.* M. Evans & Co., Inc., New York, 1974.

Otto, Herbert A.: *Guide to Developing Your Potential,* Charles Scribner's Sons, New York, 1967.

⎯⎯, and John Mann: *Ways of Growth,* Grossman Publishers, New York, 1968.

Peter, Laurence J.: *The Peter Prescription,* A Bantam Book, William Morrow & Company, Inc., New York, 1972.

Pohl, Margaret L.: *Teaching Function of the Nursing Practitioner,* William C. Brown Company Publishers, Dubuque, Iowa, 1968.

Rogers, Carl R.: *On Becoming a Person,* Houghton Mifflin Company, Boston, 1961.

    : *Freedom to Learn,* Charles E. Merrill Publishing Company, Columbus, Ohio, 1969.

Roache, Margaret Olson: "Humanistic Learning," *American Journal of Nursing,* **74**(8):1453–1456, August 1974.

Rokeach, Milton: *Beliefs, Attitudes, and Values,* Jossey-Bass, Inc., Publishers, San Francisco, 1970.

Satir, Virginia: *Conjoint Family Therapy,* Science and Behavior Books, Inc., Palo Alto, Calif., 1967.

Spitzer, Robert S. (ed.): *Tidings of Comfort and Joy,* Science and Behavior Books, Inc., Palo Alto, Calif., 1975.

Towle, Charlotte: *Common Human Needs,* National Association of Social Workers, Inc., New York, 1965.

Williams, Roger J.: *You Are Extraordinary,* Random House, Inc., New York, 1971.

Chapter 4

Focusing on Communities

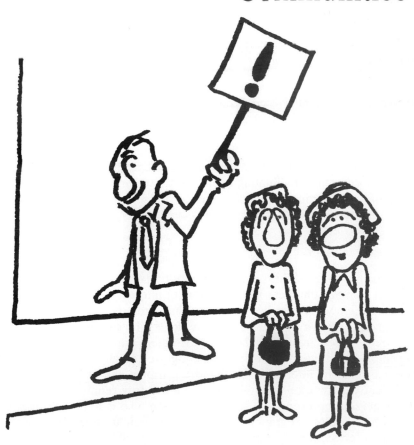

"Oh Harry isn't for or against anything in particular he just likes to occasionally demonstrate his community involvement . . ."

Since community health nurses are practicing in a variety of geographical locations, the setting of the local community and factors affecting it must be studied in addition to the health needs of the local residents. Each community, whether urban, suburban, or rural, has its own unique characteristics, strengths, and limitations. As the nurse becomes knowledgeable about the community in which she is working, she enhances her ability to play a significant role in developing awareness of and improving the health practices of its people. As stated by Remillet and Reading, the community health nurse must know the community she serves. She must have accurate knowledge of the age-group percentages, ethnic differences, the dominant culture and subcultures, sociological factors that spawn health problems, and the resources for finding solutions once problems have been differentiated from cause. Accumulation of data is only the beginning; application of the findings in order to assess needs further and to participate in realistic decision making to improve the environment for better living follows in logical sequence.[1]

By looking at the field of health as a generalist in nursing, the community health nurse must be prepared to know multiple facets of the community; the health problems, needs, and desires of consumers; health resources, personnel, and facilities; and methods for integrating the health-care system so that all parts complete a whole. When viewed as wholeness of individuals, families, and groups, health opens up many new avenues of approach and responsibility which the community health nurse can meet if she is creative, ingenious, enterprising, and seeks to act as a coordinating, facilitating agent. In these times of rapid change, the role of the community health nurse must also reflect change to keep up with the requirements of our progressive society.

THE COMMUNITY

For the purposes of this book a *community* is defined as a group of people with a common characteristic, location, or interest living together within a larger society. Generally, a geographic area is considered to be a community; however, groups of individuals who gather together because of their interest in a particular health problem are also a community. For example, an individual may live in a congested neighborhood of a city and be particularly interested in the drug traffic and drug abuse of the residents and work actively in developing a drug rehabilitation program. This person represents a responsible citizen who is living in a particular neighborhood or geographic setting and participating in one aspect of a health interest, namely drugs. Therefore, the word "community" refers to

[1]June Remillet and Sadie Reading, "Adapting to Changing Community Health Needs," *Nursing Outlook,* 18(10):47, October 1970.

a geographic location and/or an association of interests. A citizen can live in and work with a variety of communities, dependent upon his or her dwelling place and scope of interests.

The nurse can focus on all behavior within a community from three points of view: (1) maintenance of the physical and social environment; (2) securing of help and support at times of stress; and (3) strengthening of individuals to gain a sense of self and social worth.[2] The emphasis of her work will be gauged by her perception of the diverse needs of the community citizens with whom she is working. For example, from the first point of view, she may work mainly with the elementary school population in terms of safety and immunizations. The second point of view will be directed toward young married couples with newborn infants who are entering the family system. Low-income families living within a specified housing project may be responsive to the emphasis on the third point of view, particularly when they are ready to participate in community planning and action directly affecting them.

THE COMMUNITY HEALTH NURSING PROCESS IN THE COMMUNITY

Community health nursing is a synthesis of nursing practice and public health practice applied to promoting and preserving the health of populations. In community health nursing practice the consumer is the client. Consumers include individuals, groups, and the community as a whole.[3] To become acquainted with a given community or selected populations, the nurse must determine the factors for which more data needs to be secured in order to make an adequate assessment. A realistic assessment of the health and status of the community is systematic and continuous. It takes note of the present and future health of individuals, families, and communities in terms of human-environment interrelationships. An assessment is done for the purpose of deciding the efficacy of a nursing action. If the health status data provide a basis for believing a nursing action will promote beneficial growth or change in the community, then a nursing diagnosis derived from the health status data is determined. The nursing diagnosis delineates the kind of nursing action considered to be appropriate in the selected community. Planning is essential for engineering actions which will produce desired outcomes. Implementing the plan means "doing it." Evaluation determines how well objectives were accomplished, if outcomes demonstrated success, if omissions or unanti-

[2]Donald C. Klein, *Community Dynamics and Mental Health,* John Wiley & Sons, Inc., New York, 1968, p. 10.
[3]American Nurses' Association, *Standards of Community Health Nursing Practice,* Kansas City, Mo., 1973.

cipated factors were disclosed, if satisfaction of consumer groups was gained, and if a need was revealed for continuing study and community involvement.

COMMUNITY HEALTH NURSING PROCESS—ASSESSING

Data collection is prerequisite to a realistic assessment of a community and establishment of a proposed nursing diagnosis. Securing accurate data can be done by multiple means, some of which include (1) observing the community, (2) visiting community facilities, (3) interviewing key community leaders, and (4) becoming knowledgeable about reference materials and resources which describe different factors about the community.

Observation of a Community

For the nurse who wants to study unofficially a community new to her, a first activity for gaining data is to obtain a map and drive around the local community to gain impressions of the housing, spacing of residences, business establishments, industrial establishments, neighborhood services such as grocery stores, transportation facilities, shopping centers, educational facilities, recreational facilities such as parks or playgrounds, health facilities such as hospitals, physicians' offices, safety of the environment, number of churches, and the faces of the people. Some of the questions which may come to mind are: How do the people support themselves? Is there evidence of pride in this community? How did this community come into being in the first place? Is there a "mix" of population such as several nationalities and races, extremes of wealth and poverty, extremes of young and old? Do the people seem preoccupied, busy, impersonal, friendly, prosperous, poor, old, young?

After gaining early impressions, a suggested second activity is to purchase a local newspaper and scan the contents. Does it reflect national, state, and local news or does it concentrate on folksy items? What is the nature of the advertisements in the paper? Are there editorial comments that give a sense of the attitudes of the residents? Are there any health items reported? Are there announcements of local meetings or reports of local agency activities? Are there meetings or facilities that the nurse may want to visit?

By getting a "feel" of the appearance and interests of the community, the nurse can map out subsequent activities she wishes to engage in. She can formulate questions in her mind for which she wants answers so that the ultimate goal of getting well acquainted with the community includes purposeful and informative activities. A well-informed community health nurse must know the characteristics, idiosyncrasies, and attitudes of her community. It takes time for a new nurse to become well informed but a carefully planned, informal study facilitates the process.

When visiting the homes of consumers of health services, the nurse must take note of space, safety factors, water, heating, sewage disposal, light, cleanliness, sanitation, ventilation, furnishings, food-storage facilities, bathing and toilet facilities, sleeping arrangements, play areas, yards, and gardens. The assumption must never be made that the possession of an automobile or a television set signifies evidence of an adequate income. At one time a television set was considered a luxury item; however, the appearance of one in the home is no longer a criterion for determining the solvency of the consumer.

Community Facilities within a Community

The nurse must be cognizant of the numbers and locations of educational, religious, business, industrial, and recreational facilities within a community, but the *health facilities* are of particular interest to her. Many communities have booklets or directories compiled by a coordinating or planning agency which list the names, telephone numbers, and addresses of a wide variety of community resources, the purpose for which they were formed, the services they offer, the source of financial support, the eligibility requirements for consumers, and the fees. Such a booklet or carefully compiled handbook organized with health-services information is essential data for the community health nurse to have at her disposal at all times. Frequently the directories have a classified index, which assists in locating needed services according to a given category, such as welfare assistance, services for unmarried mothers, handicapped children and adults, vocational training, special education for special conditions, services for the aging, and many more categories. The classification is done to facilitate the location of needed information with a minimum of time.

By visiting those community facilities in which the nurse is particularly interested, she becomes personally acquainted with professional workers, the implementation of health services, and the referral system, and she has the opportunity to initiate a reciprocal relationship that will give impetus to future teamwork with allied disciplines. Until the nurse has a comprehensive knowledge of available community resources and facilities, she often does not feel adequately prepared to practice her role of coordination and referral.

Key Community Leaders

Every community has formal and informal leaders who hold positions of power, influence, or status in terms of facilitating or hindering community actions. It behooves the work of the community health nurse to become acquainted with the key community leaders, because they have influence in the field of health. The leaders can be found in local government as elected or appointed officials, businesses, educational systems, religious structures, or health and welfare organizations. When investigating a local community structure it is clarifying to secure an organization chart which outlines the lines of authority and position. From the chart formal leaders of the specific organizations under scrutiny may be identified, such as the local mayor, sheriff, judge, school principal, health officer, or welfare director. Informal but significantly influential leaders may also be found in occupations or professions such as industries, banks, clergy, medicine, and law. Associations representing service clubs, labor unions, political party organizations, communication media, community councils or boards, voluntary health organizations, housing authorities, fraternal groups, cultural groups, and minority groups are additional sources for finding key community leaders.

With timing and a sensitivity for gaining appropriate knowledge from all available sources, the power structure of the local community can be determined, and future plans for activities involving the services of key citizens can be filed mentally as the nurse becomes oriented to the community. As the need arises, she is then able to contact appropriate samples of individuals to organize, plan, implement, and evaluate needed health programs, provide effective and successful services to consumers, and broaden the interpretation of nursing services to the general public. An example of a direct method which was used by one student nurse to become acquainted with the leadership of a small rural community involved a visit to the local bank and inquiring of the banker, "Who represents the power structure in this town?" The banker thought momentarily, then replied, "I guess you would say that I do!"

Reference Sources about a Community

Depending upon the type of data desired, sources of information about a local community can be found in the library, books, periodicals, historical societies or archives, newspaper offices, directories, diaries, public records, town records, community development or planning agencies, church records, vital statistics offices, and other reference locations. An additional means for securing data is to interview older residents, key community leaders, and political figures or to question a cross section of local citizens or consumers about health services.

Demographic data about a community is secured from census bureaus and vital statistics offices. Census bureaus provide information on the number and characteristics of persons living in a specified area at a particular time. Information on vital events is obtained from official registration of births, deaths, marriages, and divorces.[4] Epidemiological data is obtained from the departments of communicable disease or epidemiology which are situated in local health departments. Up-to-date statistics are generally available about the occurrence of diseases which are of concern to the local agency. Gathering descriptive data about the local community gives the nurse a preliminary basis for considering potential health programs. For example, if the nurse is thinking of initiating a prevention program for hypertension, she will want to know the numbers and locations of middle-aged persons living in the community who may be responsive to a preventive health education program regarding exercise, relaxation, and low cholesterol diets.

"Mini" studies are another way of obtaining data. They can be conducted in a variety of ways, such as constructing two or three pertinent questions and asking a selected portion of the local population about a selected interest area. For example, the data collector might ask a small sample of consumers living in neighborhoods surrounding an airport, "Are you acquainted with the term, noise pollution? Are you concerned about noise pollution in your neighborhood? Of the following resources, in your opinion, which would have the greatest influence in reducing the noise pollution in this neighborhood? The mayor? The city council? The airlines? The local newspaper? An organized group of consumers?"

By securing answers to these questions from a representative sample of consumers living in neighborhoods surrounding an airport, the data gatherer would know the concerns of the residents regarding noise pollution and the resource they regarded as most influential for securing change. The investigator also may want to survey citizens living in most distant neighborhoods to compare data of respondents based on residential proximity to the airport. The findings of such a ministudy would give an indication for further investigation and action on the selected community health problem or redirection toward a health issue more compelling to the local population.

The Health System within the Community

In many communities, according to Sanders, there are five types of health structures found within the health-care system.[5] However, a sixth type has emerged in recent years which is designed to meet the needs of consumers who have not been serviced adequately by the five existing systems. The sixth structure includes the proliferation of free clinics,

[4]Lenor S. Goerke and Ernest L. Stebbins, *Mustard's Introduction to Public Health,* The Macmillan Company, New York, 1968, p. 84.
[5]Irwin T. Sanders, "The Community: Structure and Function," *Nursing Outlook,* 11(9):642–643, September 1963.

community service centers, and neighborhood health stations which have come into being, often with the assistance of the Office of Economic Opportunity, and focus primarily on the needs of minority or low-income groups. The six health structures are closely intertwined, yet distinct enough to be studied separately by those nurses who wish to serve as coordinators and collaborators with all the structures. The five health structures described by Sanders are (1) private office practice of professionals, namely the physician or group of physicians working in the office or clinic setting; (2) group health care, in which consumers buy medical and health services by becoming members of facilities set up for that specific purpose; (3) large hospitals and clinics with their own boards and clientele; (4) public health agencies that protect, administer, and perform more preventive than curative health services for the consumer; and (5) those facilities and personnel who sell treatment products and appliances required, such as pharmacists, orthopedic supply houses, and similar establishments. Each of the health subsystems requires a different network of organized activity and therefore operates within an individualized organizational structure, which may be loose-knit or tightly coordinated.

Each health structure fulfills community expectations of a specified sort and conducts its affairs within certain codes of operation.[6] Nurses work in most of the health subsystems and give special services concurrent with the health structure and abide by the code of operation expected within that particular structure. Each health subsystem has basically similar expectations for the functioning of the nurse, but the manner in which she performs her tasks varies according to the structure and setting. In the sixth health structure, which was described as a burgeoning number of community health centers, neighborhood multiservice centers, free clinics, or similarly named stations which have come into existence because of needs of consumers, nurses either volunteer their time or are employed by organizations or consumers who receive funding from governmental sources. In the centers in which consumers are participating actively in the determination of health services, nurses play a different role than in any of the other five health structures. Primarily they are working *with* the consumer of health services, rather than *for* him, and this entails a redirection in focus in many ways, As described by Milio, the nurse sometimes must play a subtle role, or nonvisible one, in order to accomplish a desired objective.[7] Or the nurse must be able to account for her activities in a way that makes sense and is relevant to the consumer.[8]

[6]Ibid., p. 643.

[7]Nancy Milio, *9226 Kercheval: The Storefront that Did Not Burn,* The University of Michigan Press, Ann Arbor, 1970, p. 31.

[8]Kate R. Lorig, "Consumer-Controlled Nursing." *Nursing Outlook,* 17(9):52, September 1969.

It is an important task of the community health nurse to be cognizant of all facets operating within the health-care system in her given community, to be knowledgeable about coordination practices and procedures with other nurses and professional personnel working in the health structures, and to be able to interpret and link all six health structures in an understandable and intriguing way to the consumer.

An Experiential Exercise for Getting Acquainted with a New Community

Initially, nursing students tend to feel shy about entering a new community as a community health nurse. They fantasize an image in which they see themselves as imparting "pearls of wisdom" to clients—speaking with authority and great knowledge! Obviously, upon entering a community for the first time, students do not possess the essential knowledge which is implied in the fantasy. An exercise which propels students to enter the new community on a "discovery" basis has been found to be helpful in broadening their knowledge base, securing data about the community and its resources, experiencing the climate of a given setting, and building confidence in self to perform independently and assertively. The exercise is an experiential one, whereby students are asked to pretend to *be* a described person in need of particular services. For example, students may be given a written situation and assignment which will give a general direction for their exploration of community resources. Suggestions of situations which can be given to students are described briefly as follows.

> You are a young wife and mother who recently arrived in the local community. Your husband is out of work but is making the rounds regarding job possibilities. Your child is sixteen months old, is developing normally, but tends to have too many bouts of U.R.I. You wish to rent an apartment or home and want to find one today. According to the welfare worker, you can pay up to _____ a month for a place.
>
> You are a seventy-year-old widow who is hardy, curious, and full of energy. You want to volunteer your services wherever there seems to be a need. You want to visit community facilities that may be interested in receiving volunteer services from an elderly lady.

After reading the situations, students are encouraged to work in pairs or trios and venture forth into the new community as explorers. Providing the students with local directories of community resources, a people's yellow pages directory, the telephone book, the local newspaper, and maps will give them basic reference sources from which to draw a plan of action.

Students are amazingly resourceful and learn about a variety of valuable community facilities while doing this exercise. By working in pairs or trios, they support each other in taking the initiative to enter new agencies, make purposeful inquiries, and enact a pretended role. They tend to like to discover by themselves! They sometimes learn that if they present themselves as described by their situation, they are treated differently than if they introduce themselves as nursing students. They learn about the reality of supply and demand of low-cost housing, adequacies and inadequacies of community facilities, and concern for prospective clients. As a consequence of this exercise, students serve as reference persons for each other as they work with families and ask each other for information about available resources for specific health problems.

Commentary by students about their experiences give some idea of diversity of reactions and viewpoints:

> Today has helped us to see more realistically some of the problems of low-income families and alternatives for assistance. Coming from a middle-class suburban background, frankly, I never really considered the problems of this population. Until now it had no personal relevance for me.

> If I learned nothing else today, I experienced the frustration the family in question would feel in being homeless after a day's search. I'm also three times as glad for the roof over *my* head tonight.

> We presented our seventy-year-old widow as though she were flesh and blood, which, of course, she is—though we haven't met her yet—and she was soon as real to us as she was to those who were so anxious to give her a niche to fill. When on a couple of occasions we thought it best to admit we were nursing students with a hypothetical case, we were just as warmly received.

> After spending the entire day on my feet, I have to say I am really impressed with my community. I was met with consideration and kindness wherever I visited. Of course, I am prejudiced toward one particular facility—the senior citizens center of _____. I took a nice long look around before ever going up to the building. Was I ever suprised to see tables full of old women making quilts as fast as their hands would travel. I wanted to sit right down and get started working with them.

HEALTH-CARE DELIVERY IN THE UNITED STATES

The health-care delivery as it exists in the United States today is made up of providers of care from the public and private sectors. Health-care providers represent public health agencies and/or city/county health departments, voluntary and proprietary hospitals, medical schools, physicians, health maintenance organizations, philanthropies, and public and social service organizations. They provide care and treatment for the population dependent on the ability to pay a fee for service. Traditionally, there has always been a dual system of health care in the United States. The private sector has provided care for those who have been able to pay for services in either an out-of-pocket way or a third-party prepayment plan. The public sector has provided care for those who are classified as medically indigent. Up to the present, these people have been characterized as welfare, medicare, and medicaid recipients. They have come predominately from the lower socioeconomic levels of income.[9]

It is important for the community health nurse to be cognizant of the present system of health-care delivery. At the same time, it is vital to keep up-to-date and knowledgeable about pending health-care legislation which may be in the process of being authorized and funded by national and state legislative bodies. Decisions about health-care delivery are influenced increasingly by national and governmental policy. New directions for health care, health standards, accessibility, and financing of health care are all subject to changes which will have direct consequences for the consumer and health professional. The community health nurse who keeps current with legislative news and proposals is in the position of preparing for health-care delivery as changes occur, of devising health-supporting patterns of living, and raising the consciousness of consumers about access to health services.[10]

SOCIOECONOMIC LEVELS IN THE COMMUNITY

Many specific health problems in the United States are thought to be related directly to poverty, yet affluence also contributes to unhealthy conditions. Socioeconomic levels have a bearing on health status and must be studied in terms of the effect that money, education, living patterns, and life-styles have on the well-being of consumers. For example, conditions of poverty such as poor housing, inadequate nutrition, and frustration of unemployment can set the stage for pneumonia, influenza, tuberculosis, obesity, apathy, depression, accidents, and chronic disabilities. Affluent individuals who succumb habitually to self-indulgent attributes are vulnerable candidates for coronary heart disease, diabetes, alcoholism, and diagnosed psychiatric maladies.

The composition of each community has its own structure and personality which is not duplicated by any other community. Citizens generally have a vague awareness of the composition of their community but, upon questioning, reveal a lack of specific knowledge about any aspect under inquiry. They often will deny the existence of social classes yet acknowledge the presence of families of different socioeconomic

[9]Herbert Harvey Hyman (ed.), *The Politics of Health Care,* Praeger Publishers, New York, 1973, p. 160.

[10]Nancy Milio, *The Care of Health in Communities: Access for Outcasts,* Macmillan Publishing Company, Inc., New York, 1975, p. 298.

levels residing in segregated neighborhoods, either voluntarily or without choice. Socioeconomic levels are differentiated by their degrees of prestige, education, income, residence, and access to products and services in the community. They are unorganized groups. People are born into them, marry into them, or otherwise enter them from adjacent socioeconomic levels. Within them, people tend to associate with each other more than with others outside their socioeconomic level. On the average, people of different socioeconomic levels vary in aesthetic tastes, in the type of books and magazines they read, the way they vote, the size of their families, the way they spend their leisure time, and even in their sex morality.[11]

In our changing society, the characteristics identifying socioeconomic levels are constantly fluctuating, and clearly defined criteria for determining socioeconomic levels are becoming less distinct. For the purposes of community health nurses, it is valuable to maintain a curiosity about the changing nature of the social-class system, to keep up to date with current events, happenings, and research studies, in order to meet health needs of new groupings of citizens as they occur and to relate with understanding, acceptance, and readiness to the wants of the consumer.

Of import to the nurse is awareness of (1) her own method for classifying families in terms of socioeconomic level and avoiding the stereotyping based on unvalidated data, (2) her own feelings of withdrawal and superiority based on past personal experiences, and (3) the family's receptivity cues to her general services. When she is cognizant of general behaviors and attitudes representative of each socioeconomic level and her own personal reactions to a social-class image, she is better able to identify strengths and weaknesses of a given family with objectivity and work in an effective, understanding, and facilitative manner. By recognizing the family as possessing characteristics representative of an identified socioeconomic level, but also exhibiting unique characteristics which cannot be classified, the nurse is helped to view the family as a distinct entity rather than squeezing it into a poorly fitting, stereotyped mold.

Community health nurses are commonly thought to come from a middle-class orientation and do much of their health practice with people of lower socioeconomic levels. Of interest are the great variety of studies that have focused on the nurse image as seen in the context of social-class perspective. Simmons reported that in general the evaluation of nurses becomes consistently more favorable as the opinions move from higher to lower socioeconomic groups.[12]

[11]Roland L. Warren, *Studying Your Community,* The Free Press, New York, 1965, p. 351.

[12]Leo W. Simmons and Virginia Henderson, *Nursing Research, a Survey and Assessment,* Appleton-Century-Crofts, Inc., New York, 1964, p. 179.

Watts compared selective characteristics of people of lower and middle socioeconomic levels and described the person of lower socioeconomic level as being oriented to the present rather than the future and taking pleasures as they are available rather than planning for a future he cannot visualize. The person of middle-class orientation looks to the future and is willing to defer gratifications by planning ahead and saving for desired goals. He values cleanliness, work, and self-discipline.[13]

In regard to health activities, studies have been reported in professional health journals and books indicating that members of the lower socioeconomic levels have a high percentage of illnesses and are dissatisfied with the medical care available to them.[14] They have less information and knowledge about disease and are more likely to hold irrational ideas about illness, rely on folk medicine and fringe practitioners, and delay seeking medical treatment.[15] It is generally accepted that medical care is not as readily accessible to persons of the lower socioeconomic levels in the present health-care system. Members of the middle and upper socioeconomic levels know more about the dynamics of illness and health and are more aware of medical care resources for prevention and treatment of sickness. They make use of available resources in a climate of social acceptance.[16]

There are general differences of behavior required of the nurse when associating with the different socioeconomic levels of people. Some of the perceptions of the nurse are described as follows. When working with people of lower socioeconomic levels, nurses often prefer the families who are responsive to suggestions, seem to value her teaching and friendship, and demonstrate changes in health practices concurrent with her influence. The apathetic families described in Chap. 5, such as low-income families, tend to be frustrating to the nurse because she is unable to determine if her work with these families has any influence whatsoever. A greater, more intensive effort must be made by community health nurses to study families of lower socioeconomic levels and having multiple problems because the health needs are so great and new, innovative methods for giving nursing services to these families are so greatly needed. The use of role-playing techniques has been strongly recommended by many professional workers because it is appropriate to the style of this population. Role playing is action-oriented, concrete,

[13]Wilma Watts, "Social Class, Ethnic Background, and Patient Care," *Nursing Forum,* 6(2):155–162, Spring 1967.
[14]Evelyn Millis Duvall, *Family Development,* 2d ed., J.B. Lippincott Company, Philadelphia, 1962, pp. 85–86.
[15]David Mechanic, "Illness and Cure," in John Kosa, Aaron Antonovsky, and Irving Kenneth Zola (eds.), *Poverty and Health,* Harvard University Press, Cambridge, Mass., 1969, p. 207.
[16]Duvall, op cit., p. 85.

visual, and sometimes gamelike.[17] It is certainly a method with which nurses are acquainted, yet it is used little with families. In Chap. 5 an elaboration of ways for working more effectively with low-income families is given. When working with families of middle socioeconomic levels, nurses again prefer the responsive families who are interested in health information and teaching on a curing and prevention basis. The fact that these families are often better educated than families of lower income requires the nurse to be prepared always to give an intellectual explanation of any symptom within her domain of knowledge about which there is an inquiry. When a family member of middle-class orientation is better educated than the nurse, this sometimes causes anxiety feelings within the nurse which may deter her effectiveness in creating a professional image. With families of upper socioeconomic levels, the nurse is sometimes relegated to the status of servant or domestic and responds according to her perception of this station in life. With all socioeconomic levels, it helps to be thoughtfully prepared before making a contact, so that the best approach is used. If alternative options are ready, in case a change of plan is required, the nurse feels prepared and comfortable in giving the needed health services.

COMMUNITY HEALTH NURSING PROCESS—DIAGNOSING A COMMUNITY HEALTH PROBLEM

After an initial appraisal of a selected community, the nurse is cognizant of the presence of many health facilities, resources, assets, and concerned leaders. Gaps and inadequacies are recognized as existing in conjunction with some health resources and neighborhood settings. When health needs are apparent, what can the community health nurse do to remedy the problems that are seen?

First, a conceptualization of the meaning of community health must be internalized. By viewing health as a total life process, including the adaptation of the individual to the stresses in his internal and external environment, one inevitably recognizes that societal forces or social problems have a strong influence on the health of individuals and communities. One is led to conclude that to improve the health of communities, correction of adverse social factors which perpetuate or accentuate maladjustment in the environment is required.[18] Some community health problems in general which profoundly affect man's well-

---

[17]Salvador Minuchin, Braulio Montalvo, Bernard G. Guerney, Jr., Bernice L. Rosman, and Florence Schumer, *Families of the Slums,* Basic Books, Inc., Publishers, New York, 1967, p. 37.

[18]Lee M. Howard, *Key Problems Impeding Modernization of Developing Countries,* Agency for International Development, Washington, D.C., 1970, p. 50.

being include poverty, urban crowding, inadequate sanitary and waste disposal, pollution, insecurity, and food shortage. In addition, as described by Milio, when a full array of health services are not located where people are—the intended consumers—or when prices or other program characteristics intervene as barriers, people become outcasts of health care. Social groupings who are identified as outcast are those of low income, poor living areas, old age, minority race, or majority sex.[19]

Secondly, the nurse must seek an "outcast" group or health conditions revealing inadequacies. In most communities, there are several consumer groups or health deficiency areas which can be identified by the nurse. It is only a matter of personal preference and selection. Some questions the nurse might consider are:

Do all people in this community have equal access to health care? If not, who are the ones who do not have easy access? What are the barriers preventing easy access?

Does the health-care delivery system in this community give preventive services? If not, are there strategies that might change or improve the system?

Are low-income people in this community concerned about health problems? If not, can they be motivated to become active participants for improved conditions?

Are consumers in this community responsive to health education programs? If not, how might health education programs be made to seem more stimulating and attention-getting?

Is there malnutrition in this community? If so, where does it exist? Is it due to lack of education, inadequate funds, personal beliefs and values?

Do people in this community see nurses as community organizers, facilitators, consumer advocates, or social activists?

Some statements about health conditions in the United States are offered for the purpose of stimulating investigation whether these same conditions exist in the local community. Even though the United States is an affluent nation, infant mortality is high statistically, particularly for races other than Caucasian. There is evidence of malnutrition, particularly among blacks and persons of Spanish origin, living in low-income neighborhoods. The poor have more disability and limitation of activity because of chronic disease. Even though the overall death rate in the United States has changed little since the 1950s, increased deaths in the middle years (ages 15–65) have occurred. Young adults are dying primarily from accidents, homicide, and suicide, and older adults are dying from the diseases of affluence—heart disease, cancer, and stroke.[20] Two-thirds

[19]Milio, op. cit., p. 63.
[20]Ibid., pp. 43–50.

of all accidental deaths occurring from age one through thirty-five involve automobiles.[21] Eating patterns for citizens in the United States emphasize high concentrations of refined sugars and starches which lead to conditions such as dental caries, diabetes mellitus, gastric ulcers, and obesity. Occupationally induced diseases kill 100,000 persons annually.[22]

Any of the above named problems, to cite only a few, can be selected for study by the nurse and preventive measures of some type instituted. Any effort, no matter how small, is worth the energy expended. In-depth exploration and analysis of any selected community health problem in relationship to existing social conditions and the health-care delivery system as practiced in the United States is essential in order for the nurse to acquire a knowledge base sufficient for making a diagnosis and deciding future strategies for action.

The following example illustrates how nursing students can assess a selected community, identify a problem area, and diagnose a nursing activity. On a visit to the kindergarten rooms of the local school, a nurse noted obvious dental caries and poor oral hygiene practices of the children. In a subsequent conference with the principal of the school, she secured the numbers of kindergarten children, learned that a high proportion of families were low-income, ascertained that no health screening was done routinely at this school, was informed that health education sessions were wanted but not always carried out, because the teacher felt unprepared in teaching about health practices. The nurse's thought process went like this: (1) My selected community is this kindergarten. (2) I must look into the mouths of all the children and assess the extent of dental caries. (3) I must talk with the teacher to find out her interest in oral hygiene and health practices. (4) I must determine if parents will support a program promoting dental services of some kind. (5) I must decide on an activity that will be most beneficial—finding dentists for the children, finding methods of payment for dental care, teaching good oral hygiene and prevention of caries, promoting a fluoride program in this school, having a dental clinic made up of volunteer dentists and dental hygienists. At this point the nurse was ready to assess the selected problem area in depth, determine alternatives which would be most appropriate and acceptable for the kindergarten, consumers, and school population, and decide on the nursing diagnosis of choice.

INTRODUCTION TO COMMUNITY ACTION

Involvement in any kind of community action is a learning experience. A nursing student may start with a simple idea of improving health

---

[21]Committee on Ways and Means, *National Health Insurance Resource Book,* U.S. Government Printing Office, Washington, D.C., 1974, p. 82.
[22]Milio, op. cit., p. 51.

conditions in a local neighborhood, such as eliminating safety hazards from a playground for children. However, as suggestions for change are offered to individuals presumed to have control of the playground, the student soon learns that the mechanism for instituting change is complex, slow, and oftentimes frustrating. If the student persists with the idea, she learns about the existence of power, authority, influence, leadership, organizational structures, politics, vested interests, and strategies. She learns how important it is to have the necessary data accumulated and documented as gained during the assessment period; how expeditiously an influential person can secure results; how chances for success are greater if a group of concerned citizens are involved, rather than one lone individual seeking to be heard; how necessary it is to know how the "local system" works, communicates, and operates.

For purposes of assisting the beginning student in entering the complex community arena, guidelines, as proposed by Ross, are presented. The guidelines are easily grasped and give one perspective for comprehending community action "as we would like it to be" compared with "what it turns out to be." The guidelines also are analogous with the community health nursing process, yet offer broader dimensions for exploration. Table 4-1 shows the interrelatedness of the community health nursing process with the community organization process.

Community Organization Process

Community organization, as defined by Ross, is a process by which a community identifies its needs or objectives, orders these needs or objectives, takes action in respect to them, and in so doing, extends and develops cooperative and collaborative attitudes and practices in the community.[23] One primary purpose for engaging in the community organization process is to build and strengthen community integration. When the process is separated into steps and essential principles are clarified in conjunction with each step, the process is easily understood and translated into practice.

1   *To identify health needs* there must be evidence of discontent with existing conditions. This discontent must be focused into specific concerns which are shared by many in the community and for which factors can be explored regarding possible solutions. When exploring ideas with citizens, it is advisable to discern their health wants, as opposed to their health needs, so that support from a substantial number of citizens is gained regarding any potentially selected health issue. Ideally, the movement toward a health objective should be instigated by the citizens or at least receive their enthusiastic endorsement, so that motivation toward action is already inherent.

[23]Murray G. Ross, *Community Organization*, Harper & Row, Publishers, Incorporated, New York, 1955, p. 39.

Table 4-1   Interrelating the Community Health Nursing Process with the Community Organization Process

Community health nursing process	Community organization process

1 Assessing
  a Diagnosis
    (1) Documentation
       of a health need
	1 Identifying needs or objectives
	  a Discontent with existing
	    conditions
	2 Ordering or ranking of needs
	  or objectives

2 Planning
  a Goals and objectives
    to be attained
  b Theoretical rationale
	3 Developing the will and
	  confidence to work at the
	  needs or objectives
	4 Finding the resources (internal
	  and external) to deal with the
	  needs or objectives
	  a Finding acceptable
	    leaders (formal and informal)

3 Implementing
  a Strategy
	5 Taking action
	  a Activities with emotional
	    content
	6 Extending and developing
	  cooperative and collaborative
	  attitudes and practices in
	  the community
	  a Utilize goodwill
	    existing in the community
	  b Active and effective
	    lines of communication
	  c Positive reinforcement
	    of strengths

4 Evaluating
  a Criteria for evaluating
    terminal objectives
	7 Evaluating

2 *The ordering of needs or objectives* is primarily setting priorities and focusing on the most urgent health need or desire first. When a health issue is selected that represents the citizens' wants, commitment and action will be secured early with minimum prompting from any health expert. People have always known of health *needs* which would be beneficial for them, but few individuals respond to "You should have this" or "You need this" unless they *want* it. For example, a community may tend to be apathetic and unconcerned about the general drug traffic problem on which the communication media is concentrating until several local high school students from respectable homes in their own community are picked up and jailed for possession of illegal drugs. Then the citizenry is truly alerted, aroused, and ready to take action in any advised direction that will resolve the problem. Progress cannot be made in the community any faster than the understanding and consent of the concerned group of citizens.[24]

3 *To develop the will and confidence* to work with a selected health concern, leaders (either formal or informal) from the community must be found and utilized. These leaders must be regarded as acceptable representatives of the interests or participating community subgroups. When local community leaders work actively with an identified health issue, participate in gathering data and planning action, their influence spreads, and other interested citizens are drawn into the work force.

4 The core of persons who are recognized and accepted as members of a citizens' committee working on a selected health issue represent the *human resources* in the community who are held accountable by the local population. It is advisable that the concerned group represent a valid cross section of citizens and agencies in the community, that some key influential persons be included, and that a professional individual with expertise in knowledge about the selected health issue be asked to serve as a consultant when needed. By expecting committee members to be involved, the gathering of a wide variety of resources within and without the community evolves in surprising directions when the group is allowed to be innovative and creative. The capacity of local citizens to solve problems and help themselves has unlimited potential, and the task of the chairperson and/or facilitator need only be aimed at exerting indirect leadership and giving support whenever required by the group. An early action of the committee is the determination of goals or objectives to be achieved. The nurse who is a member of the committee can be instrumental in assuring that the objectives are written behaviorally, are attainable, and are acceptable to the local citizenry. (See Chap. 3 for guidance in writing behavioral objectives.) When everyone on the committee is well acquainted with, understands, and accepts the goals and/or objectives of their common endeavor, a frame of reference which serves as a basis for providing consistent direction is established.

5 Members of the citizens' committee will decide on the *action* necessary and most appropriate in order to attain their objectives. To develop strength and cohesion as a working group, activities with emotional content must be recognized as essential for developing an integrative spirit. The committee will have times of hard work, serious discussions, arguments, and problem-solving endeavors, but, hopefully, they will also have times of laughter, friendship, and celebrations. If a light touch and festive spirit is maintained when the occasion warrants it, members of the committee will remember the fun activities along with the hard work and associate the whole endeavor as purposeful and valuable. When unforeseen events occur requiring changes of plan and adaptation

[24]Clarence King, *Working with People in Community Action*, Association Press, New York, 1965, p. 82.

of action, a committed and integrated citizens' committee is able to provide flexible alternatives with minimal internal opposition.

6 It is important that *collaborative and cooperative attitudes and practices* in the community be in operation during the entire community organization process. The requirement that lines of communication remain active, open, and effective is more easily stated than accomplished. The citizens' committee should aim toward utilizing the goodwill that exists in the community. This can be done in a variety of ways such as person-to-person contacts, sharing information informally, utilizing strengths and resources within the community. With an active and open communication system existing within the committee and with representative community citizens, it is probable that differences of opinions, tensions, and conflicts will occur. However, this lends life and vitality to a movement as opposed to easy consensus or *groupthink.* Groupthink refers to the mode of thinking that individuals engage in when concurrence-seeking becomes so dominant in a cohesive in-group that it tends to override realistic appraisal of alternative courses of action.[25] Members of cohesive groups must guard against groupthink characteristics such as amiability, avoidance of verbal, harsh statements in opposition to a colleague's or leader's ideas, and concurrence with all major decisions by the group, instead of voicing inner misgivings regarding an idea. Open conflict or disagreements should be allowed to occur within a citizens' committee, and when this happens, resolution of the conflict must be handled, whether constructively or destructively. If constructively, increased understanding, tolerance, and strength are developed in the committee. When the attitudes of persons allow for cooperative and collaborative work, they learn to endure, welcome, and move comfortably with diversity and tension.[26]

An effective activity and communication device is the employment of a pilot project. When a problem is worked out on a small scale, it provides the opportunity to see and hear how an idea, technique, or operation will work. It also brings out obstacles or oversights that had not been considered in the initial plan. Clarification of procedures and outcomes also is facilitated as individuals asked to participate in the pilot study give feedback regarding their responses and interpretation of the instructions.

7 Throughout the entire community organization process, mechanisms for *evaluation* of each step are essential. This can be the task of a health professional or a nurse. Gathering essential data, requesting feedback at each step, presenting a rationale or argument for the inclusion of each step, and suggesting alternative ideas are all procedures facilitating ongoing evaluation as each step of the process is examined. Success of a project is more easily assured if evaluative means are utilized throughout the process.

[25]Irving L. Janis, "Groupthink," *Psychology Today,* 5(6):43–46, November 1971.
[26]Ross, op. cit., p. 49.

The role of the health professional who is facilitating the community organization process in regard to a specific health issue is one of working *with* the citizens, encouraging the development of all the essential elements in the process, making use of consultation as necessary, serving as a worker in the background rather than the forefront, and strengthening the capacity of the local citizenry to function as a team toward accomplishment of the goals and objectives to which they have committed themselves.

It must be pointed out that the steps of the community organization process are not necessarily followed in order. Sometimes early action will hasten the development of the other elements in the process. What is essential is that all activities have a purpose, that the positive and negative alternatives are considered before acting upon them, and that the community group is continuously evaluating or judging the evolving events that occur as movement progresses toward the established goals.

THREE MODELS OF COMMUNITY ORGANIZATION PRACTICE

According to Rothman, there are three models of community organization practice designed for making change in a community. The three approaches or models can be used in pure form or can be combined. The essentialities of each approach are summarized in order for nursing students to be consciously aware of the strategies for selection in community organization practice and the roles students will utilize, contingent upon the model selected.

The Community Development Approach

The community development approach is a process designed to create conditions of economic and social progress for the whole community with its active participation and the fullest possible reliance on the community's initiative. This approach uses democratic procedures, seeks voluntary cooperation of consumers, encourages self-help measures by citizens, seeks to develop indigenous leadership of the local residents, and utilizes identified educational objectives. The change strategy may be characterized as "Let's all get together and talk this over." If a wide range of community people are involved in determining their needs or wants, it is felt that consumers will be more inclined to participate in solving their own problems.[27] The community organization process, as described by Ross, is an example of a community development approach.

[27]Jack Rothman, "Three Models of Community Organization," from *Social Work Practice. Copyright 1968 by National Conference on Social Welfare, Columbia University Press, New York, 1968.*

For nursing students who are getting started in community action, this approach is challenging and offers an opportunity to try many leadership and group development skills. Nursing students have utilized the approach on a small scale and have successfully implemented change in small, circumscribed communities. For example, after conducting a door-to-door survey of elderly citizens living in a low-income apartment complex in which questions were asked about unmet health needs, it was found that the citizens expressed a variety of needs. A meeting of the residents was arranged to determine their responsiveness to the idea of a social and health center in the apartment building. During this community meeting, it was the intent of the nursing students to identify leaders among the residents, discuss the results of the survey about unmet health needs, elicit other areas of needs, and decide on goals as agreed upon by the residents and nurses. A health clinic subsequently was initiated in which services offered by nursing students consisted of taking comprehensive health histories, blood pressure readings, vital signs, and temperatures. Simple foot care was given, health counseling was offered based on the data secured in the health history, and referrals to appropriate resources were made. Weekly meetings of the residents and nurses led to a camaraderie that was warm and freely expressed. Social needs, as well as health needs, were given attention. When new problems arose, the residents felt comfortable in talking about their concerns during the weekly meeting and, upon encouragement from the nursing students, succeeded in finding acceptable solutions. The informal leaders who evolved showed pleasure in being instrumental toward effecting desired change and realizing their newfound capabilities.

The Social Planning Approach

The social planning approach emphasizes a technical process of problem solving with regard to substantive social problems. Agencies and organizations frequently utilize this approach as they seek to bring about desired changes according to their perspective of the area of need. Planning is rational and deliberate, and controlled change is involved. Community participation may be great or small. Proposed health bills that are designed to be introduced into the legislative process may be an example of the social planning approach. The change strategy utilized can be exemplified by "Let's get the facts and proceed logically step by step." Appropriate and pertinent data are considered essential before decisions can be made about a rational and feasible course of action.[28]

The social planning approach is comprehended by nursing students as they participate actively with specific agencies studying data about

[28]Ibid.

existing social problems. For example, a multiservice center in a small community incorporated two nursing students in their planning process for gathering specific health data from residents living in the surrounding housing project area. The purpose of the center was to provide a variety of social services for any low-income person, regardless of race, creed, color, sex, or national origin. The plan was to construct a questionnaire which inquired about the needs of the low-income people and, at the same time, explain about the services available at the center. At the planning meetings, which were composed of individuals representing a variety of services, the students added their ideas to the design of the questionnaire and, at the same time, became conscious of the priorities, focus, and desires of personnel representing other disciplines. When the time came for the collection of data, the students realized with some surprise that the personnel at the center wanted the findings to bring out a need and desire for a cooperative day-care program. As it happened, the findings of the survey showed that the residents predominately supported the idea of a health clinic. Only 23 per cent of the clientele wanted a day-care program. With the passage of time, it was noted that follow-up was done selectively on health needs as expressed by the residents. The findings of the questionnaire contained valuable data and were used as a basis for planning specific health services concurrent with the goals of the center.

The Social Action Approach

The social action approach aims at making basic changes in major institutions or in community practices which are presumed to be in need of correction. For example, if disadvantaged segments of the population were organized and made their desires known through group action, it is possible that necessary and additional resources would be made available to these people. Social action seeks redistribution of power, resources, or decision making in the community and/or changing of basic policies of formal organizations. The change strategy takes the direction of "Let's organize to destroy our oppressor." By organizing a group of citizens and talking about easily identified problems, issues are crystallized and the means for bringing pressure on selected targets by mass action are devised. In the social action approach, clients are often considered victims of "the system," or "underdogs." The action mode is direct and sometimes confronting.[29]

An example of nursing students spontaneously employing the social action approach for themselves has occurred in the past and continues to be utilized whenever they become aroused. It happens when students become greatly dissatisfied with the teaching style of a selected instruc-

[29]Ibid.

tor, start criticizing all aspects of the nursing course among themselves, and insidiously build an emotional climate which eventually reaches a passionate crisis level. At that point, small groups of students organize, decide to go to the dean of the school of nursing to complain, and demand a change of conditions in the classroom. The students feel "oppressed" and seek to have a voice in the system by applying pressure on the persons with authority. Their method generally is direct and confronting as they seek change of their untenable position. Depending upon the response of the person with authority, the students are satisfied, mollified, or offended, and, as a result of the experience, learn the meaning of a social action approach from a personal perspective.[30]

When social reform in our society is the goal of the change agent, a mixture of social action and social planning is utilized. The reformer is faced with three tasks which must be considered. He must recruit a coalition of power sufficient for his purpose; he must respect the democratic tradition which expects every citizen, not merely to be represented, but to play an autonomous part in the determination of his own affairs; and his policies must be demonstrably rational.[31] Social reform involves activity by a group or coalition of interests which acts vigorously on behalf of some outside client group which is at risk. The change strategy uses employment of facts and persuasion to apply pressure on decision-making bodies and/or campaign tactics.[32] An example of an organization involved with social reform is the League of Women Voters.

The major purpose for becoming acquainted with and studying the community organizations' models leads the nurse to be prepared in making situational diagnoses and analyses that will assist in choosing the appropriate and most effective community organization method. Regardless of the method chosen, when involved in community organization practice, the nurse eventually will see all types of action—the polite formality of community committees, deliberated by Robert's rules of order; protest marches; education of client groups regarding methods for getting the attention of power organizations; use of a "cause" or client group to promote personal gain. If the nurse considers community organization practice as a learning experience, she realizes the opportunity she has for (1) learning to speak in public about an issue, (2) learning about various means for gaining attention, (3) knowing the importance of pertinent and appropriate facts, (4) planning strategy, (5) knowing the

[30]Mary C. Jones, "Confrontation in a Classroom," *Nursing Outlook,* **18**(11):47–49, November 1970.

[31]Peter Marris and Martin Rein, *Dilemmas of Social Reform.* Copyright 1967 by Peter Marris and Martin Rein. Reprinted by permission of Aldine Publishing Company, Chicago, p. 7.

[32]Rothman, op. cit.

importance of timing, (6) gathering essential support from groups and/or organizations, rather than working alone, and (7) perceiving the advantageous role of persons in power.

When seeking the ear of a person of authority, it helps to be cognizant that communication and power cannot be divorced. Information implies action.[33] When a person agrees to listen, he or she becomes committed to a response. It can be a response of agreement, a counter argument, other information, or selective inattention to the content of the message. The person with authority holds the inimitable position of governing the direction of messages people are communicating at that point in time. However, when attention is gained and messages truly heard, the potential of a realignment of power is possibly created. It is important to remember that seeds of ideas can be planted, regardless of immediate reactions of persons with authority, and that ideas can and do germinate even though dormant for a period of time.

KENT MODEL OF COMMUNITY ORGANIZATION

Kent has worked extensively with poor and disadvantaged people and has developed a community organization model which is effective with these populations. He believes that lack of opportunity, discrimination, and an unresponsive society have forced the disadvantaged person into an inflexible mold in which values and behaviors necessary for effective participation in society are discouraged. He advocates that poor and disadvantaged populations can be reached and motivated by assessing positive characteristics or strengths. For example, identified strengths of persons in poverty include the following methods of interaction: (1) They meet and talk personally and intimately in specific locations or geographical areas. (2) They are loyal to neighbors and friends. (3) Physical contact is a characteristic ingredient of interpersonal communication. (4) They maintain close contact with the extended family, particularly in certain ethnic groups. Some groups place a higher value on having a number of children rather than acquiring material goods. (5) The life-style often consists of dependency on helping persons such as a member of one's family or a friend.[34] By recognizing and accepting the existence of the above characteristics or strengths, a beginning step is taken toward working effectively with disadvantaged persons.

Kent advocates looking at situations in disadvantaged areas in a "natural" way—including the minute and seemingly unimportant facts of

[33]Marris and Rein, op. cit., p. 281.
[34]James A. Kent, C. Harvey Smith, and Sam Burns, *An Urban Strategy for Action against Poverty,* Foundation for Urban and Neighborhood Development, Denver, Colo., 1967, p. 1.

life. In other words, the individual must be prepared to examine the real and natural situation of poverty from the perspective of poverty persons, consider ways for change, discover existing resources, and identify paths toward independent action by the poor. In taking a descriptive or "discovery" approach to the disadvantaged community, the student must be cognizant of being a stranger in an unfamiliar environment and attempt to observe "what's going on in the community." Helpful questions to keep in mind are:

What are the people doing?
What kind of games are the children playing?
Are there natural paths that most people are using?
What is the housing like?
What is the prevalent mode of transportation in this community?
What is the movement of people at certain time frames of the day?
Do people congregate at specific places at certain times of the day?

By getting a natural "feel" of the neighborhood through the senses and realizing the ownership of the neighborhood as belonging to its residents, the beginning step toward assimilation into a new environment is initiated.[35] Natural problems which are of concern to the residents are the ones for which to look. Frequently, the optimal time for helping disadvantaged persons is during a crisis period, whether the crisis is health-related or not. If concrete assistance of a constructive nature is given to a person during an immediate crisis, his or her capacity for learning experientially is at an optimal level, and action toward resolution of the problem creates an acceptance and trust between helper and helpee which is essential for subsequent teaching and interventions. Natural helpers or advisors who have special skills and talents should be sought and utilized within the community at all possible times. These individuals are the natural caretakers who are the already known helpers or family members. They must be taught the advocacy role and reinforced for all successful endeavors. A system whereby residents become natural helpers for each other is one of the goals of the Kent Model, which teaches self-help measures. If a neighborhood can be mobilized into a power position so that participation in the dominant social order of the community occurs, then responsible citizenship is learned and confidence gained in becoming a part of the democratic system that has influence upon local government. Nursing students can initiate Kent's Model in neighborhoods which show potential for learning. They must first get well-acquainted and be accepted in the neighborhood before natural

[35]Mary Bayer, "Community Diagnosis—Through Sense, Sight, and Sound," *Nursing Outlook,* **21**(11):712–713, Nov. 1973.

problems will be uncovered and natural assets discovered. They must know and understand the subgroups in the neighborhood and utilize the natural internal caretaker system before any effective action can be anticipated.[36] To enter a neighborhood, utilizing Kent's Model, is an excellent learning experience which broadens the student's perspective of community organization and the problems of lower socioeconomic and disadvantaged populations.

WARREN'S MODEL FOR ASSESSING NEIGHBORHOODS

A typology of neighborhoods was developed by Warren [37] as a means for understanding and describing the variety of highly specialized roles that neighborhoods play in the lives of their residents. The typology is based on three dimensions of organization—interaction, identity, and connections. By examining a neighborhood in terms of the three dimensions, structural characteristics and differences in neighborhood organization are disclosed. The presence of social class, income, and ethnic factors do not change the basic elements of each neighborhood. Questions to ask in terms of the three dimensions are:

A. Interaction During the year do people in the neighborhood get together quite often?

B. Identity Do people in the neighborhood feel that they have a great deal in common?

C. Connections Do many people in the neighborhood keep active in political parties and other forces outside the neighborhood?

According to Warren, neighborhoods can be classified into six types, depending upon how each question in the typology is answered. A brief description of the six types of neighborhoods is summarized as follows:

1. Integral This neighborhood stands alone and is proud of its uniqueness and its ability to organize and function as an integral unit within the larger community. Prominent citizens live here and provide linkage between outside organizations and neighborhood groups.

2. Parochial Much activity and social interactions are observed in

[36]Kent, op. cit., pp. 3–19.
[37]Donald I. Warren and Rachelle B. Warren, "Six Kinds of Neighborhoods," *Psychology Today,* 9(1):74–80, June 1975.

this neighborhood. People are friendly, and a sense of belonging is evident. However, the residents isolate themselves from the outside community with a "we take care of our own" attitude.

3. Diffuse   This neighborhood has a sameness of homes, children, and attitudes. People are friendly yet place a premium on privacy. Neighbors have a good deal in common but share little. If they need help, they prefer to seek aid from their families rather than neighbors. They identify with their neighborhood but have little interaction with each other and feel little connection with the outside community.

4. Stepping-stone   This neighborhood is open, friendly, and marked with a transient characteristic. Moving vans are frequently seen in this neighborhood. Even though residents live here temporarily, there is close interaction between the people and their ties to the larger community. However, the sense of connection is not strong in this neighborhood.

5. Transitory   There is a sameness of homes and structures in this neighborhood, but there is neither interaction nor community identification. The widespread distrust within the neighborhood communicates a feeling of "no one cares."

6. Anomic   These neighborhoods lack all the predominant characteristics. There is little interaction between residents, a sense of isolation and disinterest, and little evidence of individuals engaged in activities outside the neighborhood. The attitude, "we don't like people nosing into our business," is the prevailing one.

For nurses assessing neighborhoods with the intent to organize, it is important to examine the process of influence that goes on. Every neighborhood is an information-processing center—either keeping information out, absorbing it uncritically, or filtering its content so that interpretation of meaning is controlled via the individualistic "neighborhood perspective." Nurses should look for residents who are influential in the neighborhood information process. They represent three types: (1) residents who are officers in various kinds of voluntary organizations, such as PTAs or block clubs; (2) less visible residents who belong to no formal organizations but have the reputation for getting things done; (3) residents who are "opinion leaders," and who are approached frequently by neighbors for advice on a problem or for information about where to get help. With knowledge about the three types of residents to be on the lookout for, nurses must also understand how information is disseminated through the six types of neighborhoods.

1. Integral This neighborhood picks up resources and information from many outside points. Residents have influential jobs and links with many kinds of community groups. At the same time, they are active within their neighborhood. They bring new information and techniques into the neighborhood and let outside institutions know what people in the neighborhood are thinking. These "linking persons" have a real power base. They carry messages from local residents to outside organizations and back again.

2. Parochial People interact often and have a network of neighborhood groups. But unlike the integral neighborhood, it faces inward. Information seldom passes directly into the neighborhood; it is filtered and modified by key opinion leaders. These leaders have strong commitments to their neighborhood but are less likely than integral leaders to transmit to their neighborhood the concerns of the larger community.

3. Diffuse Residents identify with this neighborhood because they find it a pleasant place to live; but they seldom get together and do not depend on the neighborhood as a basis for shaping or protecting their life-style. Information flows slowly, and the neighborhood is often relatively slow in taking action, even though there is a great deal of organizational potential. Only under conditions of crisis does this neighborhood become organizationally active.

4. Stepping-stone This neighborhood has a high degree of internal organization as well as a large number of residents with outside connections. But the residents have no strong commitment to the neighborhood. There are usually formal mechanisms to integrate new residents quickly and to tell them about neighborhood groups. However, residents usually continue to be more active in outside groups rather than local ones.

5. Transitory The population turnover is so great and the institutional fabric so restricted that there is little action in this neighborhood. It often breaks down into cliques of longtime residents who belong to the same groups and never allow newcomers in. Neighbors feel they have little in common and usually avoid local entanglements. There may be pockets of intense activity, but there is no cohesion.

6. Anomic This neighborhood has virtually no leadership structure. A few residents may have connections to outside groups but remain inactive on their home turf. Individuals and families are on their own, confronting outside institutions without any kind of support from their neighbors. Usually they are distrustful of outside groups, but almost

Table 4-2 Guide for Neighborhood Action

| Assessing the neighborhood | Taking action | | | | | | |
Characteristics	Publish news-letter	Conduct door-to-door campaign	Adver-tise in mass media	Contact key neigh-bors	Use organi-zation lists	Form grass-roots group	Set up pipeline to city hall
1 *Interaction* During the year, do people in the neighborhood get together quite often?	Yes						
	✓	No	No	+	✓	✓	✓
2 *Heterogeneity* Are there many people of different backgrounds, life-styles, or social levels who live in the neighborhood?	Yes						
	✓	+	No	✓	✓	No	No
3 *Identity* Do people in the neighborhood feel they have a great deal in common?	Yes						
	+	✓	✓	No	✓	✓	✓

4 *Mutual aid* Yes ✓ ✓ ✓ No No No No +

When someone has a problem, are neighbors willing to help?

5 *Privatism* Yes No No + ✓ ✓ No No No

Do people in the neighborhood place more value on their family privacy than on being in touch with neighbors?

6 *Insulation* Yes ✓ + No ✓ ✓ No No

If a bill collector came around asking about a neighbor, would people in your neighborhood refuse to give out any information?

7 *Connections* Yes ✓ No ✓ ✓ + ✓ ✓

Do many people in the neighborhood keep active in groups outside the neighborhood?

8 *Turnover* Yes + ✓ ✓ ✓ No ✓ ✓

Are there many people who move in and out of your neighborhood?

never can they get help or guidance from anyone in their neighborhood. The residents are large consumers of the mass media, and the messages come through unfiltered.

Warren's examination of neighborhood structure and process provides a useful systematic description of neighborhood life in America. The following typology provides useful guidelines for nurses wanting to organize a neighborhood for action. (See Table 4-2.)

Instructions for the typology   For each "yes" answer, look across the list of strategies to find which action would be the best first step (+), which ones would be good follow-up actions ($\checkmark$), and which ones should be avoided (No).[38]

ROLE OF THE NURSE IN THE COMMUNITY

After assessing a neighborhood or local community, selecting a health problem, and becoming acquainted with community organization practices, the nurse is faced with deciding her role, in terms of her diagnosis of the health issue requiring action. She has the option of practicing as an enabler, a coordinator, a catalyst, a teacher, a data gatherer, a facilitator, an activist, an advocate, or a negotiator. To perform intelligently in any of these roles, the nurse must be completely knowledgeable about the community and the risks involved in participating in any one of the selected community organization methods. Community life is plastic, and, for the most part, consumers seek positive betterment of their environment, living conditions, and way of life. Membership in a community derives from a conscious sense of "belonging." People are friends and neighbors and interrelate according to mutual interests, common problems, common values, and common hopes. Frequently, people are aware of and dissatisfied with negative aspects of their community yet give little thought to the improvement of things. Ideas for improved health conditions or focusing on situations revealing recognized health deficiencies can be a starting point for the nurse who wishes to be an enabler, a facilitator, or a catalyst in the community. Among members of every community can be found individuals with many capabilities, ideas, and skills. All that needs to be done is finding them and giving them some direction and positive reinforcement. It is in community effort that the personal meaning of a helping hand is discovered.

The teacher role requires knowledge of the selected subject. Delving into reference books or acquiring information that will catch the attention

[38]Ibid., p. 76.

and interest of citizens is the challenge. Oftentimes, creativity is required in bringing out health issues which previously have been taken for granted. For the most part, citizens do not get excited about health education until a personal health habit has affected their lives undesirably. One method for the teacher to choose is that of a lecturer. If this method is selected, visual aids and dramatizations which attract attention and lend charisma to the instructor-lecturer frequently are ingredients for success. The teaching role also can be accomplished by behaving as a consultant and/or facilitator. Citizens who are drawn to work actively on a health issue can be encouraged and reinforced to problem-solve, implement solutions, and evaluate outcomes in a teaching-learning situation that leads them to function autonomously, independently, and confidently.

If the coordinator or negotiator role is to be assumed, knowledge of the existing community services and acquaintance with key individuals of every discipline are desirable. The role of coordinator is valuable and time-consuming, as multiple telephone calls, negotiations about optimal meeting times and places, familiarity with particular interests of clientele, recognition of the input of members of each discipline, assignment of acceptable tasks, and delegation of responsibility for the completion of assignments are undertaken.

The activist or advocate role requires willingness to risk. In many instances, the nurse advocate must be assertive, oftentimes aggressive, and willing to take the consequences of actions as they occur. A knowledge of the legislative process, bargaining and/or making compromises, political maneuvers or strategies, power as exercised by influential persons, and counterstrategies are all essential. To become an effective advocate takes time, patience, perseverance, and practice. Learning to bargain and compromise or deliberately planning a strategy aimed toward winning a desired goal are skills that nursing students are not well-prepared to do. The word "manipulation" frequently has a negative connotation; yet, manipulation is part of politics and strategy.

It is in practice and experience that the nurse learns the essence and nuances of the selected role she undertakes. Community organization work exposes the nurse to many facets of the community arena and prepares her to deal realistically with life-and-death issues affecting the life and health of consumer populations.

COMMUNITY HEALTH NURSING PROCESS—PLANNING

Planning is a process considered essential for engineering actions which will produce desired outcomes. For the nurse, the diagnosis regarding a selected community health issue contains the implication that a nursing action is appropriate and feasible as a means for attaining desired outcomes and for which planning must be done. Consequently, objectives must be written which will provide direction for the accomplishment of desired ends. Objectives which are clearly stated, explicitly descriptive of desired outcomes, realistic, measurable, and attainable give purpose and consistency to the nurse and all other individuals involved with planning. Objectives must be congruent with the desires and wants of the consumers of the community. For more information about the writing of objectives, see Chap. 3.

Health care cannot be planned without considering how economic, political, social, religious, geographic, and other factors influence its utilization. In each community the visibility of health problems differs. Also, change occurs constantly in our dynamic society regardless of whether communities plan for it or not. Identification of a health problem for which planning is necessary does not ensure resolution of the problem. Often, a plan which culminates in an outcome desired by citizens produces a new situation in which new needs are created. In other words, planning is never completed because the process produces changes which require additional planning. Because planning is a continuous process in our changing society, short-term goals which depict tangible action and specify attainable realistic outcomes are best. A short-term goal can be attached to a long-term goal; however, the long-term goal should provide mechanisms for flexibility and adaptability in reaching the ends desired.

In addition to defining objectives, the well-prepared nurse must be cognizant of the factors which shape the community organization model she has deemed appropriate. The rationale for selecting the theoretical model of community organization should be appropriate for the population with which she proposes to work. She must examine all variables of the community organization model and consciously plan strategies and role behaviors most likely to succeed. When other individuals are teammates in the planning endeavor, a knowledge of group process and group behavior is facilitative. By keeping lines of communication with the multidisciplinary team of workers open, considerate of others, active, purposeful, and supportive, a plan will emerge which generally is satisfactory to all members.

When the environment in which the action will take place is comprised of social institutions or agencies, a knowledge of the structure of the institution or agency is imperative. All institutions or agencies have a formal organizational structure and an informal one, which can be shown on paper. The formal organization depicts a structure or picture by which the efforts or functions of the people fit together logically to accomplish some purpose. The organizational structure shows how the functions of members are interrelated and integrated. The informal structure or picture reveals the efforts or functions of people that have not been formally planned but have spontaneously evolved from the needs of the members within the organization. Informal work arrangements always exist, have rules or norms for guiding the behavior of its members, have leaders and followers, and are perpetuated as a means of social life within the organization.[39] When studying the structure of a particular social institution or agency, a formal structure or organizational outline can always be elicited from the person in charge. As the investigator becomes familiar with the activities and membership of the institution, the informal structure will emerge. Pictures of formal and informal structures are graphic visual aids which are descriptive of functions, membership, and interactions characteristic of the specified institution.

Health-planning agencies within communities, such as official health-planning councils, are informative, educational, and up-to-date on health issues and health legislation that are of concern nationally and locally. Involvement in some aspect of planning in such an agency is an excellent learning experience for nursing students. Opportunity to observe group dynamics, uses of power and authority, leadership strategies, bargaining, and decision making by community experts is provided at close proximity. The purposes, benefits, priorities, and communication styles of health-planning agencies, as they are disclosed, acquaint students with business as it is conducted in the world of reality.

COMMUNITY HEALTH NURSING
PROCESS—IMPLEMENTING

Implementing a plan is the going into action phase of the nursing process. For some nurses, this is the "fun" part of the entire process. It is during the implementation phase that the nurse realizes if (1) all essential data were assessed and accumulated according to the need; (2) her diagnosis was accurate; (3) she has planned well; (4) she possesses the attributes and skills necessary for the role she has assumed; (5) she is flexible; (6) she can admit an oversight, an error in judgment, or a need for supervision and/or consultation. Implementing a plan for action in the community often involves other persons who may behave as allies, show active resistance, require constant current reports of the ongoing situation, or interfere with unexpected, restricting rules or policies. It is during these times that the nurse becomes aware of her personal capacity to be flexible, adaptable, frustrated, creative, persuasive, persistent, or firm.

When problems arise, it is well for the nurse and the members of the citizens committee to review their activities up to the moment of

[39]Joseph A. Litterer, *Organizations: Structure & Behavior,* John Wiley & Sons, Inc., New York, 1963, pp. 10–11.

intervention—their assessment of the problem, the selection of the community organization approach, the accuracy and completeness of their plan, the possibility that they overlooked a key individual or community resource, a breakdown in communication lines. Consideration should be given to what seems to be the issue of the opposition. Do opposing individuals understand the purpose of the planned action? Is clarification needed? Has language been of a superior-subordinate nature? Does the opposition have an issue that must be taken into consideration? Perhaps the selected strategy for action needs to be redirected or modified. It is possible that the gathering of more supportive groups or influential individuals may be needed. Seeking consultation from experienced experts in the community inevitably brings forth useful ideas or alternatives for consideration. It is during the implementation phase of community organization practice that individuals come face-to-face with authority, power, politics, overt or covert resistance, and obstacles, particularly if the assessing and planning processes were hasty, incomplete, inadequate, or inaccurate. The implementation phase is the time for learning, accepting and readjusting mistakes or errors in judgment, examining effective leadership styles, studying the uses of power and authority, reassessing strategies, and determining stamina and commitment regarding accomplishment of original objectives. If a project is unsuccessful the first time it is implemented, this does not mean that it is a failure. If the purpose for the project is sound, persistence and commitment in working toward the attainment of desired objectives is essential, and eventually a way is found.

COMMUNITY HEALTH NURSING PROCESS—EVALUATING

Reassessment or evaluation should be ongoing during every phase of the nursing process. If evaluation is done continuously and objectively, the attainment of goals or the success of the project is more likely to be assured. The input of new information, changes, or lack of progress require examination of the objectives and methodology and may dictate new or revised approaches for the project. If changes or modifications are required in the plan of action, objectives can be rewritten and revised. The criteria inherent in the written objectives should help to determine the success or failure of goal attainment.

The focus of evaluation can be directed toward health services given, quality of care, processes, access, satisfaction, and outcomes.[40] In evaluating the provision of health services to a consumer population, accessibility of the services for the target group must be studied. Did the

[40]Milio, op. cit., p. 260.

intended consumers make use of the services? If not, why not? Were the services relevant to the needs of the consumer group from their perspective? Did the health of the target group show measurable improvement?

Was any form of peer review utilized? How would the findings of the project compare with practices offered by other community resources? Were statistical norms changed for persons of a particular age or with a specified diagnosis? Were the results of the project as anticipated? Would case histories be descriptive of successful outcomes?

Was health behavior of consumers changed? Did the target group feel satisfied with the services as given? Were the individuals who did not utilize the services asked to contribute their views as another aspect of the evaluation study? Were results of the project interpreted accurately, objectively, realistically, and without bias? Were new, unanticipated needs created as a result of the project?

Evaluation of a project can be interpreted from a variety of perspectives—attainment of measurable objectives, change in health behavior of consumers, consumer satisfaction, use of statistical formulas showing significance of data, visual graphs, comparison of findings with projects or studies done formerly, quantitative frequency distributions, and correlation studies. Whatever the means utilized for interpreting the results of a project for selected subjects or populations, data must be clear, accurate, complete, understandable, and accountable.

SUMMARY

In becoming acquainted with any given community, the community health nurse must study its characteristics purposefully. The composition of each community has its own structure and personality, which is not duplicated by any other community. Information is gained about a community by synthesizing the community health nursing process with the community organization process. The nurse is able to identify a health-care system in every community and the existence of several social classes of citizens. Getting involved in community action requires qualities of initiative, curiosity, and persuasiveness. Several community organization models are described, including Ross, Rothman, Kent, and Warren. The role of the nurse in community action depends on the community organization model selected.

SUGGESTED READING

Adams, Richard: *Watership Down,* Macmillan Publishing Co., Inc., New York, 1972.
Bruhn, John G.: "Planning for Social Change: Dilemmas for Health Planning," *American Journal of Public Health,* **63**(7):602–606, July 1973.

Cox, Fred M., John L. Erlich, Jack Rothman, and John E. Tropman (eds.): *Strategies of Community Organization,* F. E. Peacock Publishers, Inc., Itasca, Ill., 1974.

Gentry, John T., James E. Veney, Arnold D. Kaluzny, Jane B. Sprague, and Elizabeth J. Coulter: "Attitudes and Perceptions of Health Service Providers," *American Journal of Public Health,* **64**(12):1123–1131, Dec. 1974.

Kent, James A.: *A Descriptive Approach to a Community,* Foundation for Urban and Neighborhood Development, Denver, Colo., 1972.

Kent, James A., C. Harvey Smith, and Sam Burns: *An Urban Strategy for Action against Poverty,* Foundation for Urban and Neighborhood Development, Denver, Colo., 1967, p. 1.

Kent, James A.: *Death of Colonialism in Health Programs for the Urban Poor,* Foundation for Urban and Neighborhood Development, Denver, Colo., 1972.

Kent, James A., and C. Harvey Smith: *Involving the Urban Poor in Health Services through Accommodation: The Employment of Neighborhood Representatives,* Foundation for Urban and Neighborhood Development, Denver, Colo., 1966.

Klein, Donald C.: *Community Dynamics and Mental Health,* John Wiley & Sons, Inc., New York, 1968.

Knight, Jeane Harris: "Applying Nursing Process in the Community," *Nursing Outlook,* **22**(11):708–711, Nov. 1974.

Lindberg, Helen Gray: "A Community Health Potentiator," *Nursing Outlook,* **14**(9):43–45, Sept. 1966.

Milio, Nancy: *9226 Kercheval: The Storefront that Did Not Burn,* Ann Arbor Paperbacks, The University of Michigan Press, Ann Arbor, 1970.

Milio, Nancy: *The Care of Health in Communities,* Macmillan Publishing Co., Inc., New York, 1975.

Murphy, Michael J., "The Development of a Community Health Oreintation Scale,"*American Journal of Public Health.* 65(12):1293–1297, Dec. 1975.

O. M. Collective: *The Organizer's Manual,* Bantam Books, Inc., New York, 1971.

Regester, David C.: "Community Mental Health: For Whose Community?" *American Journal of Public Health,* **64**(9):886–893, Sept. 1974.

Ross, Murray G.: *Community Organization,* Harper & Row, Publishers, Incorporated, New York, 1955.

Smolensky, Jack, and Franklin B. Haar: *Principles of Community Health,* 3rd ed., W. B. Saunders Company, Philadelphia, 1972.

Suttles, Gerald D.: *The Social Order of the Slum,* The University of Chicago Press, Chicago, 1968.

Terkel, Studs: *Working,* Avon Books, New York, 1972.

Warren, Donald I., and Rachelle B. Warren: "Six Kinds of Neighborhoods," *Psychology Today,* **9**(1):74–80, June 1975.

Warren, Roland L.: *Studying Your Community,* The Free Press, New York, 1965.

Chapter 5

Focusing on Families

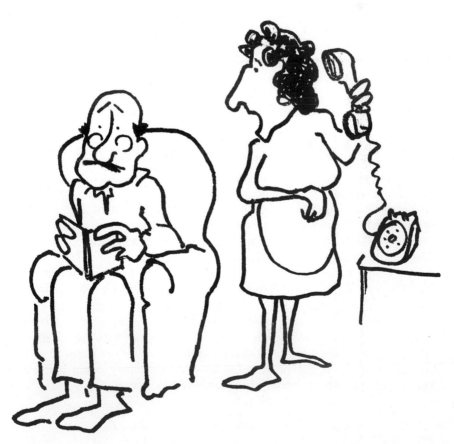

"Henry . . . what would you say—are we lower middle—middle middle or upper middle class now?"

Traditionally the family has been the unit of service for the community health nurse, However, the orientation and practice of individual nurses for years have varied on a continuum from patient-centered to family-centered, dependent upon the nature of the family system and the illness of the identified patient. Unfortunately, it is too easy to *speak* words like "family-centered," "caring," and "continuity of care" yet behave in *actions* differently from what the descriptive words suggest. Sometimes the nurse may consider that she is using the family-centered approach when she draws all the family members together for the goal of understanding and assisting the identified patient of the family to make a more satisfactory recovery. A *truly family-centered approach* is one in which the nurse meets and assesses *all* the family members, either individually or as a group, is cognizant of the developmental role, power, and influence position of each family member, identifies the interactional patterns used by the family, and works with the family, including all members, to achieve a higher level of coping ability or health. The methods used for the family-centered approach are discussed in Chap. 6.

THE FAMILY

The common meaning of the word "family" is generalized to be the nuclear family, a structural unit composed of a man and woman who are married and have children. However, in view of the living patterns and kinship systems of people of different cultures and the emerging pattern of communal living among the youth of America, the family can also be considered a primary group possessing certain generic characteristics in common with all small groups.[1] These characteristics are mainly relationships with a high degree of intimacy, extensive communication, and common goals. When viewed in this manner, the family can be seen as a miniature society, with a culture all its own.[2] The concept of family tends to be a fluid one because of the accelerating changes occurring within the societies of the Western Hemisphere. One-parent families, communal families, extended families living in a single residence, and other groups residing together in single dwellings must all be viewed in a common context, the nature of which supplies the nurse with her frame of reference, the family-centered nursing approach. For the purpose of this book, the family is the nuclear family or the primary group living and interacting together intimately in a common residence.

[1]F. Ivan Nye and Felix M. Berardo, *Emerging Conceptual Frameworks in Family Analysis*, The Macmillan Company, New York, 1966, p. 63.
[2]Ibid., p. 140.

The Systems Approach

When the family is viewed from a systems approach, its role as a basic component of society is seen as a complex, many-faceted one. A system is an organized or complex whole—an assemblage or combination of things or parts forming a complex or unitary whole.[3] The world is made up of many systems, including social, biological, physical, and environmental systems. Parsons identified a social system as a plurality of persons or social roles bound together in a pattern of mutual interaction and interdependence. It has boundaries that enable us to distinguish the internal from the external environment, and it is typically imbedded in a network of social units both larger and smaller than itself.[4] The family is an open system which sustains relationships with other systems in the total transactional field and is interdependent and independent at the same time. When using the systems approach, the family's position in society can be identified in simple or complex terms. It is helpful to visualize a system by drawing a large circle and placing elements, parts, and variables inside the circle as components.[5] Circles representing components can be separate, touching, or overlapping depending on the strength of the attracting forces in operation among the components. For purposes of simplicity, the position of the family in relation to the health-care system in the community can be illustrated as shown in Fig. 5-1. Each circle represents a subsystem which has boundaries but will admit individuals from other subsystems as necessary. It is possible for the community health nurse to act as a representative for any of the health subsystems, serve as a liaison agent with the family, and coordinate the health-care delivery system in the community so that it has meaning and purpose to the family.

From another perspective, which includes a multidisciplinary approach, the family may be drawn as one of many social systems within the community with the possibility of having transactions with other systems on a frequent or infrequent basis. The community health nurse can act as the liaison agent for a dysfunctioning family and coordinate or integrate transactions with other participating social systems so that the family's equilibrium and coping abilities are eased. The illustration of social systems from a multidisciplinary approach may be drawn as shown in Fig. 5-2. The particular role of the community health nurse as a coordinator of

[3]Fremont E. Kast and James E. Rosenzweig, *Organization and Management,* McGraw-Hill Book Company, New York, 1970, p. 110.

[4]Talcott Parsons and Robert F. Bales, *Family, Socialization and Interaction Process,* The Free Press, New York, 1955, pp. 401–408.

[5]Warren G. Bennis, Kenneth D. Benne, and Robert Chin, *The Planning of Change,* Holt, Rinehart and Winston, Inc., New York, 1961, p. 203.

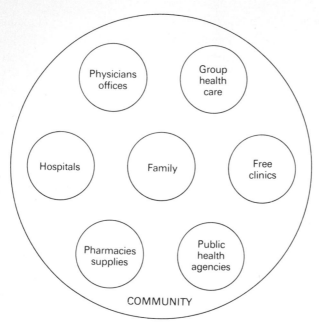

Figure 5-1   Health-care systems in the community.

services as shown in the figure can be elaborated from the following hypothetical example. The community health nurse was referred to the family initially through the department of public assistance because the mother was pregnant and was not seeking prenatal care. Following an appraisal of the family on a home visit, the nurse assessed the family as a dysfunctional one because of the evidences of marital strife, the lack of health care of older children, the lack of prenatal care for the mother, and the complaints regarding insufficient clothing and poor transportation facilities. After the nurse determined short- and long-term goals to be attained, immediate plans to talk with or make referral to personnel in each of the pictured social systems were instituted. For example, the nurse wanted to speak to the caseworker of the department of public assistance to share her observations and assessment of the family with the worker. She wanted to know if the data gathered were complete and if a cooperative effort by the caseworker and nurse would reap better results than working separately or discretely in predetermined subject areas. By conferring with the school nurse and teachers in the school system, the nurse wanted to learn if the school had been alerted to the health condition of the children of the family. Again, by a unified effort of all professionals concerned with family members, a change would be effected more easily if the family received concerted special attention. A first priority of the nurse was to refer the mother of the family to a private

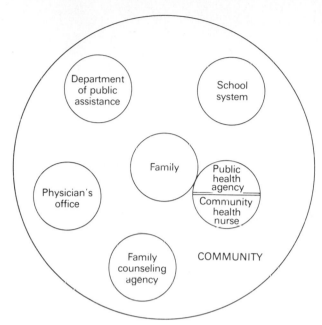

Figure 5-2 Social systems in the community.

physician for prenatal care. She planned to call the physician chosen by
the mother to advise him or her of the current health status of the mother
and the fact that continued supervisory visits would be planned during the
antepartum and postpartum periods. When the mother and father of the
family indicated a readiness to seek marital counseling, it was the plan of
the nurse to call the family counseling agency to alert them to the nature
of family problems and the fact that she had been guiding the family to
seek additional assistance. Eventually, as the designated social systems
within the community became acquainted with the family, a multidisciplinary conference of all representatives of the social systems would be
arranged by the nurse to integrate and implement the health care needed
by the family. By picturing the social systems involved with the family,
the nurse clarified the coordination aspect of her role.

Structure of the Family

The family structure is made up of individual members and the roles they
play in interacting with each other. A *role* is defined as a goal-directed
pattern or sequence of acts tailored by the cultural process for the
transactions a person may carry out in a social group or situation.[6] No role
exists in isolation but is always patterned to adjust in a complementary or

[6]John P. Spiegel, "The Resolution of Role Conflict within the Family," in Norman W.
Bell and Ezra F. Vogel (eds.), *The Family,* The Free Press, New York, 1960, p. 363.

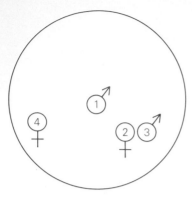

Figure 5-3 (1) Father: age 40. (2) Mother: age 38. (3) Son: age 12. (4) Daughter: age 14.

reciprocal manner with the role partner. In general, the assumption is made that a nuclear family consists of a male who enacts an instrumental role and a female who fulfills the expressive role function. The instrumental role is one which emphasizes the performance of tasks and decision making and communicates power by the thinking, logical, perceptive approach. The expressive role emphasizes support of the instrumental leader and conveys power through the ability to mediate and influence feelings and emotions of others. In every small group there are persons who demonstrate either instrumental or expressive roles. The structural relationships in a family vary according to the particular mode of family organization, social class, or culture. Thus, various manifestations of family structure are seen in terms of role behavior. The structure and role behavior of members of a given family must be determined by the nurse before she can decide intelligently on the best method for initiating a health activity. It is often clarifying for the nurse to draw her perceptions of the family structure by means of a map, particularly if she is presenting a family case study for group discussion. The map shows the number of family members in terms of their power, alignments, and boundaries. For the family that has closed boundaries, they are depicted within a closed circle, with the member demonstrating the greatest power in the center. Other family members are arranged within the circle as they relate to the person with greatest power and their alignments with other family members. The family with closed boundaries is frequently a troubled family. They communicate defensively, are judgmental and dogmatic, maintain rigid roles and rules, have secrets, try to control others, and resist change.[7] The map of a troubled family of four with a dominant father, an alignment between mother and son, and an independent daughter can look like Fig. 5-3. The space between the circles represents the psychological distance between family members.

[7]Satir, V., *Peoplemaking*, Science and Behavior Books, Palo Alto, Calif., 1972, pp. 114–116.

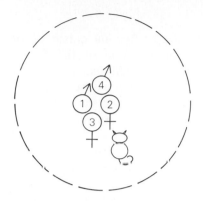

Figure 5-4 (1) Father: age 27. (2) Mother: age 26. (3) Daughter: age 4. (4) Son: age 3.

For the family with open boundaries, the map is a broken circle, allowing for outside persons to enter in as necessary. These families are considered healthy because they communicate supportively, help each other solve problems spontaneously, show understanding, share hurts with each other, have roles and rules that are flexible, give clear leveling messages, and consider changes to be normal and desirable.[8] Figure 5-4 is a diagram of a healthy family of four, in which all members work well together. The favored family cat is also included. It must be remembered that healthy families have disagreements, alignments, and variable distribution of power, depending upon day-by-day circumstances. They are considered healthy because family members are encouraged to grow and flourish in a supportive, flexible environment.

Any number of ingenious pictures of family structures can be devised by the nurse as she gathers evidence regarding the role behaviors, power, and alignments of family members. The pictures may change as the nurse's assessment of the family structure deepens. Sometimes families themselves will respond to the idea of picturing their placement in the family system when given the assignment.

Another way for presenting family structures before study groups is to do a family sculpture. Four volunteers from the study group can be requested to perform as models of the family. An assignment of a family role can be given to each volunteer, including a brief description of each one's appearance, life theme, and stance. Then, the nurse can arrange the volunteer-father, volunteer-mother, volunteer-son, and volunteer-daughter as a family unit with closeness and distance between members as she perceives it. Family members can be facing each other or standing back to back. When they assume the postures and facial expressions as described by the nurse, the visual scene of the family unit is graphic and communicates a situation with much greater impact than mere words.

[8]Ibid., pp. 114–117.

Function of the Family

In view of controversial opinions about the continuing existence of families as familiarly known in society, the function of the family assumes major importance.[9] It may be that the traditional concept of families should not be the focus of attention as much as the change or diversity of family functioning and structuring. Parsons stated that the functions of the family in a highly differentiated society are performed for the benefit of the personality rather than on behalf of the society. Families are necessary because the human personality is not "born" but must be "made" through the socialization process.[10] When babies are born and raised in their own distinct family environment, they learn to cope with the world by identifying with or in opposition to models with whom they have been intimate all their early years. Each child picks up individual characteristics from the adult models, mother and father. It is fascinating to observe small children at play and witness the behavior that is unconsciously mimicked from either the mother or the father. Children learn to perceive the world through the adult models in their environment, and they remember best the *actions* which gained their attention rather than adult words. Therefore, when adults rely on words to create an impression, they are often producing an inconsistency that is not understandable to a child. For example, when a mother cautions her child never to run across the street without first looking to the right and left for the presence of vehicles, and later runs across the street herself without following her own directives, the child takes note of this. The performed act has a much greater impact on his or her memory than the words. When the child is disciplined for running across the street without looking to the right or left, he or she tends to regard the punishment as unjust.

Hill outlined basic requirements for family survival, continuity, and growth. These included seven tasks:

1   Reproduction: planning and controlling family size
2   Physical maintenance of family members: providing food, clothing, shelter and medical care
3   Socialization of offspring into functioning adults, capable of assuming adult family roles of husband-father, wife-mother
   a   Organization of explicit expectations for children and adults
   b   Organization of family objectives to which members are subordinate
4   Allocation of resources and division of duties and responsibilities
   a   Allocation of authority, including prestige, and designation of accountability

[9]See Alvin Toffler, *Future Shock,* Random House, Inc., New York, 1970.
[10]Parsons and Bales, op. cit., p. 16.

    b   Allocation of economic income and output

    c   Division of labor: specialization of roles to secure performance of essential family jobs

    d   Division of time: scheduling of tasks and services

5 Maintenance of order within the family and between the family and outsiders

    a   Within the family: meeting the emotional needs of members and determining types and intensity of emotional-affectional ties among members; channeling of sex drives; providing means of communication among members

    b   Between family and outsiders: developing methods of articulating with other groups and the larger social structure

6 Maintenance of family morale and motivation to carry out family tasks: providing a system of rewards and punishments to keep members at family tasks; development of equilibrating and inspiring mechanisms for upset or discouraged members

7 Development of methods for orderly recruiting and releasing of group members: incorporating of adopted children, stepparents, kin, guests, and servants into family group; releasing members at adulthood to jobs and marriage[11]

The mastery of these seven tasks by families varies widely. The nurse can be of greatest assistance to families when she can identify the tasks which need strengthening, enlist the interest of family members in clarifying their own resources and methods of coping, and teach methods of problem solving and interaction skills adapted to the family and facilitative of family recuperative strengths.

Developmental Tasks

Families and individuals change and develop in different ways, according to the nature of their individual living processes, family interaction, and stimulation by the social milieu. Each family member and each family is unique in its complex of age-role expectations in reciprocity.[12] The family as a small-group system is interrelated in such a manner that change does not occur in one part without a series of resultant changes in other parts.[13] As stated by Lederer and Jackson, the family is a unit in which all individuals have an important influence—whether they like it or not and whether they know it or not. The family is an interacting communications

[11]Reuben Hill, "Challenges and Resources for Family Development," Iowa State University Center for Agricultural and Economic Development, in *Family Mobility in Our Dynamic Society.* Reprinted by permission of The Iowa State University Press, Ames, 1965, p. 255.

[12]Nye and Berardo, op. cit., p. 210.

[13]Ibid., p. 203.

network in which every member influences the nature of the entire system
and in turn is influenced by it.[14]

The family role pattern constantly changes as each member grows,
develops, and matures according to his age and cultural role expectation.
The developmental task concept takes into consideration the human
needs of the individual and the cultural demands made upon him. It is
defined as a task that arises at or about a certain period in the life of an
individual, successful achievement of which leads to his happiness and
success with later tasks, while failure leads to unhappiness in the individual, disapproval by society, and difficulty with later tasks.[15] For example,
one developmental task of the preschool child is to learn to develop
physical skills appropriate to his stage of motor development.[16] When he
learns to button his coat or tie his shoes before going to school, he gains
the approval of his mother, feels pleased with himself, and is challenged
to try new skills. A developmental task of the teen-ager is to achieve a
satisfying and socially accepted masculine or feminine role.[17] When a
teen-age girl does not perceive herself as sexually attractive or lovable,
has few girlfriends and no boyfriends, she is unhappy, and all of her
behavior reflects her dissatisfaction with herself. Her adaptation to all
subsequent events in her life is affected and often dysfunctional if the
developmental task is not satisfactorily resolved. Duvall lists in detail the
developmental tasks of individuals for each age level in the life cycle in
her book, *Family Development.* She states there are ten ever-changing
developmental tasks which are faced by every individual. They are:

1   Achieving an appropriate dependence-independence pattern
2   Achieving an appropriate giving-receiving pattern of affection
3   Relating to changing social groups
4   Developing a conscience
5   Learning one's psycho-socio-biological sex role
6   Accepting and adjusting to a changing body
7   Managing a changing body and learning new motor patterns
8   Learning to understand and control the physical world
9   Developing an appropriate symbol system and developing conceptual abilities
10   Relating one's self to the cosmos[18]

In addition to individual developmental tasks, there are family
developmental tasks, which are the responsibility of the family as a whole

[14]William J. Lederer and Don D. Jackson, M.D., *The Mirages of Marriage,* W. W.
Norton & Company, Inc., New York, 1968, p. 14.
[15]Evelyn Millis Duvall, *Family Development,* 2d ed., J. B. Lippincott Company,
Philadelphia, 1962, pp. 31–32.
[16]Ibid., p. 230.
[17]Ibid., p. 294.
[18]Ibid., pp. 40–41.

if they are going to grow and develop in a healthy, satisfying manner. The family developmental tasks keep changing as the family grows, adjusts, and matures from a beginning family, which starts with the marriage, becomes a small group when children are born, allows outsiders to enter the family system when children marry, and becomes an aging family nearing the end of the family life cycle. Duvall lists nine ever-changing family developmental tasks that span the family life cycle. They are to establish and maintain:

1 An independent home
2 Satisfactory ways of getting and spending money
3 Mutually acceptable patterns in the division of labor
4 Continuity of mutually satisfying sex relationships
5 Open system of intellectual and emotional communication
6 Workable relationships with relatives
7 Ways of interacting with associates and community organizations
8 Competency in bearing and rearing children
9 A workable philosophy of life[19]

The defined developmental task concepts for individuals and families according to their stage of human growth are extremely helpful for the community health nurse to use as guidelines when working with individuals and families. If the nurse can assist or encourage an individual or family to gain a satisfactory achievement of a developmental task that has been causing difficulties, she has facilitated growth, happiness, and movement toward maturity or self-actualization. It must be remembered that the individual himself must master the developmental tasks that he faces, but he cannot do it in isolation.[20] If an alert community health nurse identifies the juncture at which an individual or family may be stalemated in developmental task progression, she can serve as an essential, facilitating change agent when it is most needed.

FAMILIES REPRESENTING SOCIOECONOMIC GROUPS

It has been said that the community health nurse works with *all* families in need at whatever stage of development or period of adjustment they are undergoing in their family life cycle. She is a helpful assistant when the family has special problems for which they are not adequately prepared, such as illnesses, accidents, birth of handicapped children, emergence of undesirable health or social conditions, and personality disorders. Since the nurse is a generalist, she views the family objectively from the perspective of wholeness. She identifies the coping patterns of the given family, the degree of discomfort they are experiencing, and is able to

---

[19]Ibid., pp. 478–505.
[20]Ibid., p. 42.

direct their energies, when they are ready, toward community resources and facilities which most closely meet their requirements. She also directs her own energies to those professional consultants within the community from whom she needs special instruction and guidance in assisting the family to cope better with explicit problems. Families representing socioeconomic groups are described in subsequent paragraphs to alert the nurse to her style of interaction and implementation.

Low-Income Families

Community health nurses have visited low-income multiproblem families for many years, have seen little discernable changes in the behavior of these families, have felt frustrated and sometimes angry with the apathy or lack of responsiveness of members of the family. In managing these families, some nurses regard them as a challenge, some view them as an unpleasant duty contained within their caseload, and some see them as hopeless, worthless, and to be avoided, particularly if the family is resistant to any health measures offered. Obviously, these families have great need for health assistance. However, as described by a nursing student, "Low-income families are hard to move. You take health to them on a platter. You say, 'Mm, it's good.' and even though they are hungry, they hesitate to accept any of the goodies."

The community health nurse visits all socioeconomic groups, but the low-income groups receive a proportionately larger concentration of her time and services because of their high incidence of chronic diseases, multiple environmental hazards, high birth rates, high infant mortality rates, poor health standards, multiple social problems, and often inadequate delivery of health-care services. These groups are generally identified as poverty families, multiproblem families, hard-core families, disorganized families, or disadvantaged families. They are often families plagued by many serious problems, which they are unable to handle by themselves or through the services made available in the community, and they come repeatedly to the attention of community agencies in a negative connotation.[21] These families realize that health is an important reality for them but they often do not avail themselves of preventive health programs. Because community health nurses are very familiar health workers to these families, it is essential for the nurses to understand their life-styles and implement methods of approach that will be successful in changing their health practices. Much research has been done in recent years from which nurses can profit as they experiment with new ways of developing self-esteem in these families and changing destructive health patterns to more acceptable, amenable practices.

[21]L. L. Geismar and Michael A. La Sorte, *Understanding the Multi-Problem Family*, Association Press, New York, 1964, p. 33.

Families of poverty are found in every community. Many of them reflect a design for living which Lewis has characterized as the culture of poverty. Regardless of their race, creed, color, culture, or setting, they have a life-style which shows remarkable similarity in the structure of their families, in interpersonal relations, in spending habits, in their value systems, and in their orientation in time. To demonstrate the culture of poverty, the social order of a population in general must be one in which members prize the value of thrift and work toward the accumulation of wealth and property and the advancement of upward mobility. In such a society, the individuals of a low economic status tend to be seen as personally inadequate and inferior.[22]

Once the culture of poverty has come into existence in a society, it tends to perpetuate itself. The family does not cherish childhood as a specially prolonged and protected stage in the life cycle. Initiation into sexual activity comes early. With the instability of consensual marriage, the family tends to be mother-centered and tied more closely to the mother's extended family. The female head of the house is given to authoritarian rule. In spite of much verbal emphasis on family solidarity, sibling rivalry for the limited supply of goods and maternal affection is intense. There is little privacy.[23]

Irelan described four distinctive life themes which are manifested in lower-class behavior. These include (1) fatalism, (2) orientation to the present, (3) authoritarianism, and (4) concreteness. When individuals have persistent fatalistic beliefs regarding unavoidable or uncontrollable external forces in their lives, a sense of powerlessness and resignation emanates, which acts as a definite deterrent to any efforts to break a chain of unfortunate circumstances. They receive their "hard luck" as their fate. Because of their basic need for survival (physiological and safety needs), they are oriented to the present rather than the future. They spontaneously take their pleasures and discomforts immediately or in the "here and now" rather than defer gratifications to a future time. They believe in the rightness of existing systems and in strength as the source of authority. By simplifying life experiences, they classify people as either weak or strong and will use authority, rather than reason, as the basis for decision making. The theme of concreteness deals with an emphasis on material rather than intellectual things. Because these individuals are preoccupied with tangible, day-to-day problems, they understand best any activity or emotion which is concrete and visible. They value action that has results or gives tangible rewards.[24]

[22]Oscar Lewis, *La Vida,* Random House, Inc., New York, 1966.
[23]Ibid.
[24]Lola M. Irelan, *Low-Income Life Styles,* U.S. Department of Health, Education, and Welfare, Government Printing Office, Washington, D.C., 1966, pp. 7–9.

In looking at their goals in life, they want the same things that any other citizen in America wants. They want to improve their life by acquiring security, material comforts and luxuries, and social values which appeal to all individuals. Their drive toward better occupations and more income is often based on escaping the discomforts of life in poverty. They want better housing, living conditions, and education. They value the opportunity to escape routines and pressures of day-to-day existence. Their desires are similar to the desires of any other social class; however, their life experiences have been such that their expectations for reaching toward their goals have been limited drastically. It is at this juncture that the community health nurse can play an active role in eliciting the feelings and desires of family members, encouraging the development of a plan of action which is conceivable to the family, and supporting and enabling the implementation of a plan so that success is achieved. To do this, the nurse must start with minute goals that are achievable and have the strong possibility for culminating in a positive direction. Success breeds success, and families in poverty must begin at a level that they can see, understand, and trust. Oftentimes this means that the nurse must spend considerable time in developing the self-esteem and self-confidence of the individuals with whom she is working before they are ready to move toward a projected desired goal, even though it may be a minute one.

It must be emphasized that not all poor families exhibit characteristics of the culture of poverty. There are stable lower-class families who are cohesive and function as integral parts of the society. The fathers are employed in steady positions as semiskilled or unskilled workers, and have an elementary school level of education. In these homes the intellectual stimulation for the children is rather low. These families profit from the attention of the nurse but must not be managed or categorized in the same classification as the families who demonstrate the poverty culture.

It cannot be overemphasized that each family with whom the nurse comes in contact must be assessed *individually.* Textbook profiles and research studies point out important, significant data with which the nurse should be familiar to aid in her understanding and implementation of purposeful nursing actions. For example, the levels of social functioning are spelled out in detail for families classified as inadequate, marginal, and adequate by Geismar and La Sorte,[25] and descriptive characteristics which will help the nurse to work with disorganized and disadvantaged families are elaborated upon by Minuchin et al.[26] The ultimate success of the nurse's work depends on the synthesis of her knowledge of facts and

[25]Geismar and La Sorte, op. cit., pp. 205–222.
[26]Minuchin et al., op. cit., pp. 192–242.

data about families, her ability to relate, and the individuation of her nursing efforts with each family situation.

Health Perceptions of the Poor

Poverty is a health hazard because of crowded or deteriorated housing, inadequate nutrition, and insufficient medical care. Consequently, low-income families are more vulnerable to ill health and less able to cope with it. They are often ignorant about causes, treatment, and outcomes of various diseases. They are not informed or particularly concerned about preventive measures. They accept poor health conditions as inevitable, such as dental decay with ultimate loss of teeth. Physical discomfort is a way of life, and only when one becomes incapacitated and unable to fulfill daily responsibilities does he or she regard himself or herself as "sick." Therefore, treatment is sought at a late stage of development, in contrast to early detection of disease symptoms. Many low-income families do not participate in health activities or programs available in the community, including the preventive type of programs. They do not conceive of themselves as having a voice in community concerns since they lack contact with community organizations and among themselves. They tend to practice self-medication, and when they need medical advice, they ask friends, neighbors, or the druggist. They feel a distrust of physicians and clinics, particularly if they sense that they are evaluated as being inadequate or uncooperative or are treated as impersonal objects. They tend to set higher value on concrete physical improvements such as better housing, better transportation, or improved household equipment than they do on health.[27]

Working with the Poor

The nurse is better able to relate with the poor if she understands some of their behavior patterns and attitudes. She must be willing to experiment with new ways of implementing nursing activities and health teaching, since nursing actions in the past few years have not always ended in success when applied to low-income families. When knowledgeable about characteristic patterns of behavior as described by studies dealing with the poor, the nurse is better armed to adapt her approach to the specific needs of the particular family with whom she is working. When she realizes that low-income families value material things, she will readily accept the fact that they are more action-oriented than verbally oriented. When talking with an individual who uses speech as a means of direct, specific communication rather than an elaboration of thoughts or intellect, she will realize that she must create a mutual understanding which does

[27]Irelan, op. cit., pp. 51–62.

not rely on words alone. This forces her to use her ingenuity and creativity in selecting an approach which will have meaning for the family. The use of tangible rewards, demonstrations, active participation with tasks, role playing, or acting out behaviors or games are some approaches that may be more effective than words for the patient.

By being observant of the communication patterns of low-income families who are disadvantaged, the nurse can learn essential data which will have bearing on her subsequent activities. She will become aware that family members do not expect to be heard. No one really listens. If someone responds to a statement, it is not necessarily along the lines of the preceding communication. A high tolerance of interruptions and changing of subject material is demonstrated; therefore, a subject is rarely carried to any conclusion. Noise and motor activities often take precedence over the continuation of a subject being discussed. The mother is the central pathway for most transactions among family members when they are all together. Spouses rarely talk to each other but engage in a "parallel" type of conversation that is directed to a third party or to the children. The mother's messages to the children are mostly in terms of "don'ts." She rarely gives a message which emphasizes any positives to the children. Children learn to pay attention to the person rather than to the content of the message received.[28] Consequently, the children do not talk in long sentences or express their desires by words alone.

Because the intellectual stimulation at home is limited, the concepts of time, size, and shape have to be dealt with in terms of familiar objects and words. For example, children may have to be taught that a ball is a "circle," or a clock is a "square." It is not unusual that parental control is at times confusing, because of inconsistency in being at one moment completely authoritarian or at the next moment powerless. The ambivalence with which discipline and punishment of children are exercised in the home can be witnessed frequently. Often there is little evidence of commercial toys in the home, and the means by which children improvise playthings or give their attention in play can be instructive to the nurse. If no regular mealtime routine is practiced in the home, conversation at the dinner table or a parental focus on table manners is unknown.[29]

As the nurse assesses the behavior and communication patterns of a given family and synthesizes data gained from an appropriate textbook or research study, she will be prepared to try new methods of implementation which will be stimulating to the family. For example, she can set a goal to encourage spouses to talk directly to each other or alert the mother regarding her predominantly negative messages to the children. Her

[28]Minuchin et al., op. cit., pp. 201–206.
[29]Sol Adler, *The Health and Education of the Economically Deprived Child,* Warren H. Green, Inc., St. Louis, Mo., 1968, pp. 17–20.

method for drawing the attention of family members regarding her goal may be through role-playing, psychodrama, or role-reversal games. By bringing observed patterns of behavior to the attention of family members, the nurse has a starting point from which to determine if they want to do anything about it, and if so, to plan with the family regarding the best way of implementation.

It sometimes happens that family members express a desired goal which is too global, so the task of the nurse requires restricting the goal specification to a dimension possible for the family to attain. For example, a mother might express a desire for her eight-year-old son to stop wetting the bed, since this behavior causes her to be continuously annoyed and irritable with him. In order for the nurse to implement successful activities with this goal, she must elicit detailed information from both the mother and the eight-year-old son. She must be assured of the desire of both to attain the stated goal. By requesting all data related to the problem, gaining the individual perceptions of both mother and son regarding the causes of the problem, and discussing the activities each will feel able to carry out, a plan for eliminating the enuresis for one night only out of the week can be the stated beginning goal. Gathering baseline data before implementing a plan of action is always desirable. (See Chap. 6 for an elaboration of the behavior-modification method.)

Nurses must remember that the poor are distrustful of outsiders and have been exploited often, so considerable time and attention has to be given early to developing trust and a relationship in which communication has meaning for both the family and the nurse.

Middle- and High-Income Families

Many professional workers, including nurses, come from a middle-class orientation and are familiar with attitudes, values, and behavior patterns of middle-income families. Some of the characteristics descriptive of middle-class values are the desirability of the accumulation of material wealth, a belief in work and thrift as necessary attributes, an acceptance of upward mobility as indicative of success and progress, a future orientation for gratification of desires, and the importance of education. Children raised in a middle- or high-income family learn to express themselves with language which communicates observations, thoughts, and feelings. Curiosity is cultivated and questions are answered by parents. Children are raised in an environment which includes the stimuli of books, magazines, newspapers, and toys of all sizes and shapes. Mealtimes are regular and attention is given to table conversation and proper use of eating utensils.[30]

In essence, the delivery of health care in any community is structured

---

[30]Ibid., pp. 17–20.

for and utilized mainly by middle- and high-income groups because they are the people who are alert and responsive to early disease symptoms, are able to pay for services, and expend much energy in participating as planners and organizers of beneficial community services.

Working with Middle- and High-Income Families

For nurses working with middle- and high-income families, the task of encouraging preventive health services is often made easy because of the acceptance and responsiveness of the consumer. The basis for a relationship may differ from that in low-income groups because the consumer is frequently well-educated and has a cognitive understanding and natural desire to learn about any phenomenon under study which captivates his or her interest. For the consumer who prizes intellectualism, the nurse must prepare differently than for the customer who wants the concrete, pertinent facts and no more. Many middle-income family members have as great a need for strengthening their self-esteem as low-income families. However, some seem to have a high propensity for utilizing defense mechanisms, which makes the development of a therapeutic relationship difficult and time-consuming, yet essential. Defensive people respond to openness and honesty and can be convinced about an idea if it is presented in a logical manner which gives recognition to all the arguments or barriers opposing the idea. The necessity for the nurse to assess the consumer in terms of interests, personality, background, and education is vital as the nurse *plans* her teaching content and methods of approach on subsequent visits. Often it is not difficult for the nurse to recognize the need for a relationship with the middle-income family member if the consumer is friendly, receptive, and responsive—and most middle-class families are amicable. However, occasionally a family member is encountered who is hostile, openly questioning, highly educated, or unmistakably defensive, and the nurse tends to want to withdraw rather than pursue the difficult course of developing a relationship. The nurse must be encouraged to plan carefully her strategy with the challenging patient in a way that is convincing to the consumer. This requires extensive educational and psychological preparation on the part of the nurse, but she is rewarded by broadening her own educational and experiential background and by strengthening her belief in herself. If she maintains an open, honest style and refuses to react emotionally to any intentionally provocative statement by the consumer, nine times out of ten, she can "win" the patient.

FAMILIES REPRESENTING CULTURAL GROUPS

To gain an understanding of families representing cultural groups, the meaning of culture is described, followed by a discussion of selected families representing cultures upon whom the focus of attention has been centered in recent years. The overview of families of other cultures as contained in this chapter represents only a "taste" of the vast amount of information that is currently available in a cross section of popular and professional books and periodicals.

Meaning of Culture

The concept of culture refers to those specific ways of thinking, feeling, and acting which differentiate one group from another. Culture varies in its patterns and meanings as represented by different groups who have been studied. Each group has developed its own way of life based on modifications and adaptations occurring through the course of history in the particular setting in which the group lived. The design for living of any particular group is transmitted to the children of the group directly and indirectly as they grow, develop, and learn to adapt to their physical environment and the people who act as their models and teachers. Culture serves as a subtle and systematic device for perceiving the world.[31] It stands for the way of life of a people, for the sum of their learned behavior patterns, attitudes, and material things.[32]

Every culture is of paramount importance to its possessor. It is a universal tendency for human beings to accept that their way of thinking, acting, and believing is the right way and to rate one's own culture as generally superior to others. Each individual has no choice but to function in the culture of which he or she is a part. It exercises a strong influence in the way individuals perceive themselves and others. As stated by Hall, culture is a mold in which we all are cast, and it controls our daily lives and behavior in many unsuspected ways. Culture hides much more than it reveals, and it hides most effectively from its own participants.[33] It is not because of any difference in the basic nature of humankind that the cultures of different ethnic groups differ so much from one another, but because of the differences in the history of experiences which each group has undergone.[34] Because people rely on learned behavior or culture for survival, it is this acquired guidance that enables them to adapt to change.[35]

Since the community health nurse talks and works with such a wide variety of cultural groups, she must be constantly alert, consciously

[31]Benjamin D. Paul, *Health, Culture and Community,* Russell Sage Foundation, New York, 1955, p. 467.
[32]Edward T. Hall, *The Silent Language.* Copyright 1959 by Edward T. Hall. Reprinted by permission of Doubleday & Company, Inc., Garden City, New York, p. 31.
[33]Ibid., pp. 38–39.
[34]Ashley Montagu, *The Biosocial Nature of Man,* Grove Press, Inc., New York, 1956, p. 81.
[35]Benjamin A. Kogan, *Health, Man in a Changing Environment,* Harcourt Brace Jovanovich, Inc., New York, 1970, p. 34.

observant, sensitive, accepting of all differences, and curious about the behavior patterns and life-styles that are revealed in her presence. There is much to be learned about other cultural groups, and according to Hall, much about our own culture.

Cultural Shock

When an individual visits a new country for an extended period of time or returns to his own country after a long absence, he is apt to feel a "culture shock," a removal or distortion of many of the familiar cues one encounters at home and the substitution for them of other cues that are strange.[36] The person experiences great differences that seem to exist between oneself and the people with whom he or she is working. All things are regarded as strange and incomprehensible and communication is perceived as difficult because of the inconsistent response of the listener. In adapting to the new dimension in life to which the individual has been exposed, he or she must be ready to develop esteem in others who are different and at the same time maintain his or her own sense of integrity and worth. The process of developing esteem for others who are different begins with getting to know the other person, by being willing to talk his or her language, using his or her particular jargon or phrases appropriately when their meaning is understood, and finding out his or her interests. It sometimes takes effort and involves periods of frustrations, but the ultimate outcome is satisfying and broadening to one's experience when dealt with successfully.

Frequently, selected groups of student nurses undergo culture shock when they are exposed to completely new patterns of family living, an experience which often occurs in community health nursing. They see and talk with families whose culture is greatly different from their own. For many nursing students, the actual experience of entering a dirty, insect-ridden, poverty-stricken home is a highly charged one. She may have intellectualized these conditions for some time, but coming upon the actual situations at a time when she may think that she has seen all and is wise to the world and its ways can be shattering.[37] The nurses must be allowed to talk freely in discussion groups about their initial impressions, followed by encouragement to look for factors in the strange home environment that will reveal the family's strengths. As the nurses adjust to the reality of accepting differences in family living patterns, they facilitate their productiveness in implementing effective nursing services.

---

[36]Hall, op. cit., p. 156.
[37]Elaine C. Gowell, "Helping Student Nurses to Become Involved," *International Journal Nursing Studies*, 7:225–234, Pergamon Press, London, New York, Nov. 1970.

The Cultural Gap

The success of any health teaching is dependent upon the way in which it is understood, accepted, and implemented by the learner. The fact that there may be a gap or difference between the culture of the family and that of the nurse must always be remembered. Until the health worker or teacher understands the sociocultural patterns of the families she is serving, what purposes they serve, why they persist, and how they change, she will be unable to transmit health information which she believes to be desperately needed by the family. If the health teaching or activity is incompatible with the family's idea of illness and curing, the obstacle and challenge of changing their beliefs and practices must be attended to first. This necessitates many contacts with the family during which an understanding of their beliefs as the basis for their reluctance to change is gained, trust is developed as the family members accept the health worker, and the subsequent relationship of family members and health worker eases the willingness to change. Cultural values give meaning and direction to life, and it is doubtful if anyone ever really changes culture. What happens is that small, informal adaptations are continually being made in the day-to-day process of living.[38] Until the nurse has a hint of the cultural value which seems to be impeding her progress toward a desired goal with a family, she is working as though blindfolded. It is essential for the nurse to elicit the family's perception of their health problems and needs, to *avoid* making assumptions based on her *own* values, and to implement further actions based on an accurate understanding of the family's physical, mental, and emotional resources and the value they place on health. This takes effort, patience, and ingenuity. Health practices and adaptations may sometimes be initiated by appealing to pride or suggesting a gain in prestige. Long-term goals have a better chance of being implemented if they are combined with tangible measures to meet immediate health needs. For example, if the nurse has a goal for convincing the mother of a family of the necessity of immunizations for her children, she will hasten the deadline for her long-term goal if she attends to immediate illnesses, dental, clothing, or nutritional needs of the children. Early, tangible proof of her concern for the children will aid in convincing the mother of the family that the nurse is in earnest and genuinely cares about improving the overall health status of the family. Consequently, in due time the mother may be motivated to seek immunizations or practice health measures as advised by the nurse.

Sometimes the values of both the health professional and the family can be met by making use of means of adaptation and compromise. For example, for the adamant elderly Scandinavian male who stubbornly insists on the use of kerosene dressings for his leg ulcers, the nurse can

[38]Hall, op. cit., p. 90.

agree that kerosene is useful for superficial skin burns because of the property of being oil-based, but for present purposes she can indicate firmly that she will use it only around the healthy skin edges. For the leg ulcers, she will use only the prescribed medication as ordered by the doctor.

It is good to remember that an individual, regardless of his or her culture, wants to be recognized as an entity, a being who serves a purpose of some kind. When one is seen, heard, and made to feel that he or she has had an impact of some kind on the other person, then the individual feels a sense of satisfaction and fulfillment. If the nurse communicates a genuine desire to get to know the other person by learning the meaning of his or her words, which are different, his or her customs, foods, dress when different, and interests, an enduring rapport is often initiated. Universal inquiries that are responded to with warmth after two participants have established a mutual feeling of trust are "What was your early childhood like?"; "How did you meet your husband or wife?"; "Tell me about the country where you were born"; "What are your favorite foods?"; "Tell me about the holidays or celebrations that you particularly love." By eliciting descriptions of events that the patient has experienced, the nurse becomes involved in a mutual exchange which is informative of the patient's culture, habits, attitudes, and values and serves as a basis for future conversations about health practices. The nurse broadens her scope of knowledge about learned behavior and perhaps gains a curiosity which will someday prompt a desire to visit the country or locale about which the patient is speaking.

Ethnic Minority Families in the United States

Ethnic minority groups form a substantial portion of the American population. All have serious deficiencies in the areas of health, education, and welfare which are due to impoverishment, cultural differences, or combinations of both. Even though each ethnic group is unique, has a different language, life-style, and world view, this does not mean that each group is monolithic in its views. A range of characteristics, life-styles, and views exist within each ethnic group and stereotyping cannot be done based on exposure to one or two families.

A problem universal to all ethnic minority groups is the retention of their sociocultural-psychological identity existing either in harmony with or as complementary to the American culture. When discrimination is practiced by a major culture, minority ethnic groups are forced to form their own social groups or enclaves where they find belongingness and solace.[39]

[39]Kananur V. Chandra, *Racial Discrimination in Canada; Asian Minorities,* R. & E. Research Associates, San Francisco, 1973, p. 61.

Black Families

Many books have been written recently that are informative and descriptive of the black people in America. A major factor which causes the black culture to be different from that of other cultural groups who have migrated to America involves the severance of traditional ties with the native land. Black people were brought to America forcibly and were completely cut off from their past. They were robbed of language and culture. They were forbidden to be Africans and never allowed to be Americans. While other cultural nonblack groups passed on proud traditions to their children, black people were unaware of a sense of worth about the values and rituals which they shared. The culture that was born during the days of slavery passed from generation to generation, and the black people consequently developed constricting adaptations which continue to persist as contemporary character traits.[40]

The life of many blacks has been one of social chaos. Oppression and discrimination have played a major role in causing the destruction of the family structure, insecurity caused by crime, insufficient education, the lack of proper health standards, and the signs of various antisocial activities such as illegitimacy, drug usage, and alcoholism. Defense mechanisms such as apathy, self-abasement, work slowdowns, and escape into boisterous hedonism are not uncommon behaviors among blacks. Grier and Cobbs describe the black family as weak and relatively ineffective because it has not been allowed the rights and privileges of protecting its members.[41] The black male is expected to maintain a family, educate his children, and provide the normal conveniences of modern living, even though he is more likely than his white counterpart to be unemployed, earn less money, and pay more for housing. Constant failures in his attempts to be a successful provider are great blows to his manhood. Often his wife is forced to work to add to the family income.[42] As parents, the man and wife teach their children what the world is like, how it functions, and how *they* must function if they are to survive. All too often the children have the hope and desire to succeed in the world but because of futile and dangerous competition, they are unable to fulfill their ambitions. Despite these problems, the black family is first of all an extended family. Relatives share the responsibilities of child rearing and members of the family often come to the aid of a troubled member.[43]

Billingsley described in detail the three social-class groupings of Negro families. About ten percent of Negro families may be considered

[40]William H. Grier and Price M. Cobbs, *Black Rage,* Basic Books, Inc., Publishers, New York, 1968, pp. 22–24.

[41]Ibid., p. 71.

[42]A. Ludlow Kramer, *Race and Violence in Washington State,* Report of the Commission on the Causes and Prevention of Civil Disorder, 1969, p. 24.

[43]Grier and Cobbs, op. cit., p. 87.

upper-class because the men are highly educated, are in high-income brackets, have secure careers and adequate comfortable housing. About forty percent of all Negro families are middle-class as distinguished by educational, income, and occupational achievement and styles of family life. Half of all Negro families are in the lower classes. Of these, there are the "working nonpoor," the "working poor," and the "nonworking poor." The "working nonpoor" are the families with the males working as semiskilled, unionized laborers in industries. The "working poor" represent families whose males work in unskilled and service occupations with marginal incomes. The "nonworking poor" are those families who receive the most publicity and who comprise 15 to 20 percent of Negro families. These are people who are unemployed or intermittently employed, supported by relatives and friends or by public welfare.[44] The *majority* of *poor Negroes* live in nuclear families headed by men and not by women and are self-supporting rather than supported by public welfare.[45]

When studying the "nonworking poor," the lower-class Negro family, the existence of a matriarchal pattern is frequently found. Many black families are headed by the woman because opportunities for welfare payments are better for the female-headed household. The woman is often overburdened by many children and substandard living conditions. Her attitude toward her child may be one of ambivalence or indifference. Discipline tends to be inconsistent, but the child is expected to meet high standards of behavior and is severely punished when he or she fails to meet them. Activities are impulse-determined and consistency is totally absent. The children are often given more freedom outside the home and form important peer-group contacts early in life. The influence of the peer-group association often has more significance to the child than that of his or her parents because of the sense of importance and the identity of being a "gang" member.[46]

A black norm of behavior has developed which involves a profound distrust of white citizens and of the nation. The black person has learned to protect himself or herself from physical hurt, cheating, slander, humiliation, and outright mistreatment by the official representatives of society. For his or her own survival, the black individual views every white person as a potential enemy until proved otherwise and sees every social system as set against him or her unless he or she personally finds out differently.[47] This in part explains the many pent-up resentments and

---

[44]Andrew Billingsley, *Black Families in White America,* Prentice-Hall, Inc., Englewood Cliffs, N.J., 1968, pp. 8–9.

[45]Ibid., p. 139.

[46]Martin Deutsch, Irwin Katz, and Arthur R. Jensen, *Social Class, Race, and Psychological Development,* Holt, Rinehart and Winston, Inc., New York, 1968, p. 204.

[47]Grier and Cobbs, op. cit., p. 149.

latent frustrations felt by blacks and being expressed in many overt and covert ways, according to Martin Luther King.[48]

For the white nurse visiting the black family, verbal and nonverbal evidences of the resentments and frustrations are easily detected if the nurse is sensitive and alert to cues. Many of the traditional nursing behaviors in home visits, which had a logical basis for existence initially, are being interpreted in a different way by blacks. Standeven cited the example of the community health nurse's routine in placing a newspaper under the nursing bag. The blacks saw this action as indicating their home was particularly repelling and dirty, and the nurse was avoiding contamination of herself and the bag.[49] Members of the black family are particularly sensitive to cues of behavior. They do not like a friendly, charming manner if it seems phony, but respond with warmth and consideration of the nurse *after* they are convinced that she accepts them as having value and truly desires to be of assistance. There is much for the white nurse to learn about blacks, and the best teachers are blacks themselves, whether they are black nurses or black families. If the nurse concentrates first on initiating an empathic relationship, the resultant dialogue between the two involved persons will enhance their knowledges of each other, their adaptations of behavior, and result in positive exchanges which may be beneficial to both nurse and patient.

The health status of black groups is complicated by environmental conditions, unemployment, and lack of money to obtain medical treatment. Residents of racial ghettos have a high incidence of major diseases. The infant mortality and prematurity rate is higher for Negroes than for Caucasians. The rate of illegitimacy is high among the poor. One of the many tasks of the nurse is to increase the knowledge and sensitivity of black families about available health-care facilities such as medical and dental services, hospitals, and clinics dealing with family planning, abortion counseling, immunizations, child health, drug abuse, nutrition, prevention, and many other health-related problems. She also must be prepared to cope with the problems of little cash, transportation, baby-sitting problems, and erratic hours since these obstacles often stand in the way of attendance to health-care needs for blacks and their families. Black consumers have become active in exercising their right for health care and are increasingly convinced that they must do their own thing in health. In other words, they must play a major role in the design and management of health-care programs for blacks. According to Milio, blacks want to learn to be self-sufficient in meeting their health needs and

[48]Judson R. Landis, *Current Perspectives on Social Problems,* Wadsworth Publishing Company, Inc., Belmont, Calif., 1969, p. 108.

[49]Muriel Standeven, "What the Poor Dislike about Community Health Nurses," *Nursing Outlook,* **17**(9):72–73, Sept. 1969.

appreciate efforts from white persons only when the goal is directed toward independent self-care for blacks. In striving for the "black is beautiful" concept, they are building their self-respect and gaining confidence in their own abilities to successfully determine and cope with the intricacies of modern living.[50]

Indian Families

Increasing attention is being given to American Indian culture and the role of the Indian in our current society. Since different tribes live in various locations of the United States, information about local Indian families must be obtained from literature specifically describing the local tribe and from the Indian people themselves. There are a great variety of Indian tribes who have their own histories, languages, customs, religions, and traditions. In addition, strong Indian leaders and war chiefs of the past hold a revered place in the memories of their people and symbolize the great tradition of the Indian people. As described by Deloria, individual tribes show incredible differences. The single aspect of major importance is tribal solidarity. Tribes that can handle their reservation conflicts in traditional Indian fashion generally make more progress and have better programs than do tribes that continually make adaptations to the white value system.[51]

There are many differences between the white culture and the Indian culture, and also among widely scattered Indian groups. A ritual or value of one tribe may not necessarily be accepted as essential by another tribe. The different geographical settings and cultural characteristics of various tribes complicate the work of health workers because transference of knowledge about one Indian tribe will not necessarily be valuable when working with a different tribe. This fact is frustrating because the health worker must start anew with each tribe with whom she works. Consequently, the health worker when working with Indian families in a local community must become acquainted with the values and beliefs of that specific Indian community. This takes time and patience. One example of a difference between two distinct tribes in terms of their responses to the implementation of health care by professionals is cited to demonstrate that the values of each tribe must be understood and dealt with as individual to that particular tribe. In a Pueblo reservation it was found that when parents were expected to transport their own children with health problems to clinics and hospitals outside the reservation, they gained a clearer understanding of the health services provided to the children and followed through with the recommended health care much

[50]Milio, op. cit., pp. 191–195.

[51]Vine Deloria, Jr., *Custer Died for Your Sins*, The Macmillan Company, New York, 1969, p. 28.

more dependably.[52] On a Tulalip reservation, however, the community health nurse was seen as more helpful if she brought concrete health services to the Indian child on the reservation or personally transported the child outside the reservation to the clinics and hospitals providing the health services.[53]

Indian people place absolute dependence on their leaders and expect them to produce. Because leadership is taxing, physically and emotionally, the usefulness of the leader is sustained only as long as he is able to withstand the pressures of leadership over a dependent people.[54] Indians welcome the future but don't worry about it. They like to meet other tribes, have a good time, and learn to trust one another. However, they reserve the right to change their minds about an issue whenever it serves their own purposes. Indians know the human mind intimately. They savor innuendo and inference and can dwell for hours on slight nuances that others completely miss. Because of this, Indians know the Indian mind best of all.[55]

The health status of Indians in some aspects is more appalling than that of blacks. The infant mortality rate is the highest in the nation, with infants dying of influenza, pneumonia, respiratory conditions, gastroenteric and parasitic diseases. The life expectancy of the Indian is less than that of all other races, and the suicide rate is triple the national rate. Suicide alone among Indian youth has caused great concern in recent years and for one tribe in western Washington led to the development of a progressive youth program in an attempt to forestall an epidemic of suicides among teen-agers. Leading diseases among the Indians are otitis media, tuberculosis, trachoma, anemia, and dental caries. A high incidence of lethal accidents, cirrhosis of the liver, and alcoholism also occurs with Indian populations.[56] Because of crowded housing, unsafe water, unsatisfactory waste disposal facilities, lack of nutritious food, and adherence to practices hazardous to health, the nurse has much health teaching to do *after* she has overcome the initial barrier of coming into the midst of the Indian people as a helping person and gone through the long procedure of becoming acceptable.

For the community health nurse working with Indian families on a

[52]Lucille J. Marsh, "Health Services for Indian Mothers and Children," Children's Bureau, Divison of Indian Health, Public Health Service, *Children*, Nov.–Dec. 1957.

[53]Rita Hoeschen Aichlmayr, "Cultural Understanding: A Key to Acceptance," *Nursing Outlook*, **17**(7):23, July 1969.

[54]Deloria, op. cit., p. 214.

[55]Ibid., pp. 215–220.

[56]Hilda Bryant, "Bad Health Adds to Indians' Woes," *The Red Man in America*. Reproduced by the information and editorial offices of the State Superintendent of Public Instruction, Olympia, Washington, by permission of the Seattle *Post-Intelligencer*, Jan. 1970, pp. 15–17.

Western reservation, Aichlmayr brought out the importance of starting a health program based purely upon the Indians' statement of need and desire and of being accepted as equals in a mutual endeavor. The concepts of social prestige, age, anonymity, time, patience, and generosity as perceived by Indians were gradually learned by the nurses over a time period of fifteen months. Indian people value sincerity, honesty, and absolute trustworthiness.[57] Similarly, as all people on the face of the earth, Indians are human beings who respond positively to treatment by helping persons when they are dealt with as having dignity, honor, and value. Regardless of race, color, culture, or creed, human beings have the universal need to be recognized and interacted with as worthy individuals.

Families of Spanish Origin

Persons of Spanish origin are the second largest minority group in the United States and live mainly in urban areas. About one-third of the total population is under eighteen years of age. Only 4 percent of all Mexican-Americans are sixty-five years or older. Families of Spanish origin tend to be larger and include more children. Almost half of all persons sixteen years old and over have not had more than an elementary education. The rate of Puerto Rican youth who have dropped out of school is particularly high. A great disadvantage of a large proportion of Spanish origin populations is their inability to use English. This is a factor that affects the amount of education that is available in schools, and the job opportunities which have been restricted mainly to low-skilled menial occupations. Spanish-speaking people are hard-working, with over three-quarters of the males in the labor force. A quarter of all persons of Spanish origin live in poverty and struggle with the basic problems of day-to-day survival. The lack of education seems to be a critical factor but not the sole one which prevents Spanish-speaking persons from advancing into secure and well-paying employment.[58]

Mexican-Americans represent a substantial portion of persons of Spanish origin. These individuals or their parents have come from Mexico and have brought with them many customs and traditions. They speak Spanish and have a noticeable accent.[59] Chicanos are also individuals whose ancestry is from Mexico; consequently, they have similar customs and traditions. Chicanos are the activists of the Mexican-American

[57]Aichlmayr, op. cit., pp. 20–23.

[58]*A Study of Selected Socio-Economic Characteristics of Ethnic Minorities Based on the 1970 Census,* vol. 1, *Americans of Spanish Origin,* Department of Health, Education, and Welfare, Washington, D.C., July 1974, pp. 1–118.

[59]Edward Casavantes, "Pride and Prejudice: A Mexican-American Dilemma." Nathaniel N. Wagner and Marsha J. Haug, *Chicanos, Social and Psychological Perspectives,* The C. V. Mosby Company, St. Louis, 1971, p. 49.

population and are working toward attainment of the qualities of self-determination and realization of inherent worth and value. Chicanos are a part of a cultural revolution, linking the past with the future in the bicultural world in which they presently live.[60]

Problems descriptive of families of Spanish origin include (1) lack of environmental stimulation in the home, (2) bilingual, bicultural conflicts with the Anglo society, (3) displacement of parents from the home environment, and (4) lack of adequate education.[61] Even though many of these families have been residents of the United States for years, they have resisted acculturation into the Anglo culture and have remained apart from the mainstream of American citizens. They retain their own language and distinctive cultural beliefs and values. Some differences seen in the Mexican-American culture as opposed to Anglo culture are:

1 Latin culture provides an emotional security and sense of belonging to its members.

2 Work is viewed as a necessity for survival but not as a value in itself.

3 Life is lived and experienced in the present, the here and now.

4 The traditional Latin approach requires courtesy, good manners, diplomacy, and tactfulness when communicating with another individual. The manner of expression is likely to be elaborate and indirect.

5 Mexican-Americans are very sensitive to criticism regardless of the manner in which it is given.

6 Latins are highly sensitive to the environment and love sounds, action, bright colors, and spicy foods.

7 The family is likely to be the single most important social unit in life because of the emotional and material security provided. The concept of family includes members of the extended family with whom there is much communication, sharing, and closeness of relationships. Interpersonal patterns within the family are organized around two dimensions—that of respect and obedience to elders and that of male dominance of females.[62]

Many minority families of Spanish origin are low-income, maintain cohesive connections with the extended family socially and in times of need, have a close social network system with members of the same

[60]Eliu Carranza, "The Mexican-American and the Chicano," in Antonia Castaneda Shular, Tomas ybarra-frausto, and Joseph Sommers (eds.), *Literatura Chicana,* Prentice-Hall, Inc., Englewood Cliffs, N.J., 1972, p. 39.

[61]Robert Aranda, "Development Delivery and Evaluation of a Chicano Health Services Seminar," unpublished master's thesis, University of Washington School of Public Health, 1974, p. 2.

[62]Nathan Murillo, "The Mexican-American Family," in Nathaniel N. Wagner and Marsha J. Haug (eds.), *Chicanos, Social and Psychological Perspectives,* The C. V. Mosby Company, St. Louis, 1971, pp. 97–108.

culture, employ common channels of communication, and attend special events of common interest. They are a strong subculture with definite health-seeking behavior. For the most part, they believe in folk medicine and treatment as practiced by their ancestors and frequently combine the best of two belief systems—their own home remedies with the health care practices of American professionals. In general, they distrust Anglos who do not speak Spanish or show respect for the existence and practice of cultural beliefs and folk treatment for specific illnesses.[63]

For nurses who work with these families, fluency with the Spanish language is desirable. In addition, the nurse must be flexible in reconciling recommended health-care practices with folk medicine and the use of herbs and rituals. Her communication should provide clear explanations in response to family questions, suggestions for actions with positive consequences, and acceptance of positive values in ritual acts performed by the family. Understanding and respecting the ethnic culture is imperative; the nurse should not focus only on Anglo views of the nature and causation of illness. The needs of these families are many, and they accept help best from those people who allow them to retain their identity and encourage self-help measures.

Asian-American Families

Of the Asian-American population, the Japanese are the largest subgroup in the United States. Well over one-third of Asian-Americans live in the western states and 90 percent live in urban areas. The majority of Asian-American families consist of husband and wife; however, a trend toward dissolution of families with a female head of the household is on the increase. Among families of Asian-American populations, Japanese families are, on the average, the smallest. Of all Japanese males sixteen years and above, 70 percent have finished high school, and 19 percent have completed college. A quarter of the population of all Chinese males, sixteen years or older, have obtained college degrees, which is double the United States average. Asian-American men and women have a high rate of participation in the labor force, and a high proportion of the Asian-American males are employed as professionals and managers. There are great contrasts in levels of income of Asian-American populations; however, family incomes tend to be better than or on a level with incomes of United States families in general. Despite a greater tendency among Asian families to look after surviving elders, the rate of poverty among

---

[63]Joan Edna Uhl, "A Description of Lay Referral Networks and Health Care Seeking Behavior among Mexican-American Families in Seattle: The Need for an Appreciation by Health Professionals," unpublished master's thesis, University of Washington School of Nursing, 1975, p. 33.

Asian elderly is as serious as it is for the elderly in the country as a whole.[64]

Asian-American families combine two cultures which influence the magnitude of one's ethnic identity—meaning the extent of an individual's incorporation of his "Japaneseness or Chineseness" into his total ego identity.[65] As expressed by Yoshida, "Mother was wise enough to know that American children could not be reared like Japanese children, that we were products of the new world and we required freedom." My father "always spoke to us in Japanese. I could understand him, but I couldn't express myself in Japanese, so I replied in English. . . . We did all the things white kids our age did for fun, but we never forgot we were Japanese Americans."[66]

The structure and values of Asian-American families are changing; however, traditional values continue to influence the socialization of the offspring as parents interpret appropriate and inappropriate behavior. The families retaining traditional values are patriarchal, with communication and authority flowing vertically from top to bottom. The father's behavior is generally dignified, authoritative, remote, and aloof. Sons are highly valued over daughters. The primary allegiance of the son is to the family. The inculcation of guilt and shame are the principal techniques used to control the behavior of family members. The behavior of individual members of an Asian family is expected to reflect on the whole family.

The roles of family members are highly interdependent. Independent behavior which might upset the orderly functioning of the family is discouraged. If a person has feelings which might disrupt family peace and harmony, he or she is expected to hide them. Restraint of potentially disruptive emotions is strongly emphasized in the development of the Asian character. With the lack of outward signs of emotions, Asians have been stereotyped as reserved, passive, and/or inscrutable. Traditional Asian values also emphasize formality in interpersonal relations, obedience to authority, and achievement in academic and occupational life.[67]

[64]*A Study of Selected Socio-Economic Characteristics of Ethnic Minorities Based on the 1970 Census,* vol. II, *Asian Americans,* Department of Health, Education, and Welfare, Washington, D.C., July 1974, pp. 1–159.

[65]Gary M. Matsumoto, Gerald M. Meredith, and Minoru Masuda, "Ethnic Identity: Honolulu and Seattle Japanese-Americans" in Stanley Sue, and Nathaniel N. Wagner (eds.), *Asian-Americans: Psychological Perspectives,* Science and Behavior Books, Inc., Ben Lomond, Calif., 1973, p. 65.

[66]Jim Yoshida with Bill Hosokawa, *The Two Worlds of Jim Yoshida,* William Morrow and Company, Inc., New York, 1972, pp. 17, 18, 20.

[67]Derald Wing Sue, "Ethnic Identity: The Impact of Two Cultures on the Psychological Development of Asians in America," in Sue and Wagner, op. cit., pp. 140–141.

In studying the interplay of the original ethnic culture with the American culture, an emergence of three personality types has evolved, which is described as follows: The *traditionalist Asian* has strongly internalized the basic ethnic values of his or her culture. Primary allegiance is to the family into which he or she was born. Self-worth and esteem are defined by ability to succeed in terms of high educational achievement and occupational status. With success, this Asian feels respectable in American society and has brought honor to the family name.

The *marginal Asian* cannot give unquestioning obedience to traditional parental values. This Asian attempts to assimilate and acculturate into the majority society which causes him or her to suffer because of a marginal status between two cultures. The tendency to gauge self-worth as defined by Caucasians is accepted. The determination of his or her acceptability is shown by the number of Caucasian friends he or she has and by fluency with the English language.

The *Asian-American* is in the process of formulating a new identity by integrating past experiences and heritage with present conditions. He or she feels that complete obedience to traditional values limits self-growth. Parental emphasis on high achievement is too materialistic for the Asian-American who is trying to find meaning and self-identity. He or she believes in being assertive, questioning, and active in order to develop in the present environment. This Asian also faces conflicts and experiences a great deal of guilt and frustration in parental relationships. In individualistic ways, he or she is trying to help the Asian people; however, many do not understand the effort.[68]

For the nurse working with Asian families, her behavior is similar to that described for working with middle-income families. These families are intelligent, educated, courteous, friendly—particularly when the purpose for the encounter is known, accepted, and a rapport has been initiated. A recognition and respect for the distinctive culture of the family can be acknowledged when eliciting a family health history which includes questions regarding values, beliefs, customs, treatments, and health practices. Incorporation of practices important to the family is essential, along with the health measures the nurse wishes to introduce. A curiosity about the family's particular beliefs, as shown by the nurse who actively listens, demonstrates her genuine desire to assist in the way most helpful for the family and contributes to their sense of worth and identity. At times the educational process may be reversed; the nurse may learn of

---

[68]Stanley Sue and Derald Wing Sue, "Chinese American Personality & Mental Health," Tachiki, Amy, Wong, Eddie, Odo, Franklin, Wong, Buck (eds.), *Roots: An Asian American Reader*, Project of the UCLA Asian American Studies Center, 1971, pp. 72–77.

remedies and health practices which have greater healing potential than the ones she came prepared to advocate.

Families of Other Cultural Groups

In each local community there are often families representing a given culture who can be found in residential pockets, neighborhoods, or cul-de-sacs. They may be groups of Scandinavians, Filipinos, Italians, Jews, and other groups representing a country, a particular section of the United States, or a religious creed. Each group has its own distinct culture in addition to some assimilation of United States culture. The task of the nurse is to become acquainted with each cultural group and attempt to understand the manifestations of behavior about which she is curious. Each family has characteristics and behaviors which need to be assessed before any effective action or teaching can take place. To learn more about a cultural group, the nurse can begin by inquiring about their foods, since people prefer to eat their own kind of food and often enjoy sharing their particular likes and individualized patterns of eating with others. She can ask about the manner of dress and admire distinctive clothing, such as the sari of the women of India or the pina cloth of the Filipino. Historical tales can be requested about the early beginnings of the culture, such as the Puerto Rican history or the ancient civilization of the Aztecs. Descriptions of recreational festivities that have special meaning can be elicited, such as the bullfights of the Mexican and Spaniard, the Bon Odori of the Japanese, or folk dance festivals of the Scandinavian. She can request clarification of the roles of family members, such as the male dominance or machismo exercised in Mexican and Hindu homes. The meaning of religious procedures of Italians or Jews can be elicited in terms of the marriage ceremony or upbringing practices of the children. Clarification of beliefs about health practices that seem impractical, ritualistic, or incongruent to the nurse can be requested. Always, the nurse must remember that when asking additional information about a cultural group, she must transmit genuine and sincere interest in the activities and practices of the family. If she can promote a liaison with the family based on mutual understanding of existing behavior patterns, a solid base for teaching and counseling about practical and acceptable health practices is eased. Underlying the implementation of any desired health action is the implicit suggestion to both nurse and family that planned change is wanted. Consent to change is most easily acquiesced when a mutual understanding and agreement occurs between nurse and family. Preparing a family for change often takes time and patience and is most easily accomplished when a therapeutic relationship has been developed simultaneously with the strengthening of the family's readiness.

FAMILIES WITH DISTINCTIVE RELIGIOUS BELIEFS

Every nurse is obligated to develop a knowledge, understanding, and appreciation of the religious practices of the families under her care, especially as they apply to birth, marriage, illness, and death. This is particularly true for the nurse in her work in the home, where patients can carry on their religious practices more freely than in a hospital. Such a knowledge and appreciation on the part of the nurse will help to overcome some of the barriers to communication. Priests, rabbis, and clergy are always willing to explain the meaning of the religious practices of their people and to be helpful to the community health nurse.

In general, the nurse should know and understand, to some degree, the main tenets or principles of the world's major religions as they affect family health practices, such as the status of women and children in the family, diet patterns, and acceptance of medical care. An understanding and appreciation of these points by the nurse will make it easier for her to communicate with families of various religious backgrounds.

Many times nursing students find it hard to accept what they perceive as proselytizing from their clients. All nursing students as well as all individuals have a right of choice. Listening and trying to understand another's beliefs, values, or religion does not necessitate a conversion. Listening and understanding broadens a person's perspective, gives clues as to the perception and emotional status of the speaker, and opens avenues for facilitative mutual discussions regarding beliefs and values that constitute the decisions each individual makes. Being open, curious, and respectful of another's religious beliefs is facilitating of a relationship. At the same time, the listener is not required to argue when beliefs differ or one's own beliefs are attacked. Nonjudgmental, nondefensive listening gives poise and the added knowledge gained about the client is valuable.

FAMILY MIXTURES

Families who are fragmented, mixed, or "mixed-up" present a special challenge to community health nurses. Flexibility and an ability to "roll with the punches" is required of nurses practicing in today's society. All kinds of family mixtures, combinations, and compositions are encountered in addition to nuclear and extended families. The nurse must be nonjudgmental, curious, accepting, and see each family as unique and possessing potential for growth.

Single-Parent Families

Single-parent families become single-parent through death, divorce, or by choice. The number of single-parent families have mushroomed, due in part to the escalating divorce rate in the United States. Ninety-five percent of the heads of such families are women and their socioeconomic status is low-income. For example, in 1973, the average income for all families headed by a male with the wife present and at least one child under six was $12,200. The corresponding figure for father-only families was $9,500. But the income for a mother-headed family was $3,600, far below the poverty line of $5,000.[69]

A major challenge for these families is creating a growth-producing environment for children when a significant adult is absent or the parenting role is assumed by transient-type role models. In our society, fathers and mothers are extremely influential in molding and structuring the environment of their children either positively or negatively. The early experiences of children are healthy and growth-producing, destructive and self-limiting, or a mixture of both. For the single parent who has major responsibility for parenting the children in the home, the task is tremendous because that individual must fulfill roles that are usually handled by two people, one male and one female. When the single parent is female, how does she talk to the children about their father, the departed male? How do the male children view maleness if they do not have a consistent model to observe? The same questions can be asked in reverse if the father is the single parent. How do children learn about common interactions and relationships between males and females unless they can observe a living demonstration on a daily basis? Is the single parent able to assume all the mothering and fathering capacities needed by the children? Does the single parent overprotect and create dependency? Are children of single parents confused about masculine and feminine sexuality?

A one-parent family is basically incomplete. If the single parent recognizes the incompleteness of the family, ways for providing a completeness can be managed, such as having the children live with a whole or nuclear family on periodic occasions or extending family relationships to include significant males and/or females who are warm and trustworthy role models.[70]

Single parents need a great deal of outside help and support for their roles. For example, when the parent works, acceptable day-care centers or baby-sitting facilities are needed. It is generally recognized that children do not have to be with their mothers or fathers all the time; however, they need a strong reciprocal attachment with loving adults. Efforts to provide children with constant, caring adults should be the aim of the single parent. Day-care experiences can be positive ones in

[69]Pam Moore, "A Look at the Disintegrating World of Childhood," *Psychology Today*, Magazine Newsline, June 1975, p. 34.
[70]Satir, op. cit., pp. 170–172.

encouraging children to learn cooperation, sharing, and new developmental skills.

Not all single parents are prepared initially to cope with the sole responsibility, the cost, the loss of freedom and privacy, and the loneliness of single parenthood. In many instances, they need a supportive person with whom they can share their concerns. This person can be a community health nurse who is able to assist in problem solving, suggest appropriate community facilities for particular concerns, bring in helping persons and resources representing a cross section of services available in the community, and strengthen the capabilities and confidence of the client.

In many single-parent families in which the woman is the head, there frequently is a boyfriend who lives with the family, is present only occasionally, or is a brief transient-type contact. For community health nurses it is important to know if a boyfriend exists because if so, he represents an influential position in the household for the time that he is connected with the family. It is desirable to meet the boyfriend and regard him as a substitute father for the period of time he is in the home, unless the mother definitely states otherwise. Besides being a sexual partner for the single parent female, the boyfriend is a male role model and often plays a role in disciplining the children. If he has successfully gained the acceptance of the mother's children, he contributes stability to the family system. If he is not accepted by the children or is present for a temporary time only, it is often helpful for the nurse to request and arrange family conferences with the goal of encouraging all members of the family to learn to communicate openly about their daily activities, concerns, routines, or questions. Whether a situation is seen as right, wrong, good, or bad is immaterial. What is important is for all members of a family unit to feel comfortable about talking openly and giving clear messages to one another so that self-worth grows.

Blended Families

Blended families, as described by Satir, put together parts of previously existing families. Individuals in these families consist of a wide range of possibilities, such as wife, wife's children, wife's ex-husband, husband, husband's children, husband's ex-wife, children of the current husband and wife, etc. Even though all of these individuals do not live under one roof, they are in each other's lives—whether acknowledged or not. All these individuals are significant to the growth and success of the blended family.

Some problems that can occur in blended families include: (1) differing directions children receive from the various "responsible" adults concerned about their development; (2) the "hurt" of a divorce which has been satisfactorily resolved or is still unfinished business; (3) the inclination of natural mothers or fathers to be protective of their "own" children and to resist new perspectives brought into the family by the new mate; (4) the expectation of mothers that the new male spouse will take over the role of disciplining before a relationship has been developed with the children; (5) the new mate's feeling of exclusion when the family enjoys a joke or memory that is reminiscent of the former marriage; (6) the sharing of the parenting role by natural parents with stepparents; (7) the fact that some parents may be in closer contact with their stepchildren than with their natural children; (8) the difficulty of knowing how to manage rituals, traditions, holidays, birthdates, visits with in-laws, and grandparents; and (9) the uncertainty of children that they are free to love whomever they want to regardless of the shadows of the past.[71]

A major task of community health nurses is to encourage open communication in blended families, bring out the concerns or problems that are troubling family life, be supportive of problem-solving attempts, and strengthen the resources of all family members so that they are able to learn, accept, and grow. This is most easily done by means of family conferences or talking with both parents of the new marriage. The nurse performs the facilitative role of suggesting potential problem areas, eliciting feedback from each parent of the new marriage, and encouraging open, honest discussion of all implications, alternatives, and consequences of behavior. For guidelines about a family conference see Chapter 6.

Potentially Abusing Families

Child abuse is a family affair. Everyone in the family knows about it, but no one talks about it. When abuse is known to have occurred, it is not so important to find out which parent did the abusing, as it is to counsel both parents to assess the basis for trouble in the family and the precipitating factors that led to the abuse. When potential for abuse is suspected, a family history elicited by the nurse is helpful for determining early interventions before anything happens. If the nurse decides to ask for a family history, she must attempt to help the parents to relax and be comfortable with her. She must be person-centered and initiate the interview by indicating her concern for each parent's feelings. For example, the nurse might say, "I sense that your life is pretty difficult at times. Do you see it that way?" Be honest at all times, and give concrete examples of what you want to communicate. For example, *do not say,* "I think you punish your child when she cries too long." (Too threatening.) *Do say,* "When your daughter cries for a long time, it must be frustrating and hard to know how to stop it."

For actual abuse to occur, there are three qualifications that must be met. There must be (1) potential for abuse, (2) a special kind of child

[71]Ibid., pp. 173–195.

(either obnoxious or passive), and (3) a crisis. In assessing the potential for abuse, the nurse must perceive how parents see themselves, their spouse, their parents, their child, and other people. Some questions that may be helpful in eliciting the information you want are as follows:

1 Feelings about self
    a How were you punished as a child when you did something wrong?
    b Would you say you had a happy or unhappy childhood?
    c Were you close to either parent as a child?
    d Did you feel your parents were pleased with you?

Many "abusing" parents feel isolated, have low self-esteem, and had a primarily negative childhood. These individuals were not "mothered" or nurtured lovingly and may not know how to nurture others.

2 Feelings about parents
    a Do you think the way your parents punished you is the best way to get children to behave?
    b What kind of relationship did you have with your mother when you were a child?
    c How would you describe your relationship with your mother now?
    d Do your parents help you out in any way now when you need it?

Frequently, "abusing" parents communicate the feeling that they were not regarded as worthwhile by their parents, and they believe their parents were justified in that viewpoint. They strove to please their parents but never quite made it. Seldom were their needs as children understood by their parents.

3 Feelings about spouse
    a What happens when you and your spouse disagree on how to handle the children?
    b Does your spouse recognize when you are "uptight"?
    c Does he (she) help you out at these times?
    d In what way is your spouse helpful with the children?
    e Is there anything in your marriage that could be better?

The relationship with the spouse is extremely important. Frequently, an individual will marry a person with similar feelings of low self-esteem. "Abusing" parents do not always know how to be supportive of each other, particularly when one is "uptight."

4 Feelings about other people
   a Do you ever feel helpless and want help from others when problems with the children occur, such as crying, disobedience, or misbehavior?
   b Who do you turn to at times like this?
   c How do you reach this person?
   d Do you use a baby-sitter? How often? Who?
   e What do you do when you are concerned about your children?

"Abusing" parents rarely have coping mechanisms or solutions with which they are satisfied. If they do not turn to other persons for help, or do not know how to reach others, the following information assists in determining the risk for abuse:

5 Feelings about their child
   a Are you having any problems with your child's behavior?
   b What kind of things make you feel really nervous and upset?
   c How do you handle accidents when they happen to your child?
   d How do you feel inside when your child cries?
   e How well do your children understand your feelings?
   f Do your children know when you are upset, and do they help you then?
   g Do your children live up to your expectations?

Parents who abuse tend to have unrealistic expectations of their children. They anticipate the attainment of certain developmental tasks based on their own desires rather than on the readiness or ability of the child. A rigid, righteous attitude of the parent should be watched for, if present.

For abuse to occur, the child must be a special kind of child who is either the wrong sex, was born at a wrong time, looks or behaves like someone the parent dislikes. The fussy baby or ornery little kid is more vulnerable to abuse than the "good" baby or child. It is helpful for the nurse to watch the behavior of a child when a parent is in a period of stress. If a child comforts and meets the parent's need, this often suggests that the child doing the comforting may be the one at risk.

Finally, for abuse to occur, there must be a crisis or precipitating factor. Perhaps, the crisis was triggered in this particular family because the child did something that taxed the patience or tolerance of the parent at a time when the parent was feeling particularly "low" anyway. The parent wanted reassurance or nurturing, and instead, it was at this time that the child did something wrong—triggering an emotional reaction. In such families, it may be that stress and recurring crises are a normal way of life, and abuse is one way of releasing feelings of frustrations and incompetence.[72]

For the nurse suspecting abuse in a family, it is necessary to initiate a relationship of trust with the parents before eliciting a detailed family history. The nurse must focus attention on parents and demonstrate a genuine concern for their thoughts, feelings, and actions. If she is allowed to do tangible activities with the children, she can interact sociably with them, read to them, have them draw pictures for her, and demonstrate caring concern based on each child's level of understanding and readiness. In all interactions with each parent, reinforcement must be given for positive behaviors or actions so that self-esteem starts to build. If a homemaker or babysitter is needed in the home, the nurse can assist in finding appropriate resources for these services. Parents Anonymous groups are excellent resources for families willing to go to such groups. At all times, members of other disciplines who are working with the "abusing" family must be called by the nurse and all activities coordinated in such a way that goals are similar, congruent, and attainable.

When the nurse suspects abuse and feels that her interventions have made no difference in the activities of the family, it is advisable to discuss her observations and data regarding potential for abuse with her nursing instructor or supervisor. Dependent upon the policies and rules of the local agency, the correct procedures for reporting child abuse in that community will be explained.

Families with Suicidal Members

Often community health nurses inadvertently learn that persons to whom they are giving service have formerly threatened suicide or are giving it serious thought because of their feelings of despair and helplessness and a belief that nothing can be done about their lives. In order to be responsive to any "cry for help," the nurse must be cognizant of prevention or follow-up phases of suicide. Prevention of suicide involves the identification of high-risk groups and/or individuals; the ready availability of responsive services, such as crisis clinics; the dissemination of information, particularly about prodromal clues; the lowering of taboos so that citizens can more easily ask for help; and the sensitization of professionals and ordinary citizens to the recognition of potential suicide. Follow-up activities are those that occur after a suicidal event, such as (1) working with an individual after he has made a suicide attempt or (2) working with survivor victims of a committed suicide to help them with their sense of anguish, guilt, anger, shame, and perplexity.[73] Life has two aspects, its

---

[72]C. Henry Kempe and Ray E. Helfer, *Helping the Battered Child and His Family,* J. B. Lippincott Company, Philadelphia, 1972, pp. 55–64.

[73]Edwin S. Shneidman, *On the Nature of Suicide,* Jossey-Bass, Inc., Publishers, San Francisco, 1969, pp. 20–21.

duration—length or shortness—and its scope—richness or aridity.[74] Community health nurses have frequent opportunity to enable others to see life as having meaning and richness, provided they recognize early behavioral clues of ambivalence regarding the value of life in their patients.

McLean defined a suicidal crisis as a period of time during which a person experiences an extremely strong wish to die, which conflicts with the wish to live. The crucial element that makes suicide prevention possible is the ambivalence. The nurse must utilize all her knowledge and relationship skills to keep a potentially suicidal patient focusing on the desire to live. Crisis intervention in suicide prevention is outlined in detail by McLean, consisting essentially of the following elements:

    1   Establishing a relationship, maintaining contact, and obtaining information
    2   Identifying and clarifying the focal problem or problems
    3   Evaluating the suicidal potential
    4   Assessing strengths and resources of the patient
    5   Formulating a therapeutic plan and mobilizing the resources of the patient and others.[75]

When the nurse tells the patient contemplating suicide, "Don't do it," she is communicating that she cares. If she is able to extract a promise from the patient which is purposely designed to be fulfilled at a later time, she has probably assisted the patient in overcoming his or her existing ambivalence of the moment. Few persons contemplating suicide renege on a promise. By being aware of the nature of suicide, in either the prevention or follow-up phase, the nurse adds another dimension to her intervention skills.

SUMMARY

The family has traditionally been the unit of service for the community health nurse as a means for focusing on all members of the family toward achieving higher levels of health or wholeness. The family was defined as a nuclear family or primary group living and interacting together intimately in a common residence. From the perspective of a systems approach, one of the roles of the community health nurse was described as that of coordinating the health-care systems and social systems within the community with the health needs of the family. The nurse also assesses

[74]Ibid., p. 29.
[75]Lenora J. McLean, "Action and Reaction in Suicidal Crisis," *Nursing Forum*, 8(1):28–41, 1969.

the structure of families, the functions, and developmental task levels of families and individuals within the family. Interacting with families representing different socioeconomic positions requires careful preparation by the nurse, as she plans to implement successful activities with each family according to their values, beliefs, and culture. Low-income families frequently cope with multiple health problems and health hazards of a different nature than middle- and high-income families. The existing health behavior and health needs of families representing cultures unfamiliar to the nurse are studied in order to facilitate changes of health practices which will be desirable, acceptable, and beneficial to the family.

SUGGESTED READING

Ackerman, Nathan W.: *The Psychodynamics of Family Life,* Basic Books, Inc., Publishers, New York, 1958.

Angelou, Maya: *I Know Why the Caged Bird Sings,* Bantam Books, Inc., New York, 1970.

Bell, Norman W., and Ezra F. Vogel: *The Family,* The Free Press, New York, 1960.

Billingsley, Andrew: *Black Families in White America,* Prentice-Hall, Inc., Englewood Cliffs, N.J., 1968.

Craven, Margaret: *I Heard the Owl Call My Name,* Doubleday & Company, Inc., Garden City, N.Y., 1973.

Deloria, Vine, Jr.: *Custer Died for Your Sins,* The Macmillan Company, New York, 1969.

Duvall, Evelyn Millis: *Family Development,* J. B. Lippincott Company, Philadelphia, 1962.

Geismar, L. L., and Michael A. La Sorte: *Understanding the Multi-Problem Family,* Association Press, New York, 1964.

Ginott, Dr. Haim G.: *Between Parent & Child,* The Macmillan Company, New York, 1965.

Grier, William H., and Price M. Cobbs: *Black Rage,* Basic Books, Inc., Publishers, New York, 1968.

Hall, Edward T.: *The Silent Language,* Doubleday & Company, Inc., Garden City, N.Y., 1959.

Henry, Jules: *Pathways To Madness,* Random House, Inc., New York, 1971.

Herzog, Elizabeth: *About the Poor: Some Facts and Some Fictions,* U.S. Department of Health, Education, and Welfare, Children's Bureau, 1967.

Hymovich, Debra P., and Martha Underwood Barnard: *Family Health Care,* McGraw-Hill Book Company, New York, 1973.

Irelan, Lola M.: *Low-Income Life Styles,* U.S. Department of Health, Education, and Welfare, Government Printing Office, Washington, D.C., 1966.

Kempe, C. Henry, and Ray E. Helfer: *Helping the Battered Child and His Family,* J. B. Lippincott Company, Philadelphia, 1972.

Kerr, Lorin E.: "The Poverty of Affluence," *American Journal of Public Health,* **65**(1):17–20, January 1975.

Langsley, Donald G., and David M. Kaplan: *The Treatment of Families in Crisis,* Grune & Stratton, Inc., New York, 1968.

Lederer, William J., and Don D. Jackson: *The Mirages of Marriage,* W. W. Norton & Company, Inc., New York, 1968.

Leininger, Madeleine M.: *Nursing and Anthropology: Two Worlds to Blend,* John Wiley & Sons, Inc., New York, 1970.

Lewis, Oscar: *Five Families,* Basic Books, Inc., Publishers, New York, 1959.

Lynn, David B.: *The Father: His Role in Child Development,* Brooks/Cole Publishing Company, Monterey, Calif., 1974.

Messner, Gerald: *Another View: To Be Black in America,* Harcourt Brace Jovanovich, Inc., New York, 1970.

Minuchin, Salvado, Braulio Montalvo, Bernard G. Guerney, Bernice L. Rosman, and Florence Schumer: *Families of the Slums,* Basic Books, Inc., Publishers, New York, 1967.

Nye, F. Ivan, and Felix M. Berardo: *Emerging Conceptual Frameworks in Family Analysis,* The Macmillan Company, New York, 1966.

Otto, Herbert A. (ed.): *The Family in Search of a Future,* Appleton-Century-Crofts, Meredith Corp., New York, 1970.

Patterson, Gerald: *Families: Applications of Social Learning to Family Life,* Research Press Company, Illinois, 1971.

Rogers, Carl R.: *Becoming Partners: Marriage and Its Alternatives,* Dell Publishing Co., Inc., New York, 1972.

Satir, Virginia: *Peoplemaking,* Science and Behavior Books, Inc., Palo Alto, Calif., 1972.

Shneidman, Edwin S.: *On the Nature of Suicide,* Jossey-Bass Inc., Publishers, San Francisco, 1969.

A Study of Selected Socio-Economic Characteristics of Ethnic Minorities Based on the 1970 Census, vols. 1 and 2, Department of Health, Education, and Welfare, Washington, D.C., July 1974.

Sussman, Marvin B.: *Sourcebook in Marriage and the Family,* Houghton Mifflin Company, Boston, 1968.

Shepard, Katherine F.: "Family Focus," *American Journal of Public Health,* **65**(1):63–65, January 1975.

"The Changing Family Scene," *American Journal of Nursing,* **75**(10):1647–1666, October 1975.

"The Sick Poor," *American Journal of Nursing,* **69**(11):2423–2454, November 1969.

Tachiki, Amy, Eddie Wong, Franklin Odo, and Buck Wong, (eds.), *Roots: An Asian American Reader,* Project of the UCLA Asian American Studies Center, 1971.

Tapia, Jayne Anttila: "The Nursing Process in Family Health," *Nursing Outlook,* **20**(4):267–270, April 1972.

Toffler, Alvin: *Future Shock,* Random House, Inc., New York, 1970.

Wagner, Nathaniel N., and Marsha J. Haug: *Chicanos: Social and Psychological Perspectives,* The C. V. Mosby Company, St. Louis, 1971.

Chapter 6

Working with Families

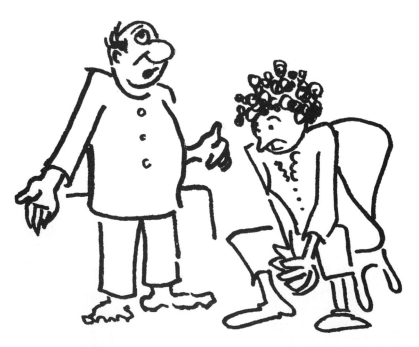

"Alice! How long can you brood over missing a developmental task?"

For years the home visit has been the principal means by which community health nurses interacted with families. Recently, however, the uncertainty about the efficacy of outcomes and costs of home visits have been critically questioned. As a result, many agencies have required a severe reduction of visits to homes. It must be realized that families can be worked with in a variety of settings, including the home, office, school, industry, job, clinic, neighborhood center, and any other location that is acceptable to the family and the nurse. Careful consideration of the environmental aspects of the selected setting must be taken into account by the nurse. Because she wants the family to be relaxed and comfortable, she must check the setting for noise, distractions, privacy, lighting, warmth, arrangement of furniture, facilities for refreshments, if wanted, and availability of site for family, transportation, and parking requirements.

For nursing students, the home continues to be a desirable setting for working with families because of the learning opportunities existing in the home for observing family interactions, patterns of coping, and life-styles. Families are the most natural in their own familiar territory. Nursing students learn that the implementation of the nursing process seems different in territory away from institutions. To become comfortable in a community environment, the nurse must familiarize herself with the great variety of health facilities; the differences in settings, atmospheres, and helpfulness of personnel; and the feeling of practicing as an independent agent for health promotion.

Community health nurses increasingly are making use of telephones and group meetings in place of home visits on a one-to-one basis. Group meetings are advantageous for reaching and educating numbers of people and providing stimulating health teaching in a practical manner. (For more discussion about groups, see Chap. 7). The nurse must be prepared to do both individual and group work and sometimes may wish to diversify her methods of working with the family by talking with individual members occasionally, on a one-to-one basis, and meeting with the entire family at other appointed times.

COMMUNITY HEALTH NURSING PROCESS

The community health nursing process consists of five steps. They are (1) assessing—identifying the need for the act, (2) planning—arranging for the methods and techniques necessary to meet the assessed need, (3) implementing—taking the action required to carry out the plan to meet the need, (4) evaluating—testing the outcome of the actions against previously determined criteria and (5) studying and researching—searching for knowledge in a systematic way. A model which summarizes

Table 6-1   Community Health Model for Nursing Process

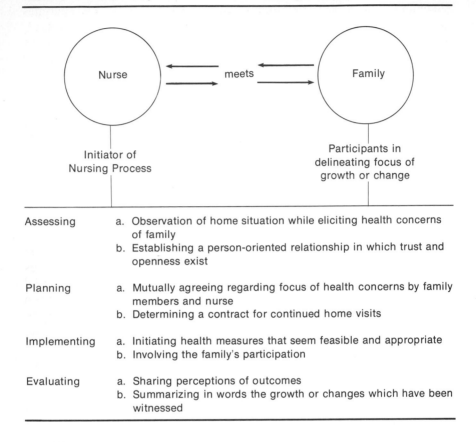

Assessing	a. Observation of home situation while eliciting health concerns of family
	b. Establishing a person-oriented relationship in which trust and openness exist
Planning	a. Mutually agreeing regarding focus of health concerns by family members and nurse
	b. Determining a contract for continued home visits
Implementing	a. Initiating health measures that seem feasible and appropriate
	b. Involving the family's participation
Evaluating	a. Sharing perceptions of outcomes
	b. Summarizing in words the growth or changes which have been witnessed

the meaning of the first four steps of the nursing process as applied to families in community settings and discussed in this chapter is shown in Table 6-1. The nurse and family are mutual participants in moving toward therapeutic outcomes. The nurse initiates the nursing process and works with the family as they are ready to grow, learn, and become responsible for attainment of desired goals. For more discussion about study and research, see Chap. 10.

COMPONENTS OF A VISIT

When making a visit, the community health nurse is faced with many functions, immediate or latent, which include preparation for the visit, her introduction to the family, contract with the family, assessment, plan, implementation, evaluation, and written summary. These functions occur on every visit, but the depth of purpose and emphasis changes as movement toward an agreed-upon goal by family and nurse becomes more resolute. The ultimate objective of the nurse is to assist the family's advancement toward wellness or an acceptance of their present reality as exemplified by their improved coping skills, increased self-confidence, and attainment of better levels of health. *Wellness*, as defined by Dunn, is an integrated method of functioning that is oriented toward maximizing the potential of which the individual and family are capable, within the environment where he or they are functioning.[1] When the family and nurse agree that essential and desired goals have been reached satisfactorily, then the nurse has accomplished her purpose as a helping change agent.

PREPARATION FOR A VISIT

There are two acceptable methods used by nurses when preparing for a visit. The first method consists of thorough preparation and assimilation of all data before making the first visit, and the second method postpones the gathering of related data until the first visit has been made and initial impressions have been received by the nurse. The first method requires a careful reading of the family folder in order to become familiar with the family constellation and the unique considerations of cultural, ethnic, religious, and social conditions. By reading all the nursing notes thoroughly, an impression is gained about the past events and successful and unsuccessful maneuvers which have occurred between the family and former nurses. Talking with other nurses or personnel from related fields who know the family also helps the nurse to form a mental image of the situation for which she is becoming prepared. The second method consists of a brief perusal of the family folder to make note of the family constellation and reason for the referral or continued visits. A conscious effort is made to avoid reading nursing notes or talking with personnel who are acquainted with the family before making the first visit. When the second method is used, the nurse is dependent upon her individual skills of on-the-spot observation, assessment, and the family's feedback of events that have occurred in the past as seen from their perception. After gaining a picture of the situation from the family's point of view and her own appraisal of cues which occurred on her first visit, the nurse consequently reads the family folder and nursing notes thoroughly and talks to all individuals who are acquainted with the family to ascertain if all viewpoints coincide. It is a matter of individual preference and knowledge of one's own style of proceeding which determines the method

[1]Halbert L. Dunn, *High Level Wellness*, R. W. Beatty Co., Arlington, Va., 1961, pp. 4–5.

selected by the nurse. The nurse who prefers to make her own assessment believes that the first method gives an unconscious predetermined bias, which may be deceiving and difficult to overcome. The nurse who relies on the first method believes she is more thoroughly prepared for any occurrence which may arise and will respond more successfully with tactics that may be attempted by the family.

When the family has a telephone, the nurse has the opportunity to call and arrange for a visit at an appointed time. She introduces herself and gives the reason why she wants to meet the family. By making an appointment in advance, the nurse and family member become psychologically prepared for the visit. Also, the nurse is assured that someone will be available when she makes the visit, and the family has been allowed the courtesy of arranging a time interval most suitable for them.

INTRODUCTION TO THE FAMILY

When the time comes to knock on the door or ring the doorbell, it always is a moment of uncertainty for the nurse. She knows *why* she is making the visit but never is certain what tableau will be revealed when the door is opened. Feelings vary as the nurse waits for the door to open. One student nurse described her thoughts as follows:

> (knock, knock) As I stood outside the door, I could hear the radio playing within, and various images of stubborn, suspicious, frightened, or confused countenances flashed across my mind; I hoped to meet any or none of them as best I could.

Unless the nurse is well known to the family, the first step in her visit is to introduce herself, stating clearly her name and that of her agency. She explains the reason for her visit and the source of the referral for the visit if that is necessary, e.g., "Good morning, Mrs. Brown, I am Miss Jones. I am the community health nurse from the Ocean County Health Department. Your physician, Dr. Smith, asked that we call on you about your pregnancy." Or, "Good morning, Mrs. Brown, I am Miss Jones, the community health nurse from the Ocean County Health Department and Ocean City Visiting Nurse Service. I came in response to your telephone request this morning to visit your little boy who has a cold." The introduction or social phase will vary with the situation, but warmth, friendliness, and expressed interest on the part of the nurse will help her to establish rapport with the family and to develop a relationship on which to base effective teaching later.

The social phase of the visit cannot be overemphasized, because it is during this time that the family member becomes acquainted with the nurse as having the potential for being a warm human being and not another official professional entity who must be treated with awe, respect, and compliance. When anxiety is moderately high for the nurse and the family member, recall of all the words that were spoken during the home visit is limited. When comfort and relaxation occur, facilitated during the social phase of the visit, then the professional content of the visit has more possiblity of being remembered and the family member and nurse are better able to absorb the implications of subsequent interactions.

On early contact the nurse must become acquainted with all the members in the household. She must learn their ages and be observant of interactional patterns between family members whenever feasible. It is extremely important to meet the father or head of the household, since he often holds an influential role in the family. In the past, many nurses have not made a practice of meeting the man in the family because they do not know how to cope with him for one reason or another.[2] However, when the organizational makeup of any family is studied, the conclusion reached is that the man holds an important position of influence and power and therefore must be involved. Sometimes, in order to meet the man in the family, special arrangements have to be made, such as a visit in the evening or an appointment visit near the father's place of employment. Generally when the nurse expresses a desire to meet the man of the family, the response of family members is favorable. Until all members of the household are met and actively involved, a truly accurate assessment of a complex family health situation cannot be accomplished.

When entering a home, the nurse must consciously greet all the family members present. If she recognizes by verbal or nonverbal means all members of the household, she is making her presence known and is in a position of catching their attention even though the initial response of individual family members may be one of indifference or withdrawal. Even the family's pets should be acknowledged, particularly if they seem to hold a position of esteem. For example, a staff nurse who was visiting a young couple with a new baby recognized early that the friendly Dalmatian held an important position in the affections of the new mother. It was not until several visits had been made that she came to the realization that the dog was treated as a firstborn and the new baby was regarded in attitude very similarly to that of a second-born child. By making this assessment of the dynamics of family life, the nurse was able to give more appropriate, cogent assistance to the young mother.

If the household contains a sick member who is unable to respond verbally or tangibly, the nurse should make a point of speaking directly to the patient, in a manner which indicates her belief that the patient

---

[2]Rosemary Pittman, "The Man in the Family," *Nursing Outlook,* 16:62–64, April 1968.

understands. By recognizing the existence of the patient, the nurse communicates a respect for the patient's dignity and serves as a model to family members regarding the appropriate attitude to assume toward the sick person.

Beginning Relationship with a Family

By recognizing all the members of the household and being cognizant of the interrelationships and family dynamics, the nurse is in an excellent position of soliciting and gaining cooperation from family members and eliciting health goals which will be beneficial to all. When she wants to meet with the family as a whole, she must purposefully make an appointment with the family, specifically stating that all are to be present. When the appointed time arrives, she should take the initiative for starting the conversation by introducing her reasons for wanting to talk with all the family members. She should consciously create a setting that is relaxed and aimed to put family members at ease. Encouragement of each individual to state a particular view of the health issue should be done by asking direct questions in a nonthreatening manner. She should realize that her presence in the family group is essentially that of an outsider or a third party, and this role will enable her to facilitate conversation between family members which is not usually openly expressed. She should give feedback to individuals within the family about their verbalizations as perceived by her. She should be accepting of positive and negative information and, by listening carefully, should request further information which is clarifying and factual. She should be cognizant of assets and express recognition of individual and family strengths as they become apparent. By engaging the family as a whole, the nurse is able to assess the family situation, enable the family to focus on the issue of the moment, and provide the impetus to move toward stated, desired, unified goals. Because all family members have been brought together and encouraged to discuss a health situation openly, and decisions regarding goals to be achieved have been elicited and perhaps decided upon, the predictability of a favorable outcome for future events is much more assured.

To cite an example, a student nurse who was visiting on a regular basis a family with multiple problems frequently discussed with the mother the current problems of the father's unemployment, finances, transportation, school adjustment of the four children, and discipline in the home. There was no noticeable progress in the family's ability to cope with their daily problems as reported by the mother until the nurse conceived the idea to meet the father and arrange a family conference. An appointment was made to meet the entire family and an open discussion of their situation was aired. No issues were resolved as a consequence of the meeting other than a complete reassessment of the family by the nurse. After three more meetings, during which several health issues were discussed, the family demonstrated much more unity, a happier and more secure attitude, a better insight into some of their behaviors, and an improved ability to cope with daily events. Because of the positive change in the family's functioning, the nurse felt that she benefitted most because she learned that all families are a dynamic whole, made up of individuals who must be met and involved as participating members, and resolution of health needs is facilitated with the least amount of nurse energy.

CONTRACT WITH THE FAMILY

When working with a family, it is essential that the family members and the nurse know the purpose of the nurse's visits, that there is a mutual agreement to work toward a desired end or goal, and that both family members and nurse will direct their activities or abilities toward the achievement of the mutually determined goal. In essence, a *contract* is made in which the family and the nurse are involved. As a consequence of the contract, both know the goal or goals toward which they are striving, both realize what is expected of them as participants, and both will know when the contract has been completed.

If the word "contract" seems too officious, the word "agreement" can be substituted. What is important is that the family and nurse have a contract or an agreement which has been mutually determined. The first agreement or contract can be a "small" or nonthreatening one such as, "the nurse will visit weekly to inquire regarding the health status of the family." Very often, the nurse must "sell" services she is prepared to offer, such as doing Denver Developmental Assessments on children; explaining and interpreting birth control measures that are contained in kits; bringing explanatory and appropriate audiovisual aids, books, and pamphlets; checking blood pressure and temperatures; looking into throats.

There are four patterns of responses from family members when faced with making a decision regarding a contract: (1) They know what they want help with and say so; (2) they know their own needs and priorities but are reluctant to say anything for fear the nurse might not indicate approval; (3) they are uncertain of their own needs and priorities and want others to tell them what to do;[3] (4) they cannot think of any needs or priorities at the moment of the inquiry but if given a time span in which to reflect (one week) will be able to state their desires at the appointed time.

One must be aware that there are also three states of mind when it

[3]Nena O'Neill and George O'Neill, *Shifting Gears*, M. Evans & Co., Inc., New York, 1974, p. 149.

comes to an agreement or contract. A client may state "I want to know how to stop my six-year-old boy from wetting the bed." This client may be stating (1) an intention—"I want to," (2) a decision—"I will," or (3) a commitment—"I will do it." If the nurse can determine the state of mind of the client accurately, it will help in setting up a workable contract.

If the family needs suggestions about suitable and desirable contracts, it may be helpful for the nurse to explore their perceptions of their current life-style. Is there anything that they would like different? Perhaps one child is annoying the mother, but she is not thinking of it as a health need. With some suggestions from the nurse about possible ways to change the behavior of the child, an agreement or contract may evolve.

The contract can be renegotiated every week, if necessary. Perhaps the first agreement was too easily attained, was not really what the client wanted, was not specific enough, was not realistic, or was not focused on the client's greatest need.

When a satisfactory agreement has been negotiated verbally between family and nurse, it is desirable for the goals and/or contract to be written in understandable language. It can be written by the client or by the nurse. If written by the nurse, the client should read the contract and sign his or her consent. A contract can be written as follows:

1 John will say one word clearly (other than Daddy and Momma) by the end of two months.
2 Children will go to bed routinely at 8:30 P. M. for five consecutive evenings without protest.

Initially it helps if the contract is small, specific, attainable, and reasonable. For a goal to be reachable, small "steps" must be taken which show the family that movement and progress toward the desired goal is possible and within their capabilities. The nurse must be patient, persistent, and reinforcing of the family as they move slowly and sometimes hesitantly toward the desired goal.

The ability to implement a planned goal is facilitated for the nurse when the contract is written, has specific desired terminal behaviors, and has a time limit. A methodology or theoretical framework can be easily integrated into the learning situation when terminal goals are mutually agreed upon and accepted by both family and nurse. Psychological readiness is present. Designating a time limit for specific goals is particularly important for nursing students, since their time period for working with families is generally fixed. When families are forewarned that the nursing student will be working with them for two months, that a terminal behavior can realistically be achieved within the stated time period, and when discernable progress becomes apparent, excitement and hope are engendered. The nurse learns to believe in her own ability to be an influential change agent, and feels satisfied and rewarded.

For families who have had nursing visits in which contracts have not been made, there is often an uncertainty about the reason for nursing visits. They find the nurse a pleasant person, attempt to meet her needs by telling her about their past illnesses or reasons for failure to attend clinics, and after her visit, resume their life patterns as always.

THE NURSING PROCESS: ASSESSING

Nurses are accustomed to assessing the patient's needs based on a medical and nursing model and can often identify many more needs than can a patient. However, unless a patient also sees a need as one that exists and for which help is desired, there is little point in making the assessment.

Assessment is a continuous process which becomes more accurate as knowledge of the consumer deepens. As defined by Harpine, *nursing assessment* is the continuous, systematic, critical, orderly, and precise method of collecting, validating, analyzing, and interpreting information about the physical, psychological, and social needs of a patient, the nature of his self-care deficits, and other factors influencing his condition and care.[4] While determining patient needs, the nurse will concentrate only on those needs which she can influence or change by her nursing intervention. She will seek to know the patient as a distinctive person so that she may utilize herself and her abilities as a therapeutic agent as effectively as is possible.

All persons have needs, but which needs will the patient confirm as indeed existing and with which he will accept assistance from the nurse? For low-income families, the needs which have to be focused upon early are often the physiologic and safety needs, whereas with middle- and high-income families the needs for love, belonging, esteem, or self-actualization may be the ones that are most urgent and in need of attention. All persons, regardless of social class, periodically regress in their individual fashions toward seeking satisfaction for the more basic physical needs when they indulge in overeating or lose their appetite, seek additional sleep or have insomnia, or reveal similar manifestations of stress.[5] The ability to assess and observe the patient with his present

[4]Frances H. Harpine, "Assessing the Needs of the Patient," in Helen Yura and Mary B. Walsh (eds.), *The Nursing Process: Assessing, Planning, Implementing, and Evaluating,* The Catholic University of America Press, Washington, D. C., 1967, p. 22.
[5]Sister Kathleen M. Black, "Assessing Patients' Needs," in Yura and Walsh, op. cit., p. 8.

reality makes use of the nurse's senses, her knowledge of hierarchy of needs, and her ability to relate to the patient's verbal and nonverbal cues in a facilitative manner. As she observes and makes note of cues, she must share and explore her perceptions with the patient to ascertain if he is in agreement with her perceptions.[6] Sometimes, the patient has difficulty expressing his desires and must be helped by the nurse to articulate his needs. A facilitative way to do this is to state, "You look worried. Are you concerned about something that I am unaware of?" Or the nurse may say, "Sometimes it is difficult to ask for help because we all like to think we can handle our own affairs. However, there are times when each one of us needs the help of another, and I sense that you may feel that way now. Is this true?" By admitting that we all are human beings and have moments of need, a relationship is facilitated in which each participant feels a greater freedom to exchange his own inner meanings with the other person involved.[7] When the nurse is authentic, she excludes the possibility of seeing the patient as a problem and herself as a person who can solve the problems. She tries to be responsively aware so that the patient, in turn, can be authentic and reveal his true concerns.[8]

Obstacles which tend to blunt the perceptions of nurses and deter the attainment of accurate assessments of patients and families have been experienced by all nurses and must be watched for as undesirable behaviors. The first one is taking a partial view of the person, labeling or stereotyping that person with descriptive labels such as uncooperative, slow, immature, incompetent, and so on. Once the judgment has been made or the label attached to the patient, the nurse tends to miss other positive or negative attributes which may change her mind about the person. All people have likable and dislikable characteristics, and an attempt should be made to view all persons as accurately as possible.

A second obstacle is that of viewing the patient as a thing instead of a person. All too often in nursing and medicine, patients have been referred to as a room number, a bed number, or a diagnosis. In fact, sometimes the common practice of calling a person a patient is discriminatory and not always beneficial for the person. When the person is viewed as an object, it is all too easy to deal with the individual purely as the receiver of nursing ministrations and to deny him or her the choice of accepting or refusing procedures that are designed as helpful whether the patient agrees or not.

A third deterrent is viewing the person who is the patient in terms of

[6]Harpine, op. cit., p. 22.
[7]Black, op. cit., p. 17.
[8]Ibid., p. 18.

his potential to meet the nurse's needs, rather than the nurse's potential to meet his. This obstacle has to do with the esteem needs of the nurse and her natural desire to be influential and successful with the person receiving her assistance.[9] It is difficult for the nurse to know that the patient can be helped yet have the patient refuse nursing service or observe the patient as demonstrating no improvement in spite of nursing ministrations. It is also sometimes difficult to accept the fact that the patient no longer requires nursing services and is competent to make his or her own decisions. For example, a student nurse during a routine visit to a young mother with a new baby was shown the diaper rash of the baby, which was causing the mother considerable concern. The nurse instructed the mother carefully and thoroughly about the care of the buttocks, and in the event that no improvement was demonstrated, referral to a well-baby clinic was given. The nurse promised to return in a week. Three days later, the student nurse felt a compelling urge to visit the young mother and baby to see for herself if the diaper rash was better or not. After a vigorous conflict within herself, the nurse decided that her *own* need to see the mother and baby must take second priority to the knowledge that the mother had been carefully instructed, had understood, and was probably competent to manage the situation. On the home visit the following week, the nurse received the report from the mother that the diaper rash had cleared after the mother implemented the instructions she had received from the nurse.

Factors in Assessing the Family

On the initial visit to a family many early impressions are secured, which form the initial basis for the ongoing assessment. As data are gathered and assembled continuously during subsequent visits the nurse becomes better acquainted with the family and responds to the assessment process similarly to that of assembling a jigsaw puzzle. The early pieces of the jigsaw puzzle give one an early image of the completed picture, but while sorting and trying various pieces for size, there are frequent periods of puzzlement and frustration. Until all the pieces are in place, a complete understanding of the picture is not reached. Families are like jigsaw puzzles in that sometimes it takes several months before an understanding of the mechanisms operating within families is gained by the nurse. Early impressions are important but not always accurate. Therefore, the nurse must be flexible, patient, and willing to adjust her assessment as new data are revealed over the course of time.

To make a comprehensive assessment of the family is time-consuming and must involve all the following factors on a superficial or

[9]Ibid., pp. 14–15.

detailed basis. When specialized information is needed in addition, many nursing texts and professional periodicals are available that describe more specifically the data required for special diagnoses and conditions. These factors include: (1) the family's physical and environmental status, including the medical history and present health of each family member, with special consideration of housing, number of rooms in relation to size of family, ventilation, cleanliness, sanitation, source of water supply, sewage disposal, and general safety, e.g., fire protection. (2) The family's cultural background, which is important to the nurse in her understanding and appreciation of the needs of the patient and family. What are the family's attitudes and practices with regard to religion, medical care, nutrition, and eating habits? To what degree does the family participate in the life and activities of its neighborhood and wider community? (3) The economic factors, including the occupation of the family breadwinners and the family's approximate income. The latter is helpful to the nurse when she assists with budget problems and purchasing. It will help her to determine, also, the family's eligibility for medical and dental care in clinics if it is needed and there is no medical insurance. (4) The developmental levels of family members, including ages and levels of achievement, both physical and mental. (5) The psychological factors, including family relationships both within and without the home, the emotional tone of the family life, and patterns of family behavior and intrafamily relationships, e.g., parent-child relationships and sibling rela-tionships. (6) The educational, vocational, and recreational interests of its members. Knowledge of these interests is important in the nurse's appraisal of the family because she plans her teaching according to the apparent knowledge, educational background, interests, and levels of understanding of the family members. An appreciation of the recreational needs and interests of the family and the facilities available in the neighborhood and community for meeting them is helpful to the nurse. Does the family plan its recreation together? Does their church meet some of these needs through church clubs and classes? What other community resources are available? a library? a playfield? a zoo? (7) The family's use of resources within the community. Is the family knowledge-able about resources available within the community? Are they willing to visit the resources? Are they ready to avail themselves of needed services or would they like the nurse to serve as a liaison agent initially?

In order to provide a family health service, the nurse must be alert to the health and welfare needs of all the members. For this reason she explores the many facets of family life in order to try to answer the questions, "What information do I need so that I can plan constructively with this family?" and "Which family need or needs should be given top priority immediately?"

Assessment Tools

It is always sound nursing practice to make use of screening devices, tests, or measurements whenever possible to determine more accurately what the nurse suspects based on her early observations or intuitive hunches. An essential tool for assessing the basic reflex patterns of newborns, infants, and preschool children up to three years is the reference *A Developmental Approach to Casefinding*, by Una Haynes.

This booklet describes the reflexes, how to elicit them, and how to appraise the baby during the bathing procedure. A wheel device for quick recall of developmental skills in conjunction with age in months is included with the booklet.[10]

A second excellent tool is the *Denver Developmental Screening Test*, which evaluates the gross motor, fine motor, adaptive, language, and personal-social areas of a child's functioning from birth to six years of age. It is easy to administer and utilizes participation of the parent during the testing procedure. Most parents respond with great interest to this screening device and are motivated subsequently to assist the child in practicing the skills that are in need of further development.[11]

Many more assessment tools are available for nurses to use for gaining more data about infants and children. The Neonatal Behavioral Assessment Scale as developed by Dr. T. Berry Brazelton is an example.[12] The Developmental Profile for children from birth to preadolescence by Alpern and Boll is another example.[13] Because new tools are constantly being developed, it is essential for community health nurses to maintain ongoing curiosity about research studies reported in professional journals. In this way the nurses remain up-to-date and knowledgeable about new screening devices and procedures which more accurately assess the health needs of patients and families.

HEALTH-CARE ASSESSMENT

Nursing students are learning and practicing primary nursing care skills throughout their educational program. While working in community

[10]Una Haynes, *A Developmental Approach to Casefinding*, U. S. Department of Health, Education, and Welfare, Social Rehabilitation Service, Children's Bureau, 1967. (For sale by the Superintendent of Documents, U. S. Government Printing Office, Washington, D. C. 20402.)

[11]Manual, form, and kit are available from *LADOCA*, Project and Publishing Foundation Inc., E. 51st Ave. and Lincoln, Denver, Colo. 80216.

[12]Dr. T. Berry Brazelton, *Neonatal Behavioral Assessment Scale*, J. B. Lippincott Company, Philadelphia.

[13]Gerald D. Alpern and Thomas J. Boll, *Developmental Profile*, Psychological Development Publications, Indianapolis, Ind.

settings and with families, every opportunity must be utilized for screening the health status of each family member. When a systematic screening examination is done routinely and as needed by the nurse, family members tend to respond favorably. The examination in no way approximates the physical examination of a physician. It is mainly a health appraisal in which the nurse gains a general impression of the physical status of each family member. Checking the skin, vital signs, and blood pressure; listening to heart sounds and the lungs; looking into the throat; inspecting the condition of the teeth and gums; and inquiring about essential data for the compilation of a health history for each family member is advisable. Interpretation of normal ranges of findings and the rationale underlying the systematic health appraisal impresses and educates the family as to the nurse's competence as a professional.

When a family member complains of a specific ailment, examination of the designated body system or distressed body part is essential. Physical examination techniques which include inspection, palpation, percussion, and auscultation must be done as appropriate to gain objective data along with securing a history from the patient regarding subjective data. Interpretation of the nurse's findings in language understandable to the family member is facilitative of future follow-through when advised by the nurse. Referral to appropriate resources is eased when the nurse explains the reason for the referral and the probable corrective activity that will be performed by the designated professional. Making use of physical examination skills should be given top priority by every practicing community health nurse whose objective is to educate and promote optimal health of all individuals.

NURSING DIAGNOSIS

After gaining essential data about the family and determining a contract with the patient and/or family about the need which has immediate priority, the nurse is then faced with making a nursing diagnosis that will form the basis for her plan and implementation of nursing intervention. Durand and Prince defined *nursing diagnosis* as statement of a conclusion resulting from recognition of a pattern derived from a nursing investigation of the patient or family.[14] By making a diagnosis the nurse sets the stage for her subsequent activities with the patient and/or family.

The following example very briefly illustrates an assessment of a family made by a student nurse and her subsequent nursing diagnosis.

It wasn't until after I made my initial visit that I realized that health

---

[14]Mary Durand and Rosemary Prince, "Nursing Diagnosis: Process and Decision," *Nursing Forum*, 5(4):50–64, 1966.

encompassed more than just the physical and mental, but included the social, cultural, environmental, and socioeconomic factors. . . . Identifying the medical needs of the family was not difficult since this was one of the mother's major concerns for herself and the children. The mother was very open and willing to talk about her own ailments, which were many, and the medical care needs of the children. . . . The family's economic situation was precarious, which had an effect on the follow-through of medical needs. . . . Focusing on the mental health of the family made me acutely aware of how the manner of communication can deeply affect the mental attitudes of family members toward each other. I was able to make a home visit when the mother and father were home. Even in my presence, it was quite apparent that these two people annoyed each other. The father was very intolerant of the mother's naive concepts about the subject we were discussing at the time. The mother likewise voiced her anger toward the father on a separate occasion. The mother views the father as a very egocentric individual and feels rejected by him. The problem with both of these people is that they do not have the appropriate outlets upon which to release their anger. They are unable to discuss their feelings on a rational, adult level; consequently, they use their children to release their anger on. It comes through in their communication to the children. I am sure they are unaware of how their communication is perceived by the children or anyone else. They sound intolerant, impatient, and very angry. . . . The nursing diagnosis for this family is mother and father's destructive communication patterns which affect and expand family health problems, influencing all members of the family.

NURSING SERVICES AND FEES

The nurse describes the purpose and philosophy of the agency and explains that its services are available to all in the community according to their health needs. If, however, the agency is private or nonofficial, a combination agency, or an official agency that charges for some services, she explains the fee schedule for services.

Although these services of the agency are availble to all in the community according to their health needs, today's concept (first expressed by the old woman in the London slums) that patients and families pay for services as they are able has become fairly well established and accepted. Most people wish to pay what they can, and agencies have found that patients and families tend to value nursing services and teaching more when they pay at least something for them.

In discussing the fee schedule with the family or patient, the nurse keeps the following points in mind:

1   The actual cost to the agency of the visit, including costs for travel, professional nursing services provided, equipment used, overhead expenses, e.g., rent, light, and telephone, and the necessary personnel in

addition to the nurse, i.e., administrative, supervisory, and secretarial personnel.

2   The family's ability to pay for nursing service. This is based on a consideration of the family's overall income and fixed expenditures, e.g., food, rent, utilities, and financial commitments such as insurance. When the patient is the wage earner, it is to be expected that the family income will be markedly reduced. In such situations, some families may be unable to pay the full fee but might find it possible to pay on a partial basis.

3   The type of illness and the nursing care needed. If the illness promises to be short, requiring two to three visits, a full fee might be indicated, but if it appears that the illness may be long, such as cancer or disability following a stroke, the nurse must consider the probable number of visits necessary and then evaluate with the family their ability to pay under the circumstances.

4   The fee schedule is flexible and may be adjusted easily to the family situation.

5   Many families today have certain types of medical insurance that provide for nursing services. Often they are not aware of the provisions in their policies.

When a family requests a nursing visit on an appointment basis in order to meet their convenience, the full "cost-of-visit" fee or more is charged by some agencies. On the other hand, if the family can adjust to the nurse's plans for the day, the full fee or less may be charged.

Most official agencies make no charge for visits for nursing service, demonstrations of nursing care, or teaching when the request was made because of a communicable disease; when the visit is for the purpose of supervising maternal and child health or handicapped children; when families are faced with problems of mental or emotional difficulties or mental retardation; or when the visit is a first one that has not been requested by the patient or family.

If a fee is to be charged for a first visit to a new family, and for later visits, the patient, family, and nurse discuss the fee, but before making a final decision, the nurse may wish to discuss aspects of the situation with her supervisor. Sometimes a patient or family, prompted by an appreciation of the nurse's help, will want to pay more for the services than their budget actually allows.

Generally speaking, nurses find it very difficult to discuss fees with patients and families. They recognize that their visits merit payment but are reluctant to evaluate their services in terms of monetary value. Establishing fees tends to be considered a cold, mercenary task, and talking about money conflicts with the nurses' view of themselves as warm, helping persons. For this reason, nurses have responded favorably when some official agencies have hired a person whose title is that of fee clerk. The fee clerk's primary task is to visit all new families who have been accepted for nursing services, interpret the agency's policies in regard to fees, and establish a fee for services that is satisfactory to the family. Whenever the nurse reports a change in the family's financial status after the initial encounter, the fee clerk visits again to adjust the fee according to the ability of families to pay. In many agencies a graduated fee schedule based on family income is used as a guide for determining a fair fee.

Every three to five years, community health nursing agencies conduct "cost-of-visit" studies. The findings will reflect the current cost of each visit made by the nursing agency. On the basis of this information, the fee is adjusted. Established fee schedules are helpful to the nurse as she interprets the agency services to the family.

MEDICARE

In 1973 approximately 12 percent of the nation's total health-care bill was paid in medicare benefits. Medicare (Title XVIII) is a federally administered program providing hospital and medical insurance protection for eligible elderly people. The medicare program is under the overall direction of the Secretary of Health, Education, and Welfare. Within the department, the Bureau of Health Insurance of the Social Security Administration is responsible for policy and administrative control of the program with much of the day-to-day operational work of the program performed under contract by 100-plus commerical insurance companies and Blue Cross–Blue Shield plans. These organizations have the responsibility for reviewing claims for benefits and making payments.

In each state, health officials assist the federal government in determining whether facilities that wish to provide services to medicare beneficiaries meet the conditions for participation in the medicare program. These conditions relate to the quality of patient care and various health and safety requirements.

The medicare program consists of two parts—the hospital insurance plan (part A) and the supplementary medical insurance plan (part B). Hospital insurance benefits include: (1) inpatient hospital services for up to ninety days in a benefit period, plus a lifetime reserve of sixty additional days of hospital care after the ninety days have been exhausted; (2) posthospital extended care in a skilled nursing facility for up to one hundred days in a benefit period; (3) posthospital home health services for as many as one hundred home health visits. A benefit period begins with the first day an individual is furnished inpatient hospital or skilled nursing facility services, and does not end until he has not been an inpatient in either a hospital or a skilled nursing facility for sixty consecutive days.

Supplementary medicare insurance benefits (part B) include: (1) physicians' and surgeons' services, certain nonroutine services of podiatrists, limited services provided by chiropractors, and the services of independently practicing physical therapists; (2) certain other medical and health services such as diagnostic services, diagnostic x-ray tests, laboratory tests and other diagnostic services, x-ray, radium and radioactive isotope therapy, ambulance services, and additional medical supplies, appliances, equipment, and prostheses; (3) outpatient hospital services; (4) home health services (with no requirement of prior hospitalization) for 100 visits during a calendar year; and (5) outpatient physical and speech therapy services furnished by approved providers.

Both the hospital insurance and medical insurance plans contain limitations on program benefits in the form of deductible and coinsurance amounts for which the beneficiary is responsible. The most important of these are a variable deductible with respect to part A hospital services and a deductible and 20 percent coinsurance amount with respect to most part B services.

Hospital insurance (part A) coverage is available to (1) all people sixty-five and over who are entitled to receive social security cash benefits or railroad retirement benefits; (2) social security beneficiaries under age sixty-five who have been entitled to social security or railroad retirement benefits for at least twenty-four consecutive months on the basis of a disability; (3) otherwise ineligible persons, sixty-five and older, who elect to enroll in the hospital insurance program and to pay the full cost of their coverage; (4) almost all people under sixty-five or nearly that age when the program was enacted in 1965 but who were not eligible for cash benefits.

Supplementary medical insurance is available to all hospital insurance beneficiaries and to all other people sixty-five and over, except recent immigrants.

Payment of medicare benefits is on the basis of (1) reasonable cost in the case of hospitals and other institutional providers and (2) reasonable charges in the case of physicians and other noninstitutional suppliers of services. Reasonable costs are determined on the basis of actual costs incurred by the individual provider in furnishing covered services to beneficiaries. The principles of reimbursement provide that all necessary and proper costs which maintain the operation of patient-care facilities and activities will be included in the computation of medicare reimbursement. A provision in the Social Security Amendments of 1972 now permits establishment of upper limits of "reasonableness" of costs by hospital category or type of service.

The determination of the reasonableness of charges is made by carriers pursuant to policy guidelines issued by the Social Security

Administration, which are established within the framework of general statutory instructions. In determining reasonable charges, the carrier must take into consideration the customary charges for similar services by the physician or other person furnishing the services, as well as the prevailing charges in the locality for similar services. The prevailing charge for a service is limited to the 75th percentile of the customary charges in an area. The 75th percentile amount is increased over time by a factor which takes into account increased costs of practice and increases in earnings levels in the area. Reimbursement for medicare supplies and equipment is based upon the lowest charges at which supplies of similar quality are widely and consistently available in a locality.

The hospital insurance part of the program is financed primarily through social security payroll contributions paid by employees, employers, and self-employed people covered under social security.

Of the 21-plus million people age sixty-five and older in the United States, almost 98 percent now have hospital insurance protection. Requests for medicare payment for covered services generally are submitted by the provider of services; they must be signed by the beneficiary (or someone designated, if he or she is unable to do so). The provider is reimbursed on the basis of reasonable costs of covered services and bills the beneficiary for deductible and coinsurance amounts as well as for services not covered by the program.

Claims for payment of supplementary medical insurance benefits may be submitted to the carrier either by the patient or by the physician or other supplier of services. If the patient submits a claim (an itemized bill) directly to the carrier, direct payment of benefits for covered services is received; the patient remains responsible for the physician's bill. The patient may assign the benefits to a physician or other supplier of services willing to accept assignment. In this case, the physician agrees that the allowed or reasonable charge determined by the carrier is the total charge. The physician submits the bill and is reimbursed. In this situation, the patient remains responsible for the remaining 20 percent of the allowed charges for covered services and the deductible.[15]

MEDICAID

It was in 1950 that Congress first authorized "vendor" payments for medical care—payments from the welfare agency directly to physicians, health care institutions, and other providers of medical services. In 1960 a new category of assistance recipient was established by Congress for the "medically needy" aged, whose incomes were greater than that which

[15]Committee on Ways and Means, *National Health Insurance Resource Book*, U. S. Government Printing Office, Washington, D. C., 1974, pp. 429–433.

would have qualified them for cash assistance payments, but who needed help in meeting the costs of medical care. In 1965 a new medical assistance (medicaid) program was enacted as part of the Social Security Amendments of 1965. The medicaid program had the following features:

1 It substituted a single program of medical assistance for the vendor payments under the categorical cash assistance and medical assistance for the aged programs, with a requirement that beginning in 1970 federal sharing in vendor payments would be provided only under the medicaid program.

2 It offered all states a higher rate of federal matching for vendor payments for medical care.

3 It required each state to cover all persons receiving cash assistance.

4 It permitted states to include medically needy aged, blind, disabled, and dependent children and their families at the option of the state.

5 It required that states include inpatient and outpatient hospital services, other laboratory and x-ray services, skilled nursing home services, and physicians' services, and permitted other forms of health care at state option.

In 1967 congressional concern over rapidly rising medicaid costs led to legislative action. The Congress chose as its basic method of cost control, limiting the definition of "medically needy" to persons whose income did not exceed $133\frac{1}{3}$ percent of the maximum payments for similar size families under programs of aid to families with dependent children. The 1967 amendments also included an amendment designed to focus on the health needs of medicaid children. Specifically states were required by 1969 to implement early and periodic screening, diagnosis, and treatment programs for children under twenty-one.

Increasing congressional concern with the rapidly escalating costs of the medicaid program as well as with the quality of care provided recipients led to an extensive review of the entire program. In 1972 legislation (PL 92-603) was enacted which contained a substantial number of amendments designed to control costs, strengthen program administration, and improve the delivery and review of services. Cost control amendments included provisions limiting federal participation for capital expenditures not approved by planning agencies, establishing limitations on prevailing charge levels, repealing the "maintenance of effort" and comprehensive goal requirements, and instituting mandatory and optional patient cost-sharing requirements. Amendments designed to improve program administration included provisions increasing federal matching for installation and operation of management information systems, establishing penalties for fraudulent acts and false reporting, and assigning responsibility for the establishment and maintenance of health standards to the state health agency.

Congress also focused attention on improvements in existing utilization review programs. Incentives were established for states to establish effective utilization review activities under medicaid and required coordination of these activities with those required under medicare. Congress was particularly concerned that existing utilization controls had been ineffective and that rising costs were in part attributable to the provision of medically inappropriate services. It therefore included a provision providing for the establishment of professional standards review organizations (PSROs), formed by organizations representing substantial numbers of physicians in local areas, to undertake comprehensive and ongoing review of services under medicaid and medicare. PSROs determine whether services are medically necessary and provided in accordance with professional standards.

PL 92-603 also established a supplemental security income program (SSI) which, effective 1974, replaced federal/state welfare programs for aged, blind, and disabled individuals. States were permitted to establish programs supplementing the basic federal payment. Medicaid eligibility determinations for these individuals could no longer be tied to eligibility under the old federal/state cash assistance programs. Subsequent legislation specified the requirements for mandatory and optional coverage.

Increasing medicaid costs have had a particularly severe fiscal impact on the states. Welfare costs typically constitute one of the largest items in the state budget, and vendor payments have increased 583 percent in ten years (from 1965 to 1974).[16]

Medicare and medicaid should not be considered as static programs. Their requirements have continued to develop and change, depending somewhat on the economic, social, and political climate in each state. New programs and practices have been devised to meet specific needs and new conditions and some old ones have been discarded, having proved to be ineffective. It is anticipated that legislation will be passed by Congress at some date for a national health insurance plan that will meet the medical, nursing, and health needs of the nation's entire population at a reasonable cost. This will demand a tremendous amount of comprehensive planning and thought on the part of all concerned. Nurses must utilize the opportunity to contribute their ideas because of their present experience in working with medicare, medicaid, and other federal medical programs.

[16]Ibid., pp. 487–490.

THE NURSING PROCESS: PLANNING

When sufficient data about the health needs of a patient or family have been gained and a contract with the family established, the nurse is faced with the necessity for planning. A plan is the method of action or the blueprint for activity based on the resources available and the goals desired.[17] Of primary concern is the patient with his or her knowledge, capabilities, customary patterns of coping, resources, needs, desires as he or she sees them and as the nurse sees them. The nurse must also consider her own knowledge, capabilities, ways of coping, resources, needs, desires, as well as her limitations, which may have a bearing on the attainment of the patient's desired goals.[18] The setting of the patient must be viewed from a realistic and objective standpoint to ensure that desired goals have the potential for successful fulfillment.

While talking about realistic goals the patient desires, the nurse can give valuable assistance by suggesting practical, short-term and long-term goals. The long-term goals exemplify the ultimate objectives desired by the patient, whereas the short-term goals represent the graduated steps marking progression toward the desired long-term goals. When short-term goals are attained, they build confidence that the next goal can likewise be achieved. For example, for the mother who wishes her son to be toilet trained, the long-term goal is independent self-care in toileting for the son. The short-term goals may be (1) determining the boy's physiologic and psychological readiness for toilet training; (2) ascertaining the boy's present toileting patterns; (3) setting up a toileting procedure which is feasible for the mother and son and includes rewards or positive attitudes for activities done successfully; and (4) determining a measuring method or chart for observing frequency of success. Early expectations should be minimal, then show progress as the boy develops skill in his toileting activities. Charts with gold stars can often be motivating stimuli for preschool children. When toileting accidents occur infrequently, then the mother realizes that the long-term goal has been achieved.

It is important that the family and nurse plan toward desired goals together because goals decided upon are a prelude to action for both family and nurse. Dependent upon the health-care needs of the family, the goals may be directed toward care of sickness and handicaps or health teaching and counseling.

Care of Sickness and Handicaps

For those patients needing physical care, the nurse plans her administration of nursing procedures and treatments prescribed by the physician

[17]Joan Nettleton, "Planning to Meet Patient Needs," in Yura and Walsh, op. cit., p. 44.
[18]Ibid., p. 47.

and also includes an inventory of all medications used by the patient to ensure that the drugs are being taken properly as ordered and are having the desired effect. The nurse remains up-to-date on rehabilitation and exercise measures and plans for execution of activities for daily living for those patients who desire to acquire new self-help skills. For those patients on special diets, she obtains a history of their nutritional practices and plans for implementation of ideas which seem practical and geared to the patient's needs, desires, and limitations.

Frequently the nurse will need to adapt nursing equipment and procedures to the home situation; she can encourage family members to work with her in improvising many articles to contribute to the patient's safety and comfort, such as a back rest from a cardboard carton or a wheelchair made by attaching castors to the bottom of each leg of a sturdy chair. The use of disposable, self-help, and low-cost equipment is always an important consideration. Utilizing transfer procedures which ease the difficulty of moving a patient from one object to another or from one room to another is sometimes a major feat to accomplish in the setting of some homes.

Many ideas for assisting the patient with personal grooming and eating may be found in current nursing periodicals and pamphlets. On occasion, families work out helpful ideas for the comfort and safety of the patient that will contribute to independence. They should be encouraged to do this, and appreciation should be shown for their efforts.

During bedside nursing activities, the nurse has the opportunity to observe the patient and assess his or her condition. She may note also the degree of understanding the family has for the situation. Whenever possible, she should delegate certain responsibilities to family members so that they may participate in the care of the patient, such as assembling equipment for a bath or a treatment. She shows one or more of the family members how they may care for the patient in her absence and observes them in a return demonstration. Family members will watch closely the nurse's techniques, even when she is not consciously teaching. The care she takes with the contents of her nursing bag, with her handwashing, and with the use of equipment is of great interest to them.

Patients and families like to know what is causing the patient's distress, so interpretations of the medical phenomena underlying the disease process are appreciated when explained in an understandable manner. Also, explanations of the treatment, its purpose, its length, and what can be expected as an end result are important in enlisting the intelligent cooperation of the patient and family members.[19] If the patient is faced with a choice of two acceptable treatment plans, he or she should be allowed to make the decision regarding the treatment plan desired after

[19]Letha Hickox, "Planning to Meet Patient Needs," in Yura and Walsh, op. cit., p. 65.

being made cognizant of the benefits and limitations of both plans. At all times in community health nursing, the resourceful nurse is prepared for situations requiring adaptability and flexibility. As reported in a study by Johnson, a limiting factor in the delivery of nursing care that was documented repeatedly was the variability of patients' reactions to services rendered by nurses.[20] To meet unexpected challenges successfully takes skill, planning, ingenuity, acceptance of risk, and the belief that all persons have potential talents just waiting to be tapped.

Health Teaching and Counseling

Much of the work of community health nurses consists of teaching and counseling patients and families about better ways of coping with health problems so that they are able to increase their competency in dealing with their health needs and desires. The utilization of patient and family strengths and resources requires involvement of the patient and family in the plan of care. Also, an effective relationship of the nurse with the family must be developed before success can be assured.

In health counseling the approach varies with the family. In one family, the nurse may feel the direct approach will serve the best purpose. In another family, one of the members may be able to assume leadership and make plans and decisions with little assistance from the nurse other than encouragement and support.

Anticipatory guidance is an important part of health counseling. A guided discussion of probable happenings or events provides an opportunity for clarifying ideas, for lessening anxiety, and for constructive teaching. By anticipating the occurrence of an expected event, various ways of handling the event can be explored so that when it actually happens, few surprises transpire. For instance, the nurse can explain objectively to the expectant mother the mechanics of labor and delivery, using a birth atlas or similar teaching material. This also may provide the mother with emotional support, so that she may be better prepared to accept the experience of her delivery.

New methods for teaching and counseling families appear constantly in books and professional periodicals. Some of them are easily adapted for use in community health nursing. Methods which should be considered when planning for selected families, dependent upon the nurse's assessment of the situation and her knowledge of the implementation of the method, are described briefly as follows:

1. The behavior modification or social learning approach. The behavior modification approach is used widely in schools, institutions,

---

[20]Walter L. Johnson, *Content and Dyanmics of Home Visits of Public Health Nurses,* Part II. American Nurses' Foundation, Inc., New York, 1969, p. 124.

and homes for children and adults who have special learning needs, such as those persons with distinct handicaps or who are retarded. Social learning theory is similar to the behavior modification approach, but it focuses on concepts and methods aimed at facilitating positive behavior or attitude change. The approach differs from the behavior-modification approach in its emphasis on the use of the individuals in the existing environment as the main sources for reinforcement. For the community health nurse assisting the mother in the home in helping the identified patient to acquire necessary new skills or acting as a liaison agent between special schools and the home environment, an understanding and application of behavior-modification and/or social learning methods is essential.

According to an operant point of view, an individual tends to behave in certain ways as a result of events which immediately follow particular behavior. One tends to repeat behaviors that have been rewarded. An operant response is simply a behavior which is governed by its consequences. For the nurse who is observing specific behaviors in a patient, emphasis is placed on noting those events or occurrences which immediately precede and immediately follow a behavior of interest. To become completely knowledgeable about the occurring events requires *direct observation* of patient interactions and behaviors by the nurse. As the nurse watches, she observes antecedent events, behaviors or responses of the patient, and consequent events which give her cues as to which conditions produce a positive or negative behavior in the patient.[21] By recording her observations and the frequency with which the observed behaviors occur, she has a base of knowledge from which to plan for effective intervention. The basic premise of the operant method is that behaviors can be shaped in patients by the consistent use of reinforcers. Reinforcers are rewards, behaviors, or events which increase the probability of the desired response. Reinforcers are used to strengthen, weaken, or shape behavior.

When the nurse visits a family with a child who is in need of assistance with a growth and development pattern and may respond to the behavior-modification method, she must interpret the method and its purpose to the parents, enlist their interest and cooperation, assess the child's functional level of development, and plot on a chart the variability in the child's achievement of self-help skills in daily living—feeding, toileting, dressing, play, discipline, sleep, and motor development.[22] When she has assembled the data about the child and family, it is advisable to consult with behavior modification experts, decide whether to attempt to work with the family on a concentrated basis herself, or refer the child

[21]Linda Whitney Peterson, "Operant Approach to Observation and Recording," *Nursing Outlook*, 15 (3): 28–32, March 1967.
[22]Ibid.

Table 6-2   How to Write Down the Observed Baseline Data of the Feeding Abilities of a Five-Year-Old Retarded Child during One Mealtime
SETTING: Five-Year-Old Retarded Child Was Sitting at Luncheon Table. Soup, Crackers, and Applesauce Were in Small Dishes on the Table. The Time Was 12 Noon.

Antecedent event	Behavior	Consequent event
1. Mother gave graham cracker to child.	2. Child grasped cracker with left hand and ate entire cracker.	3. Mother smiled and said, "You liked that, didn't you?"
4. Mother offered a spoonful of soup of a thickened consistency to child. (After several spoonfuls)	5. Child opened mouth expectantly, took food, and swallowed all of it.	6. Child looked expectantly for next spoonful.
7. Mother offered spoonful of soup to child.	8. Child opened mouth, took food, and held it in mouth.	9. Mother said, "You've had enough of that, hmm?"
10. Mother was talking to nurse and not feeding child for several minutes.	11. Child spontaneously picked up spoon awkwardly, dipped it into applesauce dish, and successfully maneuvered the spoon to mouth and swallowed the applesauce.	12. Mother did not notice child's behavior until nurse said, "Good girl! You fed yourself some applesauce."
13. Mother offered spoon to child and said, "Here, take another spoonful of applesauce."	14. Child refused spoon, would not touch it, and cried.	15. Mother said, "OK, I'll feed you."

and family to an appropriate community facility which will give a comprehensive and complete indoctrination of the method.

If the nurse has been encouraged to proceed with the family herself, she must confer with the parents regarding the one behavior which they would like strengthened or weakened first. By selecting one behavior, the nurse is then ready to make direct observations and write down precise baseline data about the behavior. By giving herself specific time intervals on several different days for data gathering, a base rate of the frequency of the selected behavior is gained, in addition to the antecedent events which stimulated the behavior. Also, ideas are accumulated about which reinforcers of the behavior have positive or negative results. When sufficient data have been charted, the nurse is ready to work out a plan of action with the parents regarding the shaping of the desired behavior. See Table 6-2 as an example for recording data. By showing the parents the frequency with which the behavior occurred in conjunction with the antecedent events, a plan of action can be devised where agreement will be reached whether to strengthen or to weaken the specific behavior. A reinforcer will be selected which the parents and nurse will use consistently to shape the desired behavior. At selected time intervals, the nurse will observe and chart the behavior to measure if the plan of action is demonstrating progress. The successful use of the behavior-modification method requires frequent consultation with personnel who are skilled in using the method, a team approach with the parents, and patience of the nurse, since predictability of child response is variable.

The method can be modified for use with many families who desire to change specific behaviors in "normal" children. Since the use of positive reinforcers (rewards, praise) is less common than the use of negative reinforcers (criticisms, punishment) in the average American home, the social learning method can be successfully implemented to shape desired behaviors in children by instructing parents to use effective positive reinforcers in a consistent pattern with the children. For example, to shape a desired behavior, the parents can be instructed to consistently notice and praise their son every time he hangs up his coat after school. On the days when he does not hang up his coat, the parents can be instructed to consistently give him a chore that he does not find attractive. In this way, the shaping of the desired behavior is secured as the boy realizes the consequences of the original act. An excellent self-help type of book for parents to use who want to teach their children desired behaviors is *Living with Children,* by Patterson and Gullion.[23] The ingenious community health nurse is able to adapt the use of the method to the capacities of a family after she has observed significant family behavior patterns and interpreted an attractive means for implementing the method in a way that catches the interest of parents.

2.   The family therapy approach   Family therapy is a procedure that makes use of a true group, a primary group. The sphere of intervention is not the isolated individual patient but rather the family viewed as an organismic whole.

Family psychotherapy . . . is a procedure that makes use of a true group, a primary group; the sphere of intervention is not the isolated individual patient, but rather the family viewed as an organismic whole. . . . It is developing a body of knowledge, . . . illuminating those processes by which the family supports or damages individual development and also those by which the individual supports or damages family development. . . . It is evolving a specific system of therapeutic intervention, disclosing how the

[23]Gerald R. Patterson and M. Elizabeth Gullion, *Living with Children,* Research Press, Post Office Box 2459, Station A, Champaign, Ill. 61820, 1968.

family method may be related to and combined with other means of supporting the goals of family life. . . . It merges the efforts of treatment with the goals of prevention of illness, maintenance of health, and education in the problems of family living.[24]

Community health nurses can make use of a modified form of family therapy when they accept the premise that an individual can change and adjust behavior in a healthy manner only when the family system allows it. In other words, for one person's behavior to change, the responses of family members must likewise change. The basic procedure in family therapy is to gather the family members together to talk about their relationship with each other.[25] By so doing, the nurse is able to view family interaction patterns and reactions of individual family members to each other. Until the nurse has met the entire family and made an assessment of the family's interaction system, she cannot hope to change coping behaviors of any individual family member with any pronounced degree of success.

Virginia Satir makes use of a growth model for families based on the idea that people's behavior changes through process and that the process is represented by transactions with other people. Growth occurs when the system permits it. The therapist is intimately involved in the transactions, and anything he may offer the patient or family to expedite learning and exchange is utilized to help them grow within the context of the relationship. This model requires willingness of the therapist to be experimental, spontaneous, and flexible. The goal of the growth model is to teach people to be congruent, to speak directly and clearly, and to communicate their feelings, thoughts, and desires accurately. The therapist serves as an example of an active, learning, fallible human being who is willing to cope honestly and responsibly with whatever confronts him, including his own vulnerabilities.[26] The implementation of a family therapy approach on a modified basis by the community health nurse can be an exciting learning experience for both the family and the nurse. One thing to be remembered by the nurse in the implementation of the family-therapy method is that she should not talk solely on a one-to-one basis with any member of the family; she should serve mainly as the facilitator and instigate interaction of family members with each other, and not with the nurse. If family members will direct open, honest

[24]Nathan W. Ackerman, Frances L. Beatman, and Sanford N. Sherman, *Expanding Theory and Practice in Family Therapy,* Family Service Association of America, New York, 1967, pp. 4–5.

[25]Penny Kossoris, "Family Therapy," *American Journal of Nursing,* 70 (8): 1730–1733, August 1970.

[26]Virginia Satir, *Conjoint Family Therapy,* rev. ed., Science and Behavior Books, Inc., Palo Alto, Calif, 1967, pp. 182–183.

statements to each other, communication patterns are more congruent and the nurse can interpret the intent behind the statements in such a way that they are nonthreatening and understandable to the other family members. Also, in this climate the presence of a third party, the nurse, often helps some family members to say things that they are unable to utter usually.

Whether or not the nurse actively participates in the family therapy method or acts as a coworker with a qualified family therapist, she should be able to identify family interactional patterns which are dysfunctional as described by Satir. These families should be directed or guided toward treatment with family therapists or family counseling facilities. Much of the work of community health nurses is of a preparatory nature and consists of helping dysfunctional families to become aware of ineffective or destructive interactional patterns and motivating them to seek expert help, since they are often unhappy families and have multiple health problems.

For nurses who have not practiced any form of family therapy or counseling, it feels risky to gather family members together to talk about their interactions. Oftentimes, it seems less threatening to call the meeting a family conference and to have the reason for the conference clearly labeled as helping the family member who seems to be the "obvious" one in trouble. Once the family is together in a comfortable setting with the nurse who is acting as the therapist, the procedure for managing the counseling session is outlined as follows:

1   The nurse should introduce herself to each member of the family first, shake hands, or exchange a pleasantry in recognition of each individual family member in the group.

2   Efforts should be made to assist all members of the family to feel comfortable and relaxed.

3   The nurse should state the purpose of the family conference clearly and ask family members to correct or add to the information according to their individual perceptions.

4   In getting the family to "work," the nurse should talk directly to and individualize each member of the family in a way that communicates that each one is valued.

5   Clear questions must be asked and family members expected to give clear answers. When answers are fuzzy or "gray," the nurse should seek clarification until the answer is made clear.

6   The nurse must always be in charge of the meeting. She should be a "model of confidence" whether she feels so or not. By maintaining charge, the nurse may have to interrupt, firmly silence a family member, rearrange the seating of the family, request family members to do a task such as drawing pictures, or provide a distraction of some sort.

7   When concluding the conference, it is facilitative to give the family an assignment or homework tasks which they are willing to do. It must be of such a nature that it makes sense to each family member, is fun, and gets them started in the direction of the goal toward which they are striving. The assignment can be quite simple, such as eating *one* family meal without arguments. If a family can function without arguing one time, it reveals to them the possibility that with one step at a time, future desired goals may be attainable.

Questions that are helpful and sometimes illuminating for the nurse to ask the family during the conference are as follows: "What would you like different in this family?" "What would you like for yourself in this family?" "In what way do you let other people know how you feel?" "How do you let another family member know that you are pleased with them?"

Satir described the use of "family-system games" based on her classification of interaction patterns as either open systems or closed systems. *Closed systems* are those in which every participating member must be very cautious about what he or she says. The principal rule seems to be that everyone is supposed to have the same opinions, feelings, and desires, whether or not this is true. In closed systems, honest self-expression is impossible and if it does occur, the expression is viewed as deviant or "sick" by other members of the group or family. The *open system* permits honest self-expression for the participating members. In such a group or family, differences are viewed as natural and open negotiation occurs to resolve such differences by "compromise," "agreement to disagree," or "taking turns." In open systems, the individual can say what he feels and thinks and can negotiate for reality and personal growth without destroying himself or the others in the system.[27] By the use of simulated games, Satir helps families to see and understand the nature of their own family system and experience the movement from a pathologic system of interaction to a growth-producing one. She elicits the family's feelings, responses, and body reactions to the games, each other, and the interactions. She urges family therapists to be open, flexible, enthusiastic, and innovative.[28] By being knowledgeable about Satir's approach to families and willing to try some of the suggested exercises, the community health nurse can adapt and improve her own style of interacting successfully with families. When the nurse initiates role-playing games in the family setting, unexpected insights are gained by all participating members. Often the games are fun and stimulating and create a lighthearted atmosphere, which is therapeutic in itself. New

[27]Ibid., p. 185.
[28]Ibid., pp. 188–189.

approaches and ideas are often received with enthusiasm by families, particularly if they are implemented skillfully and appropriately and if the results bring forth new insights.

3. The transactional analysis approach Transactional analysis offers a systematic, consistent theory of personality and social dynamics and an actionistic, rational form of therapy which is suitable for, easily understood by, and naturally adapted to the great majority of patients.[29] Its goal is to help people to be their true selves. Transactional analysis identifies three ego states inherent in each person. The ego states are systems of feelings which motivate a related set of behavior patterns.[30] They are called the parent, adult, and child ego states within each individual. The child ego state is represented by spontaneous, rational, and irrational feelings. The child expresses genuine feelings of joy or anger and speaks in words and thoughts saying "*I* am." The child can be a good or bad child. The parent ego state is represented by fixed feelings of right or wrong behavior, acceptance of traditional values. The parent moralizes and judges others and speaks in words and thoughts, saying "*you* are." The parent can be a good or bad parent. The adult ego state is represented by responsible, rational, and predictable feelings. The adult is nonjudgmental and always in the process of learning. The composition of each person's ego states varies according to past and early childhood experiences, but perceptible predominant characteristics can be identified by other persons when they take note of verbal transactions and nonverbal behavior. When people do not interact openly and make use of "games," these cues suggest that they are masking their true selves and are possibly unaware that they have a distinctive identity. For the person who consistently and spontaneously acts according to feelings, the child ego state is dominant. When the person tends to be inflexible and judgmental, the parent ego state is dominant.

Transactional analysis classifies four possible life positions that can be held with respect to oneself and others. They are interpreted in detail by Harris in a book which is easy reading for nurses and consumers.[31] The life positions are:

1 I'm ok—You're ok.
2 I'm not ok—You're ok.
3 I'm not ok—You're not ok.
4 I'm ok—You're not ok.

[29]Eric Berne, *Transactional Analysis in Psychotherapy*, Grove Press, Inc., New York, 1961, p. 21.
[30]Ibid., p. 17.
[31]Thomas A. Harris, *I'm OK—You're OK*, Harper and Row, Publishers, Incorporated, New York, 1969.

The life position "I'm ok—You're ok" is the healthy situation and is the goal toward which all persons in transactional analysis therapy strive. However, the predominant majority of people hold the life position "I'm not ok—You're ok." As explained by Harris, this is the universal position of early childhood, being the infant's logical conclusion from the situation of birth and infancy. Since all infants are naturally dependent and *must be* cared for by adults, the not-ok-ness is a natural conclusion about themselves. In this position the person feels at the mercy of others and seeks recognition and approval from others.[32] It is the people who hold the life position "I'm not ok—You're ok" of whom the community health nurse must be cognizant. By explaining the simple interpretation of the three ego states and the life positions that the majority of people hold, new insights often are gained which help people to understand a great deal more about themselves. They are naturally drawn to remember their early childhood, the role of parents in their lives, and the conclusions they reached about certain emphasized beliefs which had been accepted at face value once upon a time, yet later were questioned after weighing the facts rationally and thoughtfully. For example, a child may have been told by a parent that handling frogs would cause warts to appear on the hands. However, upon observing other children handling frogs and eventually venturing to pick one up, it was discovered that warts did not appear. Consequently, the child no longer believed a statement which had been accepted at face value formerly.

The belief is held by transactional analysts that each individual is responsible for his or her own feelings. Feelings are internal and cannot be manipulated by external forces unless the person allows and responds to the outside forces. The individual *chooses* feelings. When the going gets rough, each person runs back to familiar territory or familiar feelings which were used in early childhood. A necessity for all persons is "stroking," recognition, or attention. As infants and children, any stroking, positive or negative, was sought as long as attention of some kind was gained. Most persons are well aware of negative strokes, since the present society tends to be negatively oriented and criticisms are much more easily given by others than praise or recognition. As adults, symbolic positive strokes are solicited and acquired by receiving compliments, recognition of achievements. Positive strokes are better than negative ones or conditional ones. Conditional strokes are those that imply, "I'll approve of you *if*." When interacting with individuals and families, positive strokes, not conditional ones, designed to strengthen the recipients should be used at every appropriate opportunity by the nurse.

Transactional analysts make use of another idea which is practical and catches the interest of the consumer. The idea is that of trading

---

[32]Ibid., pp. 43–45.

stamps, which are collected daily in order to obtain an object or reward that one desires. The trading stamps in transactional analysis represent feelings; good feelings are identified as gold stamps and bad, hurt, or resentful feelings are brown stamps. Gold stamps are collected by giving and receiving tangible positive recognition and earning desirable achievements. Brown stamps are collected by giving and receiving insults, feeling injured or put upon. Brown stamps can be collected dishonestly and are often accompanied by a feeling of triumph. When a book of brown stamps or an accumulation of angry feelings is collected, a person is entitled to have a temper outburst free of guilt, or with several books of brown stamps, a divorce or extramarital affair can be claimed free of guilt. For those persons familiar with the trading stamp idea in transactional analysis, the labeling of a behavior as gold or brown stamping has lasting meaning and can often be conveyed in a nonthreatening manner. For the community health nurse who chooses to use a modification of the transactional analysis method with families, the interpretation of the basic beliefs and language are easily conveyed and understood and provide a nonthreatening climate for growth-promoting interaction. The goal toward which the nurse would work in using this method is assisting the patient or family to become their true, genuine selves and rely less on behaviors which mask their identity.

4. The parent effectiveness training approach In developing parent effectiveness training, Gordon wanted to provide a preventive program helping parents to communicate facilitatively with children. He was convinced that adolescents do not rebel against parents, but against certain destructive methods of discipline almost universally employed by parents.[33]

All parents have feelings about the behavior of their children which can be defined into an area of acceptance and nonacceptance. The acceptability of behavior as defined by the parent may change from day to day, may vary in terms of the individual child performing the behavior, or may show inconsistency dependent upon the parent's mood or the situation in the home. Parents cannot be wholly consistent regardless of their determination to be so because parents are people who, if they are real, have a variable area of acceptance. When parents "seem" to accept a behavior but are not genuine about it, the child invariably knows the true feelings of the parent. For parents who want to facilitate the growth and actualization of their children to the fullest potential, they must communicate their acceptance in such a way that the children *feel* the acceptance. They must learn the language of acceptance which is communicated

[33]Thomas Gordon, *Parent Effectiveness Training*, Peter H. Wyden, Inc., Publisher, New York, 1970, p. 3.

verbally and nonverbally and incorporates the skill of *active listening.* Active listening requires the listener to suspend personal thoughts and feelings in order to attend exclusively to the message of the speaker. It forces accurate receiving. To listen actively the listener must (1) *want* to hear what the speaker has to say, (2) genuinely *want* to be helpful to the speaker, (3) genuinely be able to accept the speaker's feelings, (4) trust the speaker's capacity to handle personal feelings and find solutions for problems, (5) appreciate that feelings are transitory, not permanent, and (6) see the speaker as separate from the listener. The skills of active listening may seem almost impossible for parents to practice with their children, but it can be learned and effectively utilized if earnestly tried.

Another aspect of parent effectiveness training is problem ownership. When an individual has a need that is not being satisfied, that individual owns a problem. For children, the problem can be feeling rejected by a friend, getting angry when losing a game with a friend, feeling inadequate because of acne. When the child owns the problem, the parent can assist by "active listening." For parents, the problem is owned when children's behavior potentially threatens a need of theirs. For example, when the child is tugging and interrupting while the parent is on the telephone, the child's toys are scattered all over the kitchen floor, or the child does not care properly for equipment belonging to the parent. When the parent owns the problem, the parent can try to modify the child directly, modify the environment, or modify himself or herself. However, inevitably parent-child conflicts occur, and the "no-lose" method of resolution must be employed. This is essentially a problem-solving method in which both parents and children participate. The goal is to solve their unique conflicts by finding their own unique solutions acceptable to both. This method tends to be effective because the child is a participant in arriving at a unique solution, has been required to think about possible solutions, and feels less resistant to carrying out the agreed-upon solution. Relationships between parents and children tend to be more satisfying with the use of the "no-lose" method.[34]

Community health nurses can explain the concept of parent effectiveness training to parents and children and serve as educators, consultants, and arbiters in the implementation of the method. Since nursing students are so well versed in the problem-solving method, the role of "expert" is easily assumed.

4. The epidemiologic approach Epidemiology has often been considered the study of factors determining the occurrence of communicable diseases in populations. However, the study has broadened to include *all*

[34]Ibid., pp. 15–264.

diseases, whether communicable or not, and health behavior of groups of people. Epidemiology consists of a methodological investigation of disease or health behavior occurring in human groups for the purpose of discovering factors essential to or contributing to disease occurrence or unhealthy behavior and developing methods for prevention of disease or unhealthy behavior. The epidemiologic method is closely related to the problem-solving method, which is generally used with individuals rather than with groups. Epidemiology is more a method than a body of knowledge and in essence is similar to the detective approach of gathering clues or data, making hypotheses or deductions, and finding solutions. The epidemiologist mainly uses two methods for study of data, observational and experimental. By observation the investigator simply makes note of circumstances and events in the normal pattern of life. By analysis the investigator searches for association between disease occurrence or unhealthy behavior and the possible causative influences.[35]

Customarily, the community health nurse serves as an associate with epidemiologists in the study of diseases and investigation of all related data. However, by using the epidemiologic approach on a small scale with families or groups, it is proposed that the community health nurse play the role of principal investigator in seeking out solutions for diseases or health behaviors occurring in a given family or group and stimulate family or group members to serve as associates in bringing out related data. For example, a small but effective epidemiologic study could be done of a family or group who are faced with the problem of obesity or a high incidence of home accidents. In dealing with the obesity problem, a detailed history of amounts and types of food ingested by the family or group members for a period of three days to one week would provide data that could be analyzed thoroughly in terms of nutrients and calories. In addition, characteristic habit patterns associated with mealtimes and snacktimes could be studied, and antecedent events which seem to cause undesirable consequent behaviors could be observed. If the group or family members are participating as associates in the epidemiologic study, they may be encouraged to bring out facts related to eating, such as the ingestion of more food following hostile interactions with others or early childhood training which taught them to clean up their plates rather than have food wastage. When all participants are alert for possible causative factors of eating, a great amount of significant data can be secured, which will lead to ideas of possible hypotheses to be tested. The nurse serves as the detective or agent in search of significant clues from all possible perspectives, including physical, emotional, and social. By playing the

[35]John P. Fox, Carrie E. Hall, and Lila R. Elveback, *Epidemiology, Man and Disease,* The Macmillan Company, New York, 1970, pp. 7–16.

role of detective, she must have a comprehensive knowledge about the variety of factors which may lead to obesity. When a definition of the nature and significance of the problem is obtained about all the participants and all important data are collected, classified, and appraised, a hypothesis can be tentatively formulated for testing. Future practical activities based on the hypothesis can be planned and implemented for a determined time period and ultimately, an evaluation of the results of the study can be decided. For the group studying the causation of obesity, the testing of a hypothesis focusing on mealtime practices and habits may lead to more successful results than one related to ingestion of superfluous calories. By involving all family or group members in the detective game, curiosity is stimulated and motivation to change behavior is often self-induced.

In the case of a family or group having a high incidence of accidents, the nurse can introduce the idea that accidents don't happen, they are caused by what people do or by what they fail to do.[36] This idea alone may arouse the group to do some reflective thinking and serve as a stimulus for further study. If the family or group responds with the desire to lessen the occurrence of accidents, each person can be asked to determine the frequency of individual accidents and describe completely the events occurring before and during the last accident in which he or she was involved. Environmental, psychological, and stress factors representing hazards in each described situation can be elicited and studied by the group in search of commonalities. They may formulate a hypothesis based on the relationship of stress to personal psychological characteristics which culminate in accident proneness in individuals. By becoming more knowledgeable by means of references about the characteristics of persons who seem to be accident-prone, by attempting to reduce the number of stress- or risk-producing life events, and attempting to control unsafe reactions, acts, and behavior, the group may test their hypothesis by tabulating the frequency of accidents occurring to them after four weeks of discussion and study compared to their first frequency estimates. By accepting the fact that accidents occur when alertness, efficiency, skill, or judgment of persons is temporarily impaired, subsequent behavior can be made more conscious and perhaps "safe." The epidemiologic method provides a more interesting approach to accident prevention than lectures about safety. The nurse when acting as a stimulator of ideas and promulgator of learning has more satisfactions and is more apt to see learning internalized by her family or group.

5. The paradoxical communication approach The community

[36]Albert Chapman, "The Anatomy of an Accident," *Public Health Reports,* 75:630–632, July 1960.

health nurse may make use of paradoxical communication as a last resort when all other approaches have failed or as a mode of communication to which a specific type of patient will respond best. A *paradox* is a term describing a directive which qualifies another directive in a conflicting way, either simultaneously or at a different moment in time.[37] For example, in order to persuade a patient to change undesirable symptomatic behavior, he or she must be told to do something and that activity should be related to the problem in some way. For a person complaining of persistent insomnia, a directive can be given to spend each night reading books that the patient has put off reading and, to ensure against falling asleep, to stand up at the mantle and read all night. After several nights of reading while standing up, the insomnia problem may be cured and this was accomplished by the patient. The emphasis of treatment was placed on the patient's activity rather than on the symptomatic behavior.[38] By directing the patient's attention to activities which must be accomplished and avoiding the suggestion of ceasing the symptomatic behavior, the therapist poses a paradox in the patient's mind of retaining the symptomatic behavior or following directives that are not always attractive to the patient. This method of giving action-type directives related to symptomatic behavior commits the patient to either giving up the symptom or following the directives as given by the therapist. The paradoxical communication method has interesting implications, particularly for childlike persons who want to change symptomatic behavior but cannot resist the desire to rebel when told or ordered to do something. If the nurse utilizes the paradoxical communication approach, she must know her patient well enough to predict how the patient may respond to a direct suggestion. If the nurse is almost certain that the patient cannot resist rejecting an order, she can consciously give a directive which is opposed to the goal she wishes for the patient. This method often works with small children.

A student nurse accidentally stumbled upon this method of communication with the mother of a child who was diagnosed as needing a tonsillectomy to alleviate a hearing loss. The nurse had made repeated weekly visits to persuade the mother to make an appointment for the surgical procedure. Upon each home visit the mother had some legitimate excuse which had caused a postponement in scheduling the surgery. At last the frustrated nurse gave up and told the mother to forget the whole thing. In all probability the child would manage all right without the tonsillectomy. The following week the nurse visited the home and learned that the child had had the surgery and was recuperating nicely.

---

[37]By permission of Jay Haley, *Strategies of Psychotherapy*, Grune & Stratton, Inc., New York, 1963, p. 17.
[38]Ibid., p. 49.

Planning Care and Coordination with Others

As a member of the health team serving the patient and family, the community health nurse must be constantly alert to the necessity for conferring with the other interested members of the team. These members include the physician, social workers, nurses in other settings, teachers, and any number of allied community workers and health aides. By initiating communication by means of the telephone, prearranged personal discussions, or scheduling a multidisciplinary conference, all team members can be made cognizant of agreed-upon, common objectives by which all will abide in their work with the patient and family. Planning a successful intervention with and for the patient and family involves teamwork, maintenance of an open exchange of information, sharing of resources among team members, and agreement regarding the primary responsibilities of team members and ultimate goals toward which all are working. Planning with other professional and nonprofessional workers is essential and requires time and effort expended to maintain open channels of communication. By following a carefully designed plan of action which has been individualized for the patient and family, successful interventions and satisfying relationships are more likely to be attained by all persons involved.

THE NURSING PROCESS: IMPLEMENTING

Implementing a nursing care plan implies that a careful assessment and planning process has been accomplished and activities for or in behalf of the patient and family are now available which will contribute to their comfort and well-being or facilitate their coping behaviors as related to their specific health problems. Implementation is an ongoing activity or series of activities which necessitates evaluation in order to determine the effectiveness of nursing care. Action is taken with the expectation that if the planned action is followed, an expected result will occur. The evaluation process may indicate a need for reassessment and replanning or a modification of the plan of care. Implementation of nursing care includes all the activities of the nurse in carrying out the nursing care plan designed to enhance the well-being of the patient and family.[39]

While carrying out a plan of action, the nurse must be constantly aware of (1) a therapeutic use of self with the patient and family; (2) knowledge of physical, psychological, and social manifestations of pathology, deviancy, or wellness; (3) opportunities for teaching, supervis-

[39]Mildred Wesolowski, "Implementation of the Nursing Care Plan," in Yura and Walsh, op. cit., pp. 78–79.

ing, or guiding persons toward better coping patterns of health; and (4) evaluation of the total effect of the implementation activity.

The Process of Effecting Change

A persistent goal to which all nurses are committed is to influence change in patients or families in the direction of improved health or wellness. However, what motivates people to change? Will they change when they see no reason to do so? Will they change when others want them to do so? Will they change when they believe they want to do so but cannot resist the pull of forces compelling them to pursue old habit patterns? Effecting change is much more easily talked about than accomplished. According to Wheelis, *we are what we do.* The actions that we *do* describe our character to others. The fact that the action is repeated over and over reinforces the description that others have ascribed to us. When we *say* that we are one thing but *behave* or *act* in opposition to what we say, others take note of the behavior and believe the behavior rather than the words. Because we tend to maintain behavior or actions that are familiar and customary, we resist change.

All persons have potential for change and can change when they *choose* to do so. Therefore a person who is suffering or uncomfortable with a health problem, must recognize that it is a problem that is causing him or her to suffer or be uncomfortable, and must be ready and willing to do something about the problem before a change can be effected. Since we are what we do, if we want to change what we are, we must begin by changing what we do. A new mode of action is often difficult, unnatural, unpleasant, or anxiety-provoking, and in order to sustain the change, a considerable effort of will is required. Change will occur only if such action is maintained over a long period of time.[40] Consequently, the role of community health nurses in assisting patients or families to effect change can be enumerated as follows: (1) reach an agreement with the patient or family about the health problems that are causing difficulties and they desire to change; (2) assist the patient or family in determining the new behavior or action which will help them to attain their goal; (3) provide constant reinforcement for the patient's or family's behavior or actions which have been adjusted in the direction of meeting their goal; and (4) maintain contact with the patient or family for an extended period of time and continue to encourage and strengthen them in their new behavior until their goal has been attained and maintained to the satisfaction of all concerned. At the same time that the nurse is working with the patient or family to effect change, she must also be utilizing her relationship skills, cognitive knowledge about the particular health prob-

[40]Allen Wheelis, *The Desert,* Basic Books, Inc., Publishers, New York, 1970.

lems which are the focus of attention, interactional skills, and predictive skills in anticipating the probability of success in the venture undertaken by the patient, family, and nurse.

Barriers to Change

Some barriers which may be encountered by the nurse as she attempts to effect change with patients or families may be: (1) faulty perception regarding the patients' or families' readiness to change. The nurse may believe that the patient desires to change when in reality the patient is only being momentarily compliant to the nurse's persuasiveness or wishes to appear worthy of the nurse's attention. (2) The language used by the nurse may be unfamiliar to the patient or family and rather than ask for an explicit interpretation, the consumer may elect to pretend an understanding of the issues involved. (3) The emotional content of the messages between the patient or family and the nurse may be missed, avoided, or inaccurately interpreted as being irrelevant to the issue under discussion. When the nurse detects an emotion in the consumer that is not completely understandable in terms of the words being spoken, she must state verbally her uncertainty about what she is sensing or perceiving. For example, she may say to a patient who is using bullet-like speech and staring pointedly out the window, "You seem disturbed about something and I am not sure if I understand the message you are giving me. Are you angry with me?" By so doing, the patient is given the opportunity to express or interpret his or her emotion, whether it is directed at the nurse or another target. (4) Too many suggestions for change may be offered by the nurse, resulting in an overload of information for the consumer to manage. (5) The timing may be poor, inconvenient, or incomprehensible to the consumer. (6) The patient or family may misinterpret the messages of the nurse, or vice versa. To avoid misinterpretations of messages it is good practice to request the consumer to give feedback on what he or she has heard from the nurse. This is called perception checking. When a verification of the message received is indeed the message intended by the sender, then the communication is clear to both parties. (7) The patient or family may arbitrarily desire the right to refuse, regardless of the idea, because of the element of power. If the nurse is able to accept this type of consumer and assess his or her behavior characteristics, she can engage in an encounter in such a way that the consumer retains control but is provoked to *think*. Nothing is gained if the nurse enters the game of one-upmanship with the consumer.

Stress and Crisis

An emotionally healthy person is one who has dealt and is dealing in a satisfactory manner with the conflicts inherent in each stage of human development. Inherent in this description is the implication that all persons have conflicts, problems, or stresses. In other words, life is not a bowl of cherries but a roller coaster with highs and lows. By acknowledging that all persons experience stress and crisis, the complicated task of the community health nurse is to determine when to intervene with individuals and families in need of assistance.

Stress is commonly associated with the rate of wear and tear on the body or the burden under which the individual is struggling. Rapoport referred to stress as the relation of the stressful stimulus, the individual's reaction to it, and the events to which it leads.[41] The state of crisis occurs when an imbalance between an important problem and the resources immediately available to deal with it are unsuccessful. In other words, the person in a state of crisis is unable to cope adequately with the immediate problem. The essence of crisis is struggle—a struggle to master an upsetting situation and to regain a state of balance.[42] For health professionals who utilize crisis theory, a crisis is an opportunity for respondents to try new actions or new coping mechanisms which will strengthen adaptive capacities and raise levels of emotional health.

In community health nursing, the systems approach helps the nurse to view the family as an integral unit and as made up of individuals who are influenced by all occurrences within the family. She sees the family as a source of strength or a source of stress, dependent upon the constructive or destructive influences in operation within it. When a famliy is in crisis, they are at a turning point. They are faced with problems for which their coping mechanisms seem inadequate, they feel helpless and frustrated and are uncertain of how to act effectively to solve the problems.[43] It is at this point that the intervention of the community health nurse can be most effective. If her interaction occurs during the period of crisis, she has an optimum opportunity to guide the family toward improved coping mechanisms, which will successfully restore a state of balance within the family system and promote them toward a higher level of emotional health.

There are two types of crises which families undergo, developmental and situational. As described by Robischon, *developmental or maturational crises* are those which human beings experience in the process of their psychosocial growth. They are considered stages of the normal life cycle. For families, some examples of these crises occur when a new baby is born, when the children reach adolescence, or when retirement occurs.

[41]Lydia Rapoport, "The State of Crisis: Some Theoretical Considerations," in Howard J. Parad (ed.), *Crisis Intervention: Selected Readings,* Family Service Association of America, New York, 1965, p. 23.

[42]Donald G. Langsley and David M. Kaplan, *The Treatment of Families in Crisis,* Grune & Stratton, Inc., New York, 1968, p. 3.

[43]Donna C. Aguilera, Janice M. Messick, and Marlene S. Farrell, *Crisis Intervention, Theory and Methodology,* The C. V. Mosby Company, St. Louis, 1970, p. 1.

Situational or *accidental crises* are external events or stresses. They are often more sudden, unexpected, and unfortunate.[44] For example, these crises occur when a member of the family dies, a handicapped child is born, a debilitating disease is diagnosed and seen as inevitable, or a serious accident maims a family member.

As stated by Leighton, there are three universal kinds of behavior with which individuals react to authority when subject to forces of stress that are disturbing to the emotions and thoughts of the individual. They are cooperation, withdrawal, and aggressiveness. When the nurse is watchful for these behaviors, she is better able to assess the dynamics involved in each family situation. Relief from excessive stress is assisted by the utilization of a sense of humor, observable facts, reasoned thinking, and new opportunities to achieve security and satisfactions.[45]

Some of the activities which the community health nurse can use in crisis intervention with an individual or family are:

1 Help the troubled to confront the crisis by helping him to verbalize and to comprehend the reality of the situation.
2 Help him to confront the crisis in doses he can manage. If the nurse uses cues that the individual reveals nonverbally, she may facilitate verbalization of feelings which the patient had considered to be taboo but were contributing to his state of tension.
3 Help him to find the facts of the situation and explore all possible ways of coping. Proceed at the patient's pace. When exploration is done mutually, the patient is helped to think and may devise solutions which are highly original and made possible because of the stimulus of another person engaging in the problem-solving process with him.
4 Help him by recognizing his strengths and encouraging the use of his capabilities.
5 Help him accept assistance from others as needed and as he is ready, until he has mobilized his own personal resources.[46]

By being available, patient, willing to listen, and supportive of strengths, the nurse can enable individuals or families in a state of crisis to move toward resolution of difficulties in an acceptable manner and promote their sense of responsibility and well-being at the same time.

The Social Readjustment Rating Scale

Stress affects all ages and can be measured in terms of the magnitude of life changes. A rating scale developed by Holmes and Rahe measures the

[44]Paulette Robischon, "The Challenge of Crisis Theory for Nursing," *Nursing Outlook,* 15(7):28–32, July 1967.
[45]Alexander H. Leighton, *The Governing of Men,* Princeton University Press, Princeton, N. J., 1945, pp. 252–286.
[46]Robischon, op. cit., pp. 28–32.

intensity and length of time necessary to accommodate to a life event, regardless of the desirability of the event. The scoring technique which has been tested for reliability indicates the level of stress or life changes experienced by individuals. When the number of life changes clusters, the score is high. This means that an individual with a high score has had to cope with many changes within a specified time period and is therefore likely to become sick. It does not seem to matter whether the change has desirable or undesirable aspects. By reviewing forty-three items on the rating scale reflecting life-change events and scoring as instructed, an individual can determine the amount of recent stress experienced, and the likelihood of becoming ill or having an accident within the next year. The tool is best used by community health nurses not for prediction purposes, but to give some clues to families about what activities to avoid or modify if one wants to reduce a high score with subsequent chances of illness. If presented as an interesting tool with which to measure stress, family members can be encouraged to think of preventive measures and manipulate their plans so as to lessen their total life-event scores.[47] The scale and method for scoring is shown in Table 6-3.

Homework

When working with individuals in the implementation phase of the nursing process, a simple activity or assignment is frequently accepted with keenness and ambivalence—eagerness to be doing something that may help themselves and uncertainty about their ability to carry out the assignment. These tasks or activities are called "homework," a term used by David Kupfer, a transactional analyst who stated that people like to be given homework. The assignment given must be reasonable, fairly easily accomplished, and within the context of the goal toward which the patient is working. For example, for the person who has low self-esteem, an assignment can be given for that person to write down 100 strengths about himself and to show the list to the nurse on the next visit. Or the patient may be assigned a pamphlet to read and jot down questions for discussion on the nurse's return visit. Or the patient may be requested to tally on a chart the number of times a prescribed set of exercises was performed, and the nurse will anticipate examining the chart on the next visit. The performance of an assignment sometimes relieves tension, gives a sense of movement toward a desired goal, and a feeling of accomplishment that is satisfying. The achievement of the assignment, whether partial or complete, must always be recognized and reinforced positively by the nurse.

In a study reported by Geismar and Krisberg, it was found that

[47]Thomas H. Holmes and R. H. Rahe, "The Social Readjustment Rating Scale," *Journal of Psychosomatic Research*, 11:213–218, 1967.

Table 6-3 Social Readjustment Rating Scale†

Rank	Life event	Life crisis units
1	Death of spouse	100
2	Divorce	73
3	Marital separation	65
4	Jail term	63
5	Death of close family member	63
6	Personal injury or illness	53
7	Marriage	50
8	Fired at work	47
9	Marital reconciliation	45
10	Retirement	45
11	Change in health of family member	44
12	Pregnancy	40
13	Sex difficulties	39
14	Gain of new family member	39
15	Business readjustment	39
16	Change in financial state	38
17	Death of close friend	37
18	Change to different line of work	36
19	Change in number of arguments with spouse	35
20	Mortgage over $10,000	31
21	Foreclosure of mortgage or loan	30
22	Change in responsibilities at work	29
23	Son or daughter leaving home	29
24	Trouble with in-laws	29
25	Outstanding personal achievement	28
26	Wife begins or stops work	26
27	Begin or end school	26
28	Change in living conditions	25
29	Revision of personal habits	24
30	Trouble with boss	23
31	Change in work hours or conditions	20
32	Change in residence	20
33	Change in school	20
34	Change in recreation	19
35	Change in church activities	19
36	Change in social activities	18
37	Mortgage or loan less than $10,000	17
38	Change in sleeping habits	16
39	Change in number of family get-togethers	15
40	Change in eating habits	15
41	Vacation	13
42	Christmas	12
43	Minor violations of the law	11

Source: Adapted with permission from "Social Readjustment Rating Scale," by T. H. Holmes and R. H. Rahe, *Journal of Psychosomatic Research,* 1967.

†*Social Readjustment Rating Scale Instructions:*
Add up value of life crisis units for life events experienced in a two-year period.
Score of 0 to 150—No significant problems.
Score of 150 to 199—Mild life crisis and a 33 percent chance of illness.
Score of 200 to 299—Moderate life crisis and a 50 percent chance of illness.
Score of 300 or over—Major life crisis and an 80 percent chance of illness.

families respond most favorably to communication which is focused on problem solving. The approach very frequently sought by families was the quick solution. However, when family members were encouraged to think through the problem-solving process and their strengths were reinforced, movement toward their goals was more apt to be realized.[48] The assignment of homework which is individualized to fit the situation and gives the family something to do can be one of the methods used to reinforce family members about their existing strengths and latent capacity for problem solving.

The Nursing Bag

For the nurse who gives bedside care in the home, the nursing bag has always been a necessary accessory. Historically, its contents have included equipment which the nurse needed to perform her functions. The equipment has varied dependent upon the period of history that nursing care was given. In the early 1800s, the nurse carried a satchel which contained black currant jelly for the parched throat and racking cough, Irish moss to be made into a soothing drink, chicken jelly for a nourishing broth, and perhaps an orange or a lemon.[49] In the 1900s, the nurses in New York City carried heavy "telescope" bags containing more than a dozen bottles and porcelain jars.[50] From 1900 to the present era, the bags that have been used are familiar to most nurses because of their shape and black color. The contents include equipment for handwashing, taking temperatures, giving injections, doing occasional dressings, and performing other nursing skills necessary to carry out a physician's orders. Frequently the equipment is disposable and entails a careful daily scrutiny of the bag to ensure that all needed articles for the services to be performed on that day are included, are sterile or clean, and are intact.

The manner with which the nurse uses the supplies in the nursing bag communicates much nonverbal data to families about her behavior, attitude, and skill. If the family members like what they see, their respect, confidence, and acceptance of the nurse as a skilled practitioner are increased. They may adopt unconsciously some of her practices of asepsis and cleanliness. By routinely using nursing skills which include vital signs, the nurse conveys that she is truly a nurse and is genuinely concerned about the patient's welfare. Many opportunities for teaching patients can be realized through the use of the nursing bag—and the

[48]Ludwig Geismar and Jane Krisberg, "The Family Life Improvement Project: An Experiment in Preventive Intervention," Parts I and II, *Social Casework*, 27:9, November 1966 and 28:10, December 1966.

[49]Alfred Worcester, *Nurses and Nursing*, Harvard University Press, Cambridge, Mass., 1927, p. 40.

[50]Mary M. Roberts, *American Nursing, History and Interpretation*, The Macmillan Company, New York, 1954, pp. 3–4.

teaching is often not on a verbal or a demonstration basis. The most effective teaching may be accomplished purely on the nonverbal basis, during which the nurse is performirg unconsciously as a role model.

A nursing student who did a ministudy on nurses' attitudes about the bag asked the question, "Is the nursing bag a symbol of the community health nurse?" From a very small sample of practicing community health nurses, four out of five answered, "no." The fifth nurse said that the bag was "whatever the nurse makes of it." Two nursing students out of a sample of three stated that the bag was a symbol of the community health nurse.

In view of the ongoing technological advancements in medical and nursing care, it is difficult to predict if nursing bags will continue to retain the shape, color, and size that they currently have. However, a means for carrying necessary equipment which aids in the administration of nursing care in the home will always be required.

Case Finding

Inherent in every community health nursing visit are the possibilities for case finding and referral. These are important functions of each member of the community health team and are carried out in the home, the school, the clinic, and in places of employment. During the nurse's home visit, while she is providing nursing care and health counseling, she has unusual opportunities for case finding. In her discussions with the family, the nurse must be alert to and observant of early symptoms of such conditions as cancer, diabetes, communicable diseases, birth injuries, and mental and emotional disturbances. The nurse must be perceptive; she must be alert to what the patient and other family members are saying or doing and to objective and subjective symptoms that may be revealed.

A nurse calling on a migratory farm worker's family noted that Judy, a three-year-old, had a definite limp as she walked across the bare floor. The nurse questioned the mother about it, and possible symptoms, suggestive of bone tuberculosis, came to light. A referral to a children's orthopedic clinic brought a diagnosis of bone tuberculosis. Further study of the family revealed that the father had active tuberculosis.

An ostensible purpose of community health nursing service is the early finding of pregnancy and the referral of prospective mothers for medical care. At this time, i.e., early in pregnancy, the nurse can place the mothers under nursing supervision also and teach them care of themselves and their babies. This teaching can often be related to the health needs, e.g., nutritional needs, of other members of the family.

Referral

Closely allied to case finding during the home visit is referral, i.e., the referral of the patient or family to the community agency best suited or equipped to help meet the particular problems recognized by the nurse. These might be of a health, welfare, social, or recreational nature.

Often, the major task of the nurse is not referring a family to an appropriate community agency, but getting the family *ready* to accept the services of the community resource as needed and desired. The process involved in preparing a family includes the initiation of an effective relationship with the family, the recognition that problems are existing and must be resolved, and a time period during which an exploration of problems and possible solutions can be discussed with the family. The time during which the family is searching for appropriate solutions may be extended into weeks or months, dependent upon their readiness to act. In the meantime, the nurse can be utilizing methods or ideas which will reveal the discomfort the problems are causing for the family, will communicate indirectly the family's inability to resolve the problems without competent assistance, will give promise that ultimate solutions are possible and available, and that a referral to an appropriate community resource is indeed necessary to attain a desired goal. An interpretation of the services of a designated community resource and the manner in which the personnel will work with the family must be made. Also, when the family is ready to visit a selected community resource, they should be taught how best to present their desires and goals to the agency from whom they are requesting help. Sometimes the process of preparing a family for a referral to a community resource is a lengthy one and requires a patient and persistent nurse.

In making a referral, the nurse must be well aware of the services and contributions of the community's health and social agencies. Usually lists are available of recognized agencies and their services. Some agencies have developed interagency referral forms. The simplest is a card that includes the name of the agency, its address, telephone number, and the hours that the agency is open. This is signed with the name of the nurse's agency and given to the family. Other types of referral forms may include more details. In certain instances, the nurse may send the agency a notice that the patient or family have been referred, with some pertinent information relating to the situation. Some agencies arrange to return these forms to the nurse with the findings and recommendations that were made to the family. The nurse can utilize this information on future visits.

A workable referral system is basic to any community-wide program of continuity of care of the patient. It is the initial step in the development of such a program.

Closing the Visit

The community health nurse terminates her visit with a brief review of the important points she has tried to make. She stresses the positive aspects, emphasizing family strengths, and reiterates the plans the patient and family will carry out in her absence. Together the nurse and the family plan for the next visit, establishing a date and approximate time convenient for family and nurse. Summarizing the visit can be a learning experience for the patient and family and will give the nurse an opportunity to organize her thoughts in preparation for recording the visit.

Recording the Visit—Problem-Oriented Recording

Community health agencies are continuously seeking ways to improve their family records by eliminating the writing of unnecessary detail or duplication and focusing on a succinct accounting of important information. Because the search for a satisfactory record form is elusive, community health nurses must be flexible and adapt to whatever record form is in use in the particular agency for whom they are working. By concentrating on writing only essential information, nurses can limit their recording of family situations to a few well-stated sentences, phrases, or brief paragraphs. This ability takes continuous effort and self-discipline.

Adaptations of problem-oriented recording as originally introduced by Weed have appeared in many agencies as the recording of choice. The features making this form of recording useful and desirable are its systematic approach to the recording of pertinent facts, the easy accessibility of information in an orderly and logical arrangement, and the capability of evaluating the effectiveness of services given.

The components of a problem-oriented record consist of a database, a problem list, problem assessment and plan formulation, and progress notes and flow sheets. The contention of the problem-oriented recording system is that with the delineation of a patient's or family's multiple problems at a level which is understood and can be managed, a structural framework is provided for the planning and delivery of health care. When each problem is identified and recorded and has an explicitly formulated plan for investigation and management of the problem, the result is a logically organized documentation of the course of each problem. Such a record provides easy access for a methodical analysis of a family's total health needs and services provided.[51]

Database In giving comprehensive care to a family, all health-related problems must be ascertained, including potentially threatening problems, resolved or controlled problems, socioeconomic problems and emotional problems. To elicit a complete database, the assessment and screening process of each family and its members should be as systematic

---

[51]Lawrence L. Weed (major contributor), Jay S. Wakefield, and Stephen R. Yarnall (eds.), *Implementing the Problem-Oriented Medical Record*, Medical Computer Services Association, Seattle, Wash., 1973 pp. 1–15.

and thorough as conceivable. A list of the problems that are assessed by the nurse should be jotted down. The data that describe the family's perceptions of problems, their strengths, and their limitations should be included. In securing a history regarding each family member, the nurse should be cognizant of and inquire about risk factors for certain age levels, such as frequency of URIs in infants, accessibility of household poisons for preschool youngsters, susceptibility of school-age children to peer pressures related to drug abuse, diet patterns of middle-aged persons, and medication usage of elderly citizens. As much as possible, the database should be explicit, more so than wordy.

The problem of eliciting a useful database and not acquiring volumes of interesting but irrelevant data is a difficult one for many community health agencies. Some have written guidelines for data considered to be essential; some have devised database sheets for specific health situations which suggest data considered pertinent for various assessments—family, individual, social, and environmental, mental health, antepartum, postpartum, and newborn. Other agencies have allowed the nurse to be the judge of the essentiality of information to be contained in the database regarding the assessed family.

In many instances, the nature of the visit and contract with the family spells out the extent of information recommended for the preliminary database. When episodic care is given, the nurse starts with the problem list which specifies the presenting complaint of the family. To aid in determining how to manage the problem, a minidatabase is secured. In other words, information which is relevant for the specific complaint is collected and carefully analyzed before treatment measures are instituted.

Problem list   A problem is some aspect of the patient that disturbs or endangers health (mental or physical). It is something that requires further attention for diagnosis, treatment, or just observation. A problem list should contain legitimate problems to the patient, for which the nurse has a legitimate plan, for which a legitimate goal has been set, and for which legitimate progress notes can be written. The problem list can contain currently active problems, those which have been resolved, chronic problems, psychological problems socioeconomic problems, and others.

A difficulty that some nurses have in determining a problem list for families is the family's denial that they have problems. Many families reject the word "problem" when it is used to judge their methods for managing activities of daily living. They can accept words like concern, difficulty, or worry, but the word problem conveys the meaning that they are not coping satisfactorily. For many individuals, even though problems are present, it is generally conceded that each person can manage his or her own problems. When the use of the word "problem" is a deterrent to eliciting the concerns of families, use different words which connote less judgmental inferences regarding their current mode of living.

Another difficulty that nurses face in making a problem list is assigning priority to problems according to the way the nurse or family sees them. For many multiproblem families, the nurse is able to make a lengthy and legitimate problem list but the family will not accept a contract with the nurse dealing with the obvious problems, such as lack of immunization for children, unsanitary living conditions, and abusive-type disciplinary measures used with children. Instead, the family will accept a contract which is more satisfactory to their desires such as eliminating the enuresis of a preschool child, getting the children into a headstart or preschool program, and/or securing dental care for the children. Each nurse or agency must determine how problems should be itemized. However, if problems that the family recognizes and accepts are dealt with first, the more obvious ones that are disturbing to the nurse can be managed later as the relationship between family members and nurse develops into one of trust.

Problem assessment and plan formulation   Within the body of the record, the problem is referred to by number or title. Some agencies incorporate the problem assessment and plans within their progress notes. When this is done, each note is dated and signed. Recording is structured to include information classified under the categories of "SOAP" with each progress entry.

S: Subjective data consists of statements or concerns as elicited from the family's point of view. A direct quote conveying the family member's perception of the problem may be helpful.

O: Objective data includes direct physical findings, vital signs, blood pressure readings, behavioral descriptions and observations, and test or screening results if available.

A: Assessment is the nursing diagnosis, a summary statement or conclusions regarding the subjective and objective findings, any changes in the patient's status and prognosis in terms of the identified problem. If the nurse initially is unable to write an assessment in all honesty, then write "Don't know."

P: Plan includes the plan and goal for each problem and can be written in behavioral terminology if this seems helpful for the nurse. The plan can be written in several different contexts, depending upon the status and nature of the problem. It can be immediate plans related to the problem, a plan for collecting further information and data, a plan for outlining a specific methodology or initiated procedure, a plan for educating the family as to the nature and management of the problem, a plan for measuring the progress of the family in terms of follow-up of an implementation, or a plan for stating an intent to refer to an appropriate resource. Short range plans can be variable and recorded from visit to visit.

Progress notes and flow sheets Depending upon the requirements of the agency, progress notes are incorporated with the problem assessment and plans, or they are written separately. Each progress note must be dated and signed. Each problem does not have to be written about unless important changes have taken place. For rapidly developing problems, a flow sheet is used to display data of a progressive nature, such as a graphic display of TPR, B. P., fluid intake and output, or a tabular display of medication self-administration, listing of nutritional intake, or fulfillment of task assignments.

Summary reports should be written in the progress notes in "SOAP" fashion at periodic intervals. These reports should summarize all pertinent factors related to a problem, the actions taken, interpretation of flow sheet information, the outcome, and the plans for the future.

The problem-oriented record system is a tool which facilitates evaluation of services given. Problems, plans, implementation of nursing services, flow sheet data, evidence of progress or lack of it, consistency of services, resolution or nonresolution of problems—all contribute information evaluating the efficacy of nursing intervention with a family.

Other factors to remember when recording When a correction is necessary, the nurse lines out the erroneous statement, writing the correct statement below it and initialing it. The confidentiality of patient and family records must be maintained at all times. As in the hospital, the community health record is considered a legal document and, as such, is subject to court order. Elements of good record keeping include accuracy, conciseness, legibility, promptness, and the use of standard abbreviations only.

The appropriate use of the patient and family record enables the nursing staff to provide continuity of nursing care. Because of vacation relief, emergencies, and staff absences, it is not always possible for the same nurse to visit the patient each time. However, a clear, concise, and accurate record, always complete to date, makes it possible for a different nurse to make an effective home call without disturbing the sense of security the patient had in the former nurse or interfering with the general relationship between the agency and family.

The community health nursing record is used frequently as a supervisory tool. It is helpful to both supervisor and staff nurse to review it from time to time in order to trace the nurse's growth and development and to determine where she may need additional help in her work with families. The agency also reviews the records as a basis for program planning and in consideration of budgetary needs.

When visual aids have been used during the visit, the name of the pamphlet or guide should be given, either underlined or in quotes. This will help in the planning for future visits by the nurse or another staff member who assumes the responsibility for the case load. It is frustrating to a nurse who has selected a pamphlet for use in teaching to be told during the visit, "The other nurse brought me that last time."

In recording her plans for the next visit, the nurse notes what she believes the family will be ready to accept and carry out. The plan should include a memorandum to see how much and how well the patient and family learned from the teaching done at the previous visit and how they have been able to use what they learned. The plan may include calling the physician for additional orders and listing teaching aids that might be helpful.

There is a difference of opinion among agencies as to the most appropriate time for staff nurses to write their records. Some agencies wish the nurse to complete the records before leaving the home; others prefer to have this done immediately following the visit but not in the home; still others wish the recording to be done either at the end of the day or on the following morning before the nurse goes to her district. Some agencies, particularly in rural areas, provide tape recorders or dictaphones to be used by the nurse following her visit.

In summary, skillfully written records to ensure continuity of agency contact and nursing service must be accurate, complete, concise, and promptly done as is shown in Table 6-4. They should include a data-

Table 6-4 Sample Recording

Database of B. _____ F. _____. Age—25 years

Subjective	"I want to lose weight. I'm trying not to eat candy and potato chips. I have been drinking diet pop but I'm not losing any weight. I snack a lot, particularly at night".		
Objective	Height:	5'2″	Eats three meals a day.
	Weight:	189 lbs	An alert and active young woman
	Temperature:	Not taken	who does no prescribed exercises.
	Pulse	72 reg.	Has not had a P. E. for a year.
	Respiration:	20	
	Blood Pressure:	130/82	
Assessment	Overweight woman who seems committed to losing weight. Financial resources limited.		

Table 6-4 (*Continued*)

Database of B. _____ F. _____. Age—25 years

Plan	Pt. to visit local clinic for P.E. Pt. will keep food diary for one week. Request consultation from dietitian and ask about low cost foods. Return in one week. T.K., PHN

Problem list

Date	Number	Problem	Date resolved
7/7/76	1	B. wants to lose weight	

Progress notes

7/15/76	No. 1	S:	"I was shocked when I saw how many slices of bread I eat. Keeping a food diary was not easy!"
		O:	Diet high In carbohydrates.
Weight:	89½ lbs		Supplements with a candy bar almost every day.
Bust:	38"		Takes second helpings.
Waist:	30"		Eats 6-8 slices of bread a day.
Hips:	40"		T.C. to clinic re. P.E.—Normal findings. OK for Pt. to lose weight.
		A:	Recording of food diary complete for one week. Pt. good candidate for weight reduction.
		P:	Pt. willing to eliminate candy bars and second helpings for one week. Will snack on carrot sticks. Pt. will exercise daily for ten minutes: was given some simple exercises to do. Will weigh and measure Pt. every week. Goal: lose 8 lbs in a month. T.K., PHN
7/22/76	No. 1	S:	"I didn't eat any candy, but I don't think I lost any weight. I simply cannot eat another carrot stick!"
		O:	Kept food diary voluntarily for a second week.
Weight:	188 lbs		No candy.
Bust:	37½"		Exercised every day.
Waist:	30"		Pleased with loss of 1½ lbs
Hips:	40"		Recipes given for low cost, low calorie meals.
		A:	Pt. follows through well with suggestions. Has a good chance for reaching her goal.
		P:	Pt. to continue same regime. Will snack on celery sticks and eat less bread. Pt. willing to replace diet pop with water. Show food diary to dietitian and request suggestions. Weigh and measure in one week. T.K., PHN

base, an up-to-date problem list, progress notes written according to the "SOAP" categories, the plan for the next visit, the signature of the nurse, and the current date. The same principles apply in writing referrals, memorandums, and letters to professional workers in other agencies.

THE NURSING PROCESS: EVALUATING

Evaluating the intervention of a community health nurse with an individual or family requires careful appraisal of the nurse's performance and behavior and the individual's and family's responses in terms of a temporarily or permanently changed mode of behavior. The nurse constantly must be watchful for evidences of change in individual or family behavior as an index that her plan of nursing care is indeed of value and beneficial to the patient and family. If she decides that her implementation approach is not showing any desired effects based on her appraisal of the patient's response, she frequently will change her plan of care in hopes that a new approach will produce clues indicating a desired change of response or behavior on the part of the patient or family. If the nurse accepts the fact that evaluation is an ongoing activity that is constantly present in every phase of the nursing process, she realizes how crucial her evaluative skills must be in order to intervene effectively with a patient or family.

Evaluation involves measuring behavior and interpreting the results in terms of the desired behavior change—which is complicated by the fact that all such measurement contains error.[52] Since the purpose of evaluation is to predict how the individual or family will behave in the future, it is necessary to use as many measurements of behavior as are feasible. Some current evaluative methods available for nurses in community health nursing include direct observation of patient behavior by means of tangible results or attainment of desired goals, questionnaires or rating scales designed to elicit opinions or attitudes of consumers regarding effectiveness of health services, anecdotal notes jotted down on a sequential basis by the nurse, process recording or tape recording of interactions on an intermittent basis, or written family analyses. By making use of combinations of several measuring tools, an evaluation of the results of the nursing intervention tends to be more reliable. As yet, there are too few measurement tools for determining the effectiveness of nursing intervention with patients and families. Many complex factors contribute to behavior change and the endeavor to evaluate the effect of nursing intervention alone is elusive.

[52]Barbara Klug Redman, *The Process of Patient Teaching in Nursing,* The C. V. Mosby Company, St. Louis, 1968, p. 106.

Observation of Behavior

Direct observation of the patient's change of behavior or attainment of desired goals is easy in some instances but not always possible for all situations. For example, when a patient loses twenty pounds and maintains the weight loss according to the plan of care, this result represents successful accomplishment of a desired goal and tangible evidence of a change. When a mother of a family accepts a suggestion by the nurse to perform a prescribed task consistently and several weeks later exhibits the change of behavior on a routine, casual basis, this observation may be taken as evidence of successful learning by the mother. Sometimes a sensitive observation of the patient's behavior, attitude, or action will reveal clues to the nurse alerting her to think about the effectiveness of her approach. An example is cited as written by a nursing student:

> At first I thought it very easy to see what were the needs of this family. As a community health nurse, I saw my roles to be very obvious. I saw myself helping the mother to get appointments for herself and the children for their medical care. I also saw my role to be one of a health teacher, especially to the mother concerning her condition. I began to do these things. My first two or three visits were dedicated to carrying out these objectives. Mrs. S. would listen very patiently to everything I said. She would promise to make appointments for herself and the children. However, after three visits, I evaluated my progress and found that I was really getting nowhere. I would encourage her to make appointments, which she would do, but I found that most of them she was unable to keep for a variety of reasons. Actually, other than a medical check-up for Sammy, I had accomplished nothing.
>
> It was at this point that I realized that my diagnosis and plan were all wrong. I was looking at the family from my point of view, which was that of an inexperienced community health nurse. I also realized that I had placed my values on what should be done and what was not necessary. I saw that although we had developed somewhat of a good relationship, I was not meeting Mrs. S's needs as she saw them. So in my future visits, I decided to sit and listen to her and find out what her needs were. I knew it was vital that she realize my interest and concern not only in her health problems but also in the family and its relationships. Mrs. S saw her family's two main problems to be marital and financial. Health problems were secondary. She felt the need to talk with someone about these problems because she knew so few people in whom she could confide.

When the nurse feels that observation of behavior change in the individual or family is insufficient or intangible, she can make use of other measurement tools.

Questionnaires or Rating Scales

Brief questionnaires or rating scales can be used occasionally or on an intermittent basis to elicit the opinions or attitudes of consumers about

Table 6-5

---

1 I always learn something new about health when the nurse comes to visit me. ☐ yes   ☐ no
2 It helps me to be able to talk to the nurse about things that concern me.
☐ strongly disagree
☐ disagree
☐ uncertain
☐ agree
☐ strongly agree
3 I would like to talk about the latest ideas in:
☐ low-cost buying
☐ birth control
☐ nutrition
☐ developmental problems of preschool children
☐ Other _____

---

the health services they are receiving or would like to receive. The use of a questionnaire or rating scale differs from a face-to-face oral evaluation by allowing the consumer to respond to questions or statements when the nurse is not present and providing time to think about the questions before expressing an honest opinion. The consumer can be requested to mail the completed questionnaire or rating scale to the nurse or to her supervisor or teacher, whichever course of action is desired. Examples of information that the nurse may wish to obtain from the consumer may consist of statements such as those in Table 6-5.

By carefully constructing the statements or questions, the nurse can elicit and receive information and ideas from the consumer regarding attitudes about the health services already experienced or receptivity to more comprehensive health services.

Anecdotal Notes

By jotting down casual notes in a notebook from time to time about observations of the patient or family, specific levels of patient or family activity, attitudes of the patient, family, or nurse, or goals of the patient, family, or nurse, an examination of the notes at prescribed time intervals will frequently reveal minute changes that have occurred over the course of time. All too often as the nurse works with absorbed interest in the patient or family, she forgets the initial assessment of the situation and consequently is unable to determine the changes that have taken place until she is reminded to compare the status of the patient and family with the anecdotal notes written on the first visit. To be able to evaluate changes that have occurred during a specific time period and to realize that she played a role in effecting the change is strengthening to the nurse. If she discusses the changes as demonstrating the patient's or family's progress as revealed through the use of the written anecdotal notes, the patient and family members are also strengthened and motivated positively to continue to work toward desired goals. Anecdotal notes can also be shown to instructors or supervisors as evidence of a patient's or family's progress.

Process Recording—Tape Recording

By doing a process recording or tape recording of an interaction during a visit, the nurse is enabled to evaluate her interpersonal relationship with patients and families by gaining sensitivity to her interviewing skills, her follow-up of cues, her phrasing of questions and statements, and the family's responses. If she elects to do a tape recording of an interaction, she must obtain permission from the patient or family to do so. Frequently, a signed permission form which indicates the patient's or family's willingness for the use of the tape recorder and the purpose for which the interview will be reviewed simplifies the procedure. Many families respond affirmatively to the request to do a tape recording of a visit.

When the nurse chooses to do a process recording of a visit, she must be cognizant of the desirability of writing the content of the interaction as soon as possible. Its value lies in its prompt recording, and therefore it should be written immediately after the visit, as recall of the verbal and nonverbal behavior lessens as the time interval lengthens.

Process recording has been described as a verbatim recording of all recallable verbal and nonverbal communication between the nurse and the patient or family member. The record includes introductory statements describing the family constellation and the purpose of the visit; the verbatim recording of the verbal and nonverbal communication that took place between the nurse and the patient or family member; comments and analysis of feelings the nurse experienced and those she may have noticed on the part of the patient or family member; evaluation and analysis of the interaction that took place during the visit; a summary statement evaluating the visit and making plans and objectives for ensuing visits.

Process recording requires considerable time to write, analyze, and review. To become skillful in the method requires a great deal of effort, practice, and experience on the part of the nurse. Table 6-6 is a form employed by one agency in the use of this method; other agencies use variations of this form.

Family Analysis

The best description of a family analysis was written by a nursing student as follows:

> During a home visit the community health nurse is involved with the nurse-patient interaction to the extent that it is impossible to separate out the different components of the interaction. Often recording of the home visit

Table 6-6

Process Recording Form

Family
Address
Date of Visit
Purpose of Visit
Introduction

Patient-Nurse Verbal and Nonverbal Exchange and Interaction	Nurse's Comments and Analysis

Summary

back at the office does not provide the nurse with insight of the changes that are going on in the family. Webster's definition of *analysis* is an examination of a complex, its elements, and their relations. Thus, a *family analysis* could be defined as an examination of the complex which is a family, the different elements (persons) that compose it, and the relations between the elements.

The value of a family analysis lies in its potential to improve patient care. Through doing a family analysis, the nurse is able to get a grasp on what changes are going on within the family and to see her role in relation to the initiation of support of these changes. It is exciting for the nurse to get this overview of the family to see in what areas she has been effective, how, and what further needs should be concentrated on.

An analysis gives a comprehensive view of the family under study and can be done whenever such a study seems expedient. It requires a thoughtful review of all components of the nursing process, a knowledge in depth of the family, and deliberate study of the effect and direction of the nursing intervention. A guide for writing a family analysis is suggested as follows:

I   Assessment
   A   Identify health factors.
      1   Physical factors.
         a   Chronological age and physical level of growth and development.

      b Past and present physical problems.
      c Special physical abilities.
      d Utilization of medical resources.
      e Nutritional status.
   2 Mental factors.
      a Achievement in school.
      b Ability to solve problems.
      c Presence of sense of humor.
      d Special mental abilities
      e Sense of self-esteem.
   3 Social-cultural factors.
      a Nationality and cultural influences.
      b Religious beliefs.
      c Interaction with family members.
      d Dominant attitudes toward health, education, and life.
      e Child-rearing skills.
   4 Environmental factors.
      a Characteristics and atmosphere of home, car, and neighborhood.
      b Safety hazards.
      c Attitude of community toward family.
      d Beauty in environment.
   5 Socioeconomic factors.
      a Annual income of breadwinner.
      b Occupation and employment of family members.
      c Management of money.
 B What are the interfamily relationships?
   1 What are the dynamics?
      a Interactional style of communication of family.
      b Decision-making skills.
      c Relationship of family members in seriousness and in fun.
   2 What are the strengths?
II Nursing diagnosis
 A Identify the needs of the patient or family which were focused upon. List them in order of priority. Were the family members in agreement with these needs?
 B State the contract that the family and nurse made mutually.
III Nursing plan and implementation
 A Describe your plan of action to fulfill the contract.
 B What was your rationale for the plan? State nursing principles or theories used as a basis for your actions.
IV Evaluation
 A What demonstrated fulfillment of the contract? How has the family indicated that they have achieved a higher level of health?

TERMINATING WITH FAMILIES

Many nursing students recognize that separating or terminating with families is difficult and sometimes traumatic for the family and for the nurse. When a caring, therapeutic relationship has evolved in which family and nurse trust each other, have seen and taken joy in distinct progress, and feel a genuine impending distress when the time for terminating arrives, an open talk about the feelings of both parties must take place. For many families, separation by the nurse means rejection— regardless of how well it is explained. For many nurses, it is hard to "give up" a family with whom one has worked effectively and seen excellent results. By sharing her own feelings openly, the nurse encourages family members to speak openly and creates the opportunity for explanations of the termination process. Nurses can maintain a friendly relationship with families if they so desire by sending birthday cards, accepting special invitations, and/or occasionally engaging in friendly pursuits. However, the professional relationship in which the nurse was assisting the family toward accomplishment of desired goals must be terminated and released for the next nurse to carry on. Explanation of the difference between friendly and professional relationships must be explained understandably and acceptably to the family.

In the final analysis, all relationships with significant persons have a beginning, a maintenance period, and an ending. Families and nurses must learn to give and to "release" when growth has reached a maturity that helping is no longer indicated. For nursing students, the termination frequently occurs *before* the family's growth has stabilized. In this instance the nursing student must trust that the next nurse will carry on the program with the family. In order to ensure the probability, she must discuss her contract with the family, the implementation of plans, and evaluation of results with the family and with the succeeding nurse. If the family and the succeeding nurse are prepared properly, continuity can be carried on and adjustments made, even though the next nurse is a different person from the first one. It is helpful for the succeeding nurse, who has already been informed and is prepared to deal with the family, to request and listen to the family's explanation of their situation, their interpretation of the helpfulness of the services of the previous nurse, and their sense of accomplishment regarding their growth. In so doing, acceptance is communicated and the new relationship is facilitated.

SUMMARY

Working with families is most easily done by a visit, either in the home or in another convenient setting. The components that must be considered in all visits include activities such as preparation for the visit, meeting the family, setting up an agreeable contract with the family, assessing, planning, implementing, evaluating, and recording. The objective of the nurse is consistently directed toward assisting the family to advance toward wellness.

Assessing the needs of the patient or family is a continuous process, during which flexibility and willingness to redirect goals in keeping with the family's desires are essential. Use of assessment tools is important to confirm the accuracy of nurses' perceptions. Planning the nursing intervention includes the determination of methodology and techniques required to meet the assessed and distinctive needs of the patient and family. Some methods that can be used with families, dependent upon their needs, include the behavior modification approach, the family therapy approach, the transactional analysis approach, the parent effectiveness training approach, the epidemiologic approach, and the paradoxical communication approach. Implementing the plan of care consists of taking action to meet the assessed need. By taking action, the nurse must be aware of the elements influencing behavior during the change process and stress and crisis periods. She must be cognizant of factors affecting the referral process. Evaluating the implementation of a plan consists of determining outcomes in terms of success and family and nurse satisfaction. Evaluation is an ongoing activity, which can be measured and judged by the use of various methods. Some suggested evaluative techniques include direct observation of patient and family behavior, utilization of questionnaires or rating scales, writing anecdotal notes, doing process recordings or tape recordings, and writing family analyses. Recording the nursing activities of the visit succinctly on the appropriate record form completes and summarizes the nursing process.

SUGGESTED READING

Aradine, Carolyn R., and Margaret Guthneck: "The Problem-Oriented Record in a Family Health Service," *American Journal of Nursing,* 74(6):1108–1112, June 1974.

Atwood, Judith, and Stephen R. Yarnall: "The Problem-Oriented Record," *The Nursing Clinics of North America,* 9(2):215–302, June 1974.

Auerbach, Aline B.: *Parents Learn through Discussion,* John Wiley & Sons, Inc., New York, 1968.

Austin, Barbara Leslie: *Sad Nun at Synanon,* Holt, Rinehart and Winston, Inc., New York, 1970.

Axline, Virginia M.: *Dibs, In Search of Self,* Houghton Mifflin Company, Boston, 1964.

Bach, George R., and Peter Wyden: *The Intimate Enemy,* William Morrow & Company, Inc., New York, 1968.

Barnard, Kathryn: "Teaching the Retarded Child Is a Family Affair," *American Journal of Nursing,* 68(2):305–311, February 1968.

Bates, Barbara, and Robert A. Hoekelman: *A Guide to Physical Examination,* J. B. Lippincott Company, Philadelphia, 1974.

Becker, Wesley: *Parents Are Teachers,* Research Press Company, Illinois, 1971.

Bennis, Warren G., Kenneth D. Benne, and Robert Chin: *The Planning of Change,* Holt, Rinehart and Winston, Inc., New York, 1961.

Berne, Eric: *Games People Play,* Grove Press, Inc., New York, 1964.

Berne, Eric: *What Do You Say after You Say Hello?* Grove Press, Inc., New York, 1972.

Blood, Robert O., Jr.: *The Family,* The Free Press, New York, 1972.

Chinn, Peggy L., and Cynthia J. Leitch: *Child Health Maintenance,* The C. V. Mosby Company, St. Louis, 1974.

Committee on Ways and Means, *National Health Insurance Resource Book,* U. S. Government Printing Office, Washington, D. C., 1974.

Ferber, Andrew, Marilyn Mendelsohn, and Augustus Napier: *The Book of Family Therapy,* Houghton Mifflin Company, Boston, 1972.

Fox, John P., Carrie E. Hall, and Lila R. Elveback: *Epidemiology: Man and Disease,* The Macmillan Company, New York, 1970.

Gersh, Marvin J.: *How to Raise Children at Home in Your Spare Time,* Fawcett Publications, Inc., Greenwich, Conn., 1966.

Ginott, Haim, G.: *Between Parent and Child,* The Macmillan Company, New York, 1965.

Glasser, William: *Reality Therapy,* Harper & Row, Publishers, Incorporated, New York, 1965.

Goldsborough, Judith: "Involvement," *American Journal of Nursing,* 69(1):66–69, January 1969.

Gordon, Thomas: *Parent Effectiveness Training,* Peter H. Wyden, Inc., Publisher, New York, 1970.

Haley, Jay: *Uncommon Therapy,* W. W. Norton & Company, Inc., New York, 1973.

Harris, Thomas A.: *I'm Ok—You're Ok,* Harper & Row, Publishers, Incorporated, New York, 1969.

Holmes, Thomas H., and R. H. Rahe: "The Social Readjustment Rating Scale," *Journal of Psychosomatic Research,* 11:213–218, 1967.

James, Muriel, and Dorothy Jongeward: *Born to Win,* Addison-Wesley Publishing Company, Inc., Reading, Mass., 1971.

Konopka, Gisela: *The Adolescent Girl in Conflict,* Prentice-Hall, Inc., Englewood Cliffs, N. J., 1966.

Lair, Jess: *"I Ain't Much, Baby—But I'm All I've Got,"* Doubleday & Company, Inc., Garden City, New York, 1972.

Langsley, Donald G., and David M. Kaplan,: *The Treatment of Families in Crisis,* Grune & Stratton, Iec., New York, 1968.

Levine, Myra E.: "The Pursuit of Wholeness," *American Journal of Nursing,* 69(1):93–98, January 1969.

Lippitt, Ronald, Jeanne Watson, and Bruce Westley: *The Dynamics of Planned Change,* Harcourt Barce Jovanovich, Inc., New York, 1958.

Mager, Robert F., and Peter Pipe: *Analyzing Performance Problems,* Fearon Publishers, Belmont, Calif., 1970.

Marram, Gwen, D., "Patients' Evaluation of Their Care—Importance to the Nurse," *Nursing Outlook,* 21(5):322–324, May 1973.

Menninger, Karl: *The Vital Balance,* The Viking Press, Inc., New York, 1963.

Minuchin, Salvador: *Families and Family Therapy,* Harvard University Press, Cambridge, Mass., 1974.

Montagu, Ashley: *Touching,* Columbia University Press, New York, 1971.

Murray, Ruth, and Judith Zentner: *Nursing Concepts for Health Promotion,* Prentice-Hall, Inc., Englewood Cliffs, N. J., 1975.

Murray, Ruth, and Judith Zentner: *Nursing Assessment and Health Promotion through the Life Span,* Prentice-Hall, Inc., Englewood Cliffs, N. J., 1975.

Nierenberg, Gerard I., and Henry H. Calero: *How to Read a Person Like a Book,* Pocket Books, New York, 1971.

Oelbaum, Cynthia Hastings, "Hallmarks of Adult Wellness," *American Journal of Nursing,* 74(9):1623–1625, September 1974.

Parad, Howard J. (ed.): *Crisis Intervention: Selected Readings,* Family Service Association of America, New York, 1965.

Patterson, Gerald R.: *Families: Applications of Social Learning to Family Life,* Research Press Company, Illinois, 1971.

Phaneuf, Maria C.: *The Nursing Audit: Profile for Excellence,* Appleton-Century-Crofts, Inc., New York, 1972.

Raush, Harold L., William A. Barry, Richard K. Kertel, and Mary Ann Swain: *Communication, Conflict and Marriage,* Jossey-Bass Publishers, San Francisco, 1974.

Samuels, Mike, and Hal Bennett: *The Well Body Book,* Random House/Bookworks, New York, 1973.

Satir, Virginia: *Conjoint Family Therapy,* Science and Behavior Books, Inc., Palo Alto, Calif., 1967.

Seedor, Marie M.: *The Physical Assessment,* Teachers College Press, New York, 1974.

Schutz, William C.: *Here Comes Everybody,* Harper & Row, Publishers, Incorporated, New York, 1971.

Sommer, Robert: *Personal Space,* Prentice-Hall, Inc., Englewood Cliffs, N. J., 1969.

Wright, Beatrice A.: *Physical Disability—A Psychological Approach,* Harper & Row, Publishers, Incorporated, New York, 1960.

Wu, Ruth: *Behavior and Illness,* Prentice-Hall, Inc., Englewood Cliffs, N.J., 1973.

Yura, Helen, and Mary B. Walsh: *The Nursing Process: Assessing, Planning, Implementing, and Evaluating,* The Catholic University of America Press, Washington, 1967.

Chapter 7

Working with Groups

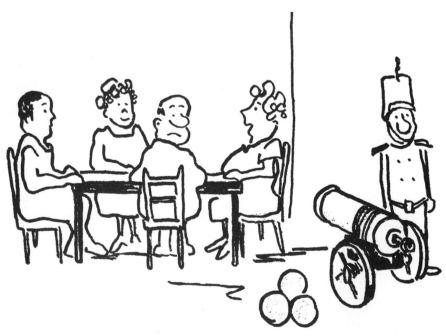

"Because of the poor attendance at our recent meetings I'd like to propose an additional amendment to the committee bylaws . . ."

With reduction of home visits which have been primarily directed toward health education and preventive health practices, community health nurses have started utilizing group approaches to reach consumers who want to learn more about content of a specific nature. In a study of McNeil and Holland, it was found that the cost of nurses serving as leaders of groups of postpartum mothers was one-third less per contact than each nurse making home visits to a comparable number of mothers.[1] The cost economy of working with groups is recognized. The added advantages of group work include the support that members give one another, the sharing of ideas and experiences, increased problem-solving capabilities and stimulation of ideas, improved reality testing, greater awareness of the universality of common problems, increased understanding and sensitivity toward others, and opportunity to test new behavior with limited consequences coming from other members of the group.

Community health nurses are learning that group work is an efficient means for facilitating growth of all consumers with whom they come in contact, for giving health education, for teaching about prevention, treatment, and rehabilitation, and for meeting other consumer needs and problems. As nurses become increasingly comfortable and confident in leading or facilitating groups, they can reach out and encourage many more people with common problems to come together to grow, learn, combine forces, give support, and resolve problems. "Nurses must know what benefits can be expected from group experiences and how to intervene in a meaningful therapeutic manner to ensure that these benefits are operant for the individuals in groups."[2] Consequently, nurses must actively seek experiences in group work, and take advantage of the vast opportunities in the community for groups of many kinds, such as prenatal, weight-watching, relaxation, mental health, child discipline, special disease conditions, geriatric, discussion, and many other groups. The opportunity for the nurse to be truly creative is potentially inherent in community group work.

The community health nurse generally has a range of membership in different professional groups such as staff, team, or in-service education meetings in agencies and multidisciplinary meetings with persons from other professions. However, she should become much more involved in community health meetings in which many of the participating members are lay people or nonprofessional representatives. By attending these

---

[1] Helen Jo McNeil and Susan Spangler Holland, "A Comparative Study of Public Health Nurse Teaching in Groups and in Home Visits," *American Journal of Public Health*, **62**(12):1629–1637, December 1972.

[2] From Gwen D. Marram, *The Group Approach in Nursing Practice*, The C. V. Mosby Company, Saint Louis, 1973, p. 5.

meetings, she will be exposed to a variety of people with a variety of expectations. She must know *why* she is a member of the group and what is to be her role and purpose. Specifically, a group may be defined as a plurality of individuals who are in contact with one another, who take one another into account, and who are aware of some significant commonality. It is essential that members have something in common and that they believe that what they have in common makes a difference.[3] Olmsted stated that there are two groups, primary and secondary. Primary groups are composed of members who are warm, intimate, and have personal ties with each other. They are usually of a small, face-to-face sort, spontaneous in their interpersonal behavior, and often have common goals. The family, gang, or friendship groups are examples. Generally a primary group is "fun," brings enjoyment of some kind, and functions in a training or supportive capacity. Secondary groups are made up of persons who are apt to be impersonal, rational, contractual, and formal. Members of these groups participate in special capacities and not necessarily as whole personalities. The groups are gathered together as a means to some end and have only intermittent contacts. Examples include a range of associations which include professional, office, community, or bureaucratic interests.[4] It is membership and functioning in secondary or community groups for which the nurse needs to become knowledgeable.

Problems in Entering a New Group[5]

When the nurse enters a new group, whether it is a professional or a community group, she is faced with four issues which must be resolved before she can be comfortable. The first is that of *identity.* She must decide on a role with which she is comfortable and which is acceptable with the group. What role should I play that is acceptable to me and to the group? The choices include that of an aggressive talker who wants to gain attention, a quiet listener who avoids all risks, a logical thinker who asks pertinent questions, the obstructionist who finds fault with all suggestions, the humorous person who gives a "light touch" to the conversation at appropriate times, and any number of other possible roles. The second issue involves *control, power,* and *influence.* Who are the persons in the group with the most power and control? Which individuals will influence me or vice versa? Therefore, initial group dialogue may be characterized

[3]Michael S. Olmsted, *The Small Group*, Random House, Inc., New York, 1959, pp. 21–22.

[4]Ibid., pp. 17–19.

[5]Adapted from Edgar H. Schein, *Process Consultation: Its Role in Organization Development*, Addison-Wesley Publishing Company, Inc., Reading, Mass., 1969, pp. 32–37.

by individuals' testing and experimenting with different forms of influence until they feel acquainted and have come to terms with the basic structure of the group. *Individual needs* and *group goals* are the third issue with which the group member is concerned. Will the group goals be such that my own personal goals are met? Can I be committed to work toward a group goal if my own need is not attended to? In many groups where group goals are decided but little action evolves, the explanation often lies in the fact that the group's needs as a whole were not requested or discussed; therefore, little member commitment was obtained. Early in a meeting group members often take a "wait and see" attitude until the direction of group activity develops, which reveals that personal interests will be met in some way. Then the members get on the bandwagon. The fourth issue that concerns the new member is *acceptance* and *intimacy*. Will I be liked and accepted by others in the group? Can I be comfortable and respectful of the others? Is the environment conducive to formal or informal behavior?

With respect to the four issues involved in entering a new group, there are generally three basic kinds of coping patterns which the membership of the group demonstrate. They are (1) the basically tough, aggressive coping, which is characterized by arguing, cutting down another's points, deliberate ignoring of others, or barbed humor. These behaviors may be manifested in an open, assertive manner or in a subtle, polite manner. Members who are resisting the authority or chairman of the group can demonstrate aggressive coping by setting up the situation with "Let's find out what the chairman wants and then *not* do it." (2) The basically tender, support-seeking coping is demonstrated by those members who try to form an alliance with another group member or who avoid conflict by being supportive of each other. Their support may be based on genuine understanding or a blindly dependent response to the person in authority, to whom they look for guidance or solution of their problems. (3) The withdrawal behavior based on denial of any feelings is characterized by the passive, indifferent kind of response. The attitude of these group members is that feelings are inappropriate in a group discussion, and they withdraw when feelings become apparent. They let others fight an issue while they sit blandly on the sidelines. However, feelings *are* a reality, and until they are brought out into the open, group tasks representative of the entire group cannot be accomplished.

When groups have worked through the four issues described and reached the point where all members realize that they are a contributing part of the group, they begin to relax and are willing to pay closer attention to each other. Their cooperation as a group becomes apparent and they are ready to attend to group tasks.

Content of Group Meetings

When an individual focuses on what the group is talking about, that is *content*. Members of the group may be working toward accomplishing some task or goal which they have established and will demonstrate specific behaviors that facilitate this end. The behaviors which aid in the group's fulfillment of its *task* include the following: (1) *Initiating:* a member proposes a task or goal, succeeds in defining a group problem, suggests an idea for solving the problem, or sets target dates for fulfillment of a task. (2) *Seeking information or opinions:* someone requests facts, asks for an expression of feelings, or seeks suggestions or ideas. (3) *Giving information or opinion:* an individual offers facts, provides information which is relevant to the discussion, or gives suggestions and ideas. (4) *Clarifying and elaborating:* a member attempts to interpret ideas and suggestions in order to clear up confusions, defines terminology, or indicates alternatives open to the group. (5) *Summarizing:* someone pulls together related ideas, restates suggestions more succinctly, reviews points that have already been considered, or offers a conclusion for the group to accept or reject. (6) *Consensus testing:* an individual may ask, "Are we ready to decide?" to test if the group is ready to make a decision.[6]

Behaviors which enable the group to survive, maintain good working relationships, and also permit maximum use of the resources of the members are called maintenance functions. These include the following: (1) *Harmonizing:* a member attempts to reconcile disagreements, reduces tension, or attempts to help people to explore their differences. (2) *Gatekeeping:* someone tries to keep communication channels open or suggests procedures that will permit sharing remarks. (3) *Encouraging:* an individual will maintain friendly, warm responses to others or will indicate acceptance of others' contributions by nonverbal means (nodding, facial expression). (4) *Compromising:* a member whose original idea was not totally acceptable will offer a compromise, may admit an error, or will modify an idea in the interest of group cohesion. (5) *Standard setting and testing:* someone will test whether the group is satisfied with its procedures or will suggest procedures that are available for testing.[7]

In all groups both kinds of behaviors are observed to some degree and are needed in order to get the job done and to keep the group in good working order. As the nurse becomes increasingly familiar with group work, she will be able to identify each behavior as it occurs.

[6]Ibid., pp. 38–40.
[7]Ibid., pp. 40–41.

Group Process

When an individual focuses on how the group is handling its communication, i.e., who talks how much or who talks to whom, that is *group process*. It refers to the "here and now" of what is happening within the group. Many groups do not wish to look at group process because they are reluctant to analyze their own and others' behavior. If individuals do not wish the group process to be studied, it should not be urged. However, if a group is willing to take five or ten minutes at the conclusion of their meeting to discuss *only* the group process as it occurred, it facilitates understanding and openness and promotes cohesion of the group. If group process is to be studied, an observer should be selected whose function is to remain objective and carefully observe the group interaction. When the group is ready to examine and reflect on their process, the observer reports personal observations to the group and discussion ensues. The observer does not provide a summary of the discussion, is free to participate in the discussion, and only reports on *process* that facilitated or inhibited the group.

Leading or Facilitating a Group

All nurses have had exposure to several group theories, such as the interpersonal framework of Sullivan; the communication framework of Watzalawick, Jackson, and Satir; the group dynamics and group process framework of Cartwright and Zander, Knowles and Knowles; the existential and gestalt frameworks of Perls, Maslow, and Rogers. As a result, most nurse leaders possibly have an eclectic theoretical orientation which, if so, is advantageous in providing flexibility and freedom for interventions with groups. If a nurse leader works with a variety of groups in a variety of settings, she has the opportunity to adapt and apply the most suitable theory with the group and intervene at the level of skill and understanding which she has mastered.[8] As she continuously studies and practices groupwork, an understanding of the concepts, principles, and assumptions of each theory becomes internalized and her effectiveness as a leader increases. In many groups the entire responsibility for leadership is expected to be taken by the chairperson. However, if the chairperson wishes to involve all members in any group, he or she can do so. By virtue of their presence in the group, all members can be seen as possessing some degree of responsibility or resourcefulness which must be ferreted out and revealed by the leader. All members ideally need and want to have a commitment toward fulfillment of the task for which the group was organized. Therefore, it is up to the leader to set the stage. Rather than

[8]Marram, op. cit., pp. 123–124.

acting as an authoritarian leader, the leader can consciously act as a *facilitator,* a person who makes sure that the task and process function of the group are carried out effectively. By doing so, the group process moves smoothly and members are reminded to continue moving toward clearly defined and mutually set goals. The leader does not dominate but encourages or facilitates all members of the group to assume responsibility for accomplishing the group goals.[9]

The task of facilitating a group takes preparation and forethought. Some of the factors and questions that must be considered by the leader are:

1. Preparation   Why is this group being formed? Will the members become interested and motivated to work toward purposeful goals? What can I say or do that will "catch" their attention? When the leader prepares for the meeting by thoroughly studying appropriate readings, reference materials, and audiovisual aids, ideas for presenting the material in an interesting and provocative way to group members can be her focus. Sometimes a short, appropriate film or tape recording will be effective or, depending on the group, a game or exercise may be the initial way of "warming up" a group and gaining their attention.[10] The ability of the leader to be resourceful, original, or creative in the beginning enhances the possibility for gaining the group's attention and ultimate commitment.

2. Getting started   What physical set-up will be most conducive to establishing a comfortable environment? Sometimes the chairs are best arranged around a table or in an intimate circle. The environment should be such that the temperature, light, and ventilation are adequate. If a blackboard, charts, or audiovisual apparatus are needed, they should be set up before the meeting begins. The leader should arrange the room so that it communicates the climate intended.

When the group members enter the meeting room, the leader should greet each individual with friendliness and make each feel welcome. When all members are gathered together, the leader should start the meeting by introducing herself and the overall purpose for being together. Time should be taken for all to become acquainted and feel a pleasant friendly atmosphere. An effective method for enabling others to relax and feel free to express their ideas is to state that a way for getting better acquainted is for all members in the group to introduce themselves and tell something about themselves. The leader should always start the introductions with a personal description and whatever information she

[9]Elwin C. Nielsen, "Process Groups for Self-Learning and Problem Solving," (unpublished).
[10]William C. Schutz, *Joy,* Grove Press, Inc., New York, 1967, pp. 117–186.

or he wishes the group to know. Dependent upon the length and extent of the leader's self-introduction will be the contribution of each succeeding member's description of self. Groups tend to conform to the norm established by the leader. If the leader divulges quite a bit of appropriate information, group members will feel more at ease in following the lead and revealing pertinent information about themselves, and general group comfort will be facilitated. Sometimes, it is a good idea to have name cards until the members are well acquainted.

3. *Purpose and objectives*   The general purpose for which the group was formed should then be expressed or reiterated by the leader, and the plan to involve the members should be executed, whether it is a game, a film, or something deliberately provocative. When the time arrives for the group members to discuss, react, or present their thoughts, the leader should ask for an expression of ideas and *facilitate* discussion from that time on. The facilitator's task involves (1) getting an expression of ideas from all members, (2) keeping the conversation centered on the issues of the meeting, (3) promoting the establishing of objectives or goals that are agreeable to all members, (4) encouraging the divulgence of each member's resources or skills, (5) promoting a commitment to the group's goals by all the members. When words or terminology are not clear, the facilitator can ask group members for clarification. If the members of the group expect the facilitator to solve an issue, she or he can return it to the group by rephrasing or reinterpreting the issue at stake. At periodic intervals summarizing statements of the discussion or important points can be phrased for the purpose of clarifying the progress of the discussion. Tolerance, patience, open-mindedness, and flexibility are important for successful meetings. As all persons in the group are encouraged to speak their ideas, thoughts are formulated and crystallized, are spread to others contagiously, and the group inevitably progresses toward new, sometimes exciting conclusions. By being willing to hear different viewpoints expressed, a flexibility and open-mindedness is facilitated and each member learns.

4. *Concluding the meeting*   The facilitator must be aware of the passage of time and stay within the scheduled limits. It may be advisable to warn the group that only five or ten minutes are remaining. Or the facilitator may summarize the progress of the discussion and ask "What have we decided to do?"; "Have we included everything?"; "What assignments or tasks do we need to do before the next meeting?" or "When shall we meet again?" If all members have participated verbally in the issues of the meeting or have demonstrated nonverbal interest, there will be a general aura of purposeful activity and involvement that denotes a successful meeting.

Criteria for Group Growth

To determine if the group is developing into an effective, workable unit which functions smoothly, the following questions can be asked and cogitated upon:

1 Does the group have the capacity to deal realistically with its tasks?
2 Is there basic agreement within the group about ultimate goals and values?
3 Does the group have a capacity for self-knowledge?
4 Is there an optimum use of the resources available within the group?
5 Does the group learn from its experience? Can it assimilate new information and respond flexibly to it?[11]

A successful and satisfying group is one in which all members participate and assume responsibility for functioning in an integrated fashion. Facilitation of such a group is a stimulating learning experience for the leader. The composition of the group does not affect the process of leading or facilitating a group. Professional groups or community groups can be facilitated by a skillful leader who consciously draws out the resourcefulness of the members, whether they have lay, nonprofessional, or professional identities. Much of what happens in groups can be attributed to the leadership, particularly if it is creative and flexible.

COMMUNITY GROUPS

Multiple groups exist in communities and can be studied from a variety of perspectives, depending on the nature of the group. Marram has identified and described the characteristics of several community groups; the ones of special interest to community health nurses include the therapeutic groups, self-help groups, growth groups, and reference groups. Other community groups with whom community health nurses are acquainted are community action groups, in-service training groups, and others.

Therapeutic Groups

Therapeutic groups are concerned with promoting emotional health and educating individuals to adjust as normally as possible to situational and developmental crises. These groups are made up of essentially "normal" people who are in need of primary prevention measures and education. They are faced with a particular crisis and can profit from learning about more satisfactory methods of coping. Community therapeutic groups are

[11]Schein, op. cit., pp. 61–63.

made up of individuals with special interests, common problems, or developmental similarities, such as juvenile delinquents, elderly persons, mothers and children, school-age children, individuals with concern for mental health, family services, chronic diseases or diagnoses, rehabilitation, cultural deprivation, and similar groups.[12]

Self-help Groups

Self-help groups are "organized and operated by group members themselves without the supervision, guidance, or leadership of professionally trained group leaders." They "solve problems of members as defined by members." They are "groups of, for, and by the client."[13] Benefits in belonging to a self-help group include support and empathic understanding from others, an impetus to change which is promoted through the use of role models who have successfully changed their life-style, and a knowledge of how to "work the system" from role models who have incorporated the essentialities required of the new life-style or environment. Examples of self-help groups are numerous and reveal the effectiveness of peer or consumer supportive systems which is not gained through other means. Successful self-help groups include Alcoholics Anonymous, Alanon groups, Parents Anonymous, Synanon, Weight Watchers, T.O.P.S., Ostomy groups (colostomy, laryngectomy, etc.), Recovery, Inc., and many others.[14]

Growth Groups

Growth groups were designed originally "to help learners incorporate the values of (participatory) democracy into their own processes of personal and collective decision making and problem-solving."[15] Emphasis on experimentation, feedback, and collective deliberation continues to be promoted in an environment which is purposely democratically free and permissive. Goals of growth groups are of an educative or therapeutic nature relating to self-awareness, self-discovery, self-enhancement, and self-actualization. Many groups directly or indirectly aim toward increasing members' ability to achieve greater skill and insights so that "take-home" knowledge will be synthesized into greater effectiveness on the job. In growth groups, the opportunity and freedom to express oneself in new ways is frequently experienced with immediate feedback from the group participants. Members often become aware of inhibitions and innate hidden capacities and gain greater sensitivity regarding their ability to relate with others. The benefits of growth groups for all participants are

[12]Marram, op. cit., pp. 24–36.
[13]Ibid., p. 39.
[14]Ibid., pp. 39–53.
[15]Ibid., p. 55.

not easily identifiable or documented. Individual reports can be found reflecting both pro and con attitudes regarding the practices of such groups. Examples of growth groups are rampant. They include T groups, sensitivity training, group dynamics, encounter, marathon, human potentiality, self- and body awareness, assertiveness training, and many, many others.[16]

Reference Groups

Reference groups designate groups which are real or imaginary and serve to influence the individual regarding perception and judgment of others, objectives, and principles which occur within his or her life sphere. As a member of a reference group, the individual behaves according to a perception of the real or anticipated beliefs and values of that group. Reference groups include religious, racial, ethnic, familial, and occupational groups. The individual can be responsive to several reference groups, but often will utilize one group in particular for evaluating behavior. Reference groups can change as the individual grows and develops through the total life process. " 'Membership' in a reference group involves a vague, yet all-encompassing identification with others in the group."[17] The individual uses reference groups as a pervasive influence throughout life and allows them to play an important role in a concept of self. It is through the eyes of referent others that a person determines who he or she is and what he or she should do.

People can be active participants of a group, but it will not be a reference group for them until they allow the group to decide for them about goals worth seeking, the manner in which to proceed, and the values and standards worth attaining. Reference groups provide individuals with positive sources of identification and security and play a role in formulating distinct identities. They give individuals a sense of belonging, a continuity and sameness with the outside world which is like others in the group but, at the same time, provide a sense of autonomy and separateness as a distinct member. Reference groups can be classified in two ways in terms of their effect on members. They can be constructive or destructive· for individuals in influencing identity formation, role adjustment, and self-concept.

Destructive reference group affiliations divide the self, instill a low self-esteem, or cause an imbalance in the satisfaction of needs for homonymy and autonomy. "Certain ethnic, racial, occupational, and religious groups have acquired a negative image in our society. Being a

[16]Ibid., pp. 55–72.
[17]Ibid., p. 75.

member of these groups elicits certain prejudices from others."[18] In Chap. 5, an explanation of identity conflicts for some ethnic minorities is explored. Constructive reference group memberships assist individuals in integrating self-perceptions, affording a balance of autonomy and homonymy, and increasing self-esteem. Members of constructive group affiliations experience feelings of knowing who they are, where they are going, and suffering few self-doubts. They are goal directed, self-assured, and self-directive. They are frequently leaders in the community.[19]

ROLE OF THE NURSE LEADER

A frequent goal of nurses who are leaders of groups "is to foster the development of the group as a whole and to enhance the growth of individuals in the group."[20] This is true particularly of therapeutic and growth groups. For self-help groups, nurses should know about them and be supportive of them. They should not expect to be members of such groups unless they are experiencing the problems common to the specified group. If called in as a consultant, they should elicit the desires of the group asking for assistance and provide information or resources as requested. Knowledge about the influence and identification of reference groups in the lives of individuals serves to broaden the assessment perspective of nurses and aids in understanding the basis for some observed behaviors.

In facilitating a climate that is nonthreatening and growth-producing for members of a group, the nurse must be knowledgeable about group dynamics, sensitive to the meaning of body language, perceptive of the behavior of each member of the group, confident in directing the activities of the group, capable in moving the group toward its stated objectives, neutral in the event an argument occurs, supportive of positive contributions or changes of behavior that occur with individual group members who are visibly anxious, knowledgeable about specific content if acting as a resource person, reinforcing of the group's successful activities, and aware of timing for summarizing and concluding meetings. For nurses who wish to become effective group leaders, frequent practice with groups must be sought, even though inner self-confidence and assurance is hesitant. The composition of all groups is different, regardless of the type of group, and learnings gained in acting as a group leader are invaluable and contribute toward development of seasoned leadership characteristics.

[18]Ibid., p. 80.
[19]Ibid., pp. 75–84.
[20]Ibid., p. 193.

CO-LEADING GROUPS

For nurses who feel unprepared to assume complete responsibility for leading a group, the option of being a co-leader is often available. A co-leader can be in the position of a subordinate to a professional leader who is recognized as having theoretical knowledge and expertise, or the co-leader can have an equal participatory role with a primary leader and share her knowledge and insights from a perspective different than that of the primary leader. Co-leading combinations are numerous, such as physician, psychologist, or social worker with nurse, male with female, superior with subordinate.

Advantages found for the nurse who engages in co-leading with a professional leader are dependent upon her needs and capabilities. Learning takes place when the expertise, technical abilities, and theoretical knowledge of the professional leader are observed and critically analyzed. Group participants are enabled to observe interactions between the master teacher and learner and translate the meaning of the behavior in terms applicable to their own situations. Opportunity for role-playing or simulating a dyad can be used for learning purposes. When she is ready, the learner co-leader can assume primary responsibility for leading the group under the supervision of the professional leader. Analyses of group process, interactions, behaviors, and decisions can be studied and discussed evaluatively following group sessions.

For the nurse who elects to co-lead on a participatory equal basis with the designated leader, experience is gained in learning to work together cooperatively. Goals, procedures, process for intervening, interrupting, and making decisions must be mutually understood between the two leaders before convening the group. With the two leaders, each has an individual perspective in observing group members, encouraging interactions, and providing direction toward the stated purpose of the session. When one leader is interacting with the group, the second leader has the opportunity to observe, actively listen, seize cues as they become apparent, intervene, and give the first leader time to reflect while temporarily relieved of the intense "heat" of responsibility for the direction of the interaction. The manner in which the co-leaders interact with each other whether in agreement or disagreement can be an excellent demonstration for group members to observe and imitate. Open, honest, spontaneous communication can be releasing and therapeutic when demonstrated well. For co-leaders who are a male and female combination, the opportunity for group members to observe instrumental and expressive roles, and modeling of interaction dynamics between a male and female, is beneficial. Also, viewpoints, insights, and supportive statements based on a sexual perspective can be freely expressed by the participatory leader of the same or opposite sex as appropriate within the context of the group discussion. Following group sessions, the two leaders can analyze their theoretical framework and share their thoughts from two perspectives regarding the dynamics that occurred, can give feedback to each other regarding their leadership characteristics and behavior, can mutually evaluate and contribute ideas for future meetings of the group.

Frequently female nurses who co-lead with a male whether from the same or another discipline, tend to be quiet and wait for the male to extend the opportunity to participate before they intervene. As co-leaders, female nurses must practice the experience of taking the initiative and interrupting when they believe the interaction can benefit from such an intervention. Nurses must gain increasing self-assurance as leaders of groups and must practice behaviors that seem initially uncomfortable (aggressive) if they truly desire to become effective group leaders and co-leaders.

GETTING THROUGH TO GROUPS

People behave differently when they are members of a group than when they are alone. Individuals join groups for a variety of reasons and are generally members of several different groups. The motivation to belong to a particular group is apparently related to an individual's sense of isolation. Individuals want to gain the security, economic and socialization advantages, sense of belonging, or sense of strength (since the group is bigger and more powerful and less vulnerable than the individual is) that a group may give. Members are exposed to the group's beliefs, values, jargon, way of dress, and other identifiable characteristics and adopt the group norm on a continuum of complete acceptance to little acceptance according to individual needs.[21] If the acceptance of a particular group is complete, the members sacrifice their own individuality and identity, and frequently are unaware that they have made such a choice. Many individuals have a more moderate commitment to groups, behaving in a given group in relationship to the benefits they derive personally. Some persons reflect the group norm only while in the presence of the group.

With the composition of groups made up of individuals who are either wholly or partially committed, or have hidden motives or personal reasons for belonging, the nurse cannot realistically expect to get through to *all* members of a group. All she can do is try to the best of her ability. When presenting an idea or activity to a group for the purpose of getting

[21]Ernst G. Beier, *The Silent Language of Psychotherapy*, Aldine Publishing Company, Chicago, 1966, pp. 152–154.

them involved, the nurse must accept and/or welcome resistance or opposition. Opposition is a sign of involvement! In order to persuade individuals to accept a new idea or activity, they must pass through a stage of resistance first—that of readjusting or giving up some of their own ideas associated with their current thinking about that subject. When people feel pressured to change their current thinking, some resistance will always be aroused.

There are three levels of listening when someone else is speaking. There is (1) the nonhearing level, where receivers are not listening at all. They may have eye contact with the speaker and give appropriate responses at right intervals such as "I see," "Mm," but their thoughts are elsewhere. (2) There is the level of hearing where individuals remember and are able to repeat the sentences the speaker said; however, there is no real absorption of ideas. (3) There is the level of hearing where listeners *think* about what the speaker is saying. Thinking means doing mental work—evaluating, comparing the thought with something else, analyzing, predicting likely outcomes, making decisions.[22]

For third-level listeners who are thinking and feeling an inner pressure in response to the speaker's ideas, resistance is inevitable. Something within them is responding to the speaker's ideas—saying that the speaker is making sense, yet they do not want to let go of their own ideas without fighting. Their resistance and struggle to convince the speaker of their own point of view means they are fully involved in considering the speaker's position. These listeners are not comfortable with their own position. They are open to persuasion. If or when the opposition becomes intense, it is best for the speaker to become neutral, objective, and no longer press the new point of view. By so doing, these listeners are given time to think about and reflect on their own and the speaker's positions, and will come to terms later with their final decision regarding the issue.[23]

In talking with groups, the nurse must be cognizant of several obstacles that impede assimilation of ideas. Members of groups have varying interests, and all are not listening equally attentively. As a group member, it is easy to release responsibility for listening and responding to the speaker when other group members are known to be consistently responsive and articulate. As a consequence, there is unequal participation and feedback from members in a group. Some individuals may take the opportunity to make an irrelevant statement or ask an irrelevant question. When doing this, they are meeting personal needs, and other members of the group lose interest if the interruption becomes prolonged.

[22]Jesse S. Nirenberg, *Gettting through to People,* Prentice-Hall, Inc., Englewood Cliffs, N.J., 1963, p. 109.
[23]Ibid., pp. 124–144.

Individual group members frequently have to suppress or control emotions which are innately aroused dependent upon the issues under discussion. When this happens, attention is temporarily distracted from active listening. Invariably within every group, there are members who respond in their unique styles and capitalize on the opportunity to perform before an "audience." There always seems to be an inhibited shy person who is afraid of saying the "wrong thing," so says nothing. For the extrovert, the temptation to talk and impress is irresistable, and the purpose of the group session is subordinated to that individual's personal needs. Or there may be group members who desire to attack the speaker as an authority figure and can generally depend on getting support from the group, either actively or passively.[24]

Awareness of the possible obstacles that can occur in groups and having a clear idea of the intended goals for group meetings helps the nurse to manage group sessions. It is frequently facilitating to orient the group's thinking at the beginning of each session. Group members should know the purpose of the meeting and what the leader intends to do. Examples should be given at every opportunity so that multiple interpretations are reduced, and feedback from group members should be encouraged. To be sure that the participants are listening and understanding, the speaker must request their ideas at intervals. This is best done with questions from the speaker designed to stimulate thought or with the encouragement of questions coming from the group. Instead of answering a group member's question immediately, it is often strategic to ask that person to elaborate further regarding personal thoughts on the subject, or wait for another group member to respond to the original question. In this way, group participation is encouraged and an environment of "freely expressed" ideas is fostered.

A certain amount of irrelevancy should be allowed during each group session since the various group members are mentally traveling along their individual routes of associated ideas at different paces. The leader can always terminate digressions whenever necessary. It is advisable to reiterate ideas by means of new applications or new examples at periodic intervals and to summarize at the conclusion of the meeting. In this way, the leader assists group members to assimilate the expressed ideas and allows time for the reinforcement of ideas to take root.[25]

SPECIAL TECHNIQUES FOR USE WITH GROUPS

Introducing new ways of dealing with the content of each meeting attracts the attention of group members, maintains interest and/or control, and

[24]Ibid., pp. 179–181.
[25]Ibid., pp. 179–188.

"gets through" to most individuals much better than the sole use of words. Introductory statements or overviews of the subject material can be presented with the use of special films, slides, graphs, statistics, or fact sheets. Short plays, skits, or short stories can be used to dramatize a problem. Poems, songs, role-playing, and psychodrama can also be utilized, or a variety of exercises or techniques can be initiated which involve the participation of group members and accelerates the process of gaining their attention.

Strengthening Exercise

An exercise that nursing students seem to need or that awakens their consciousness about personal self is Otto's personal inventory of strengths. This exercise requires each group member to write all the personal strengths which can be thought of. Usually a brief time limit for writing is given. In every group, there are always one or two participants who can think of only a minimal number of strengths. Follow this exercise with a similar one in which group members are asked to pair; the directions require each partner to write all the strengths about each other that come to mind, then share verbally with each other what was written. When the partners share, the environment becomes relaxed and much pleasure, laughter, and camaraderie is expressed. This exercise seems to have an impact of positive force with particular individuals (those who probably need it the most), and builds self-confidence and belief in one's capabilities.

Active Listening Exercise

An exercise which offers group members the opportunity to experience what "active listening" is consists of pairing, having one person talk about herself exclusively for three minutes and requesting the second person to listen attentively but nonverbally throughout the entire three minutes. In this exercise the listening person becomes aware of the difficulty of actively listening—particularly when unable to respond verbally in any way. The talking person learns how easy or how difficult it is to talk about self and may learn some new insights about self.

Many exercises or experiments described for families are contained in the book, *Peoplemaking,* by Virginia Satir. Trying these experiments in a learning situation for nursing students or for families who are willing to receive new ideas causes individuals to reflect and become consciously aware of family dynamics. Learning to cope in a structured situation differently and positively takes time, a conscious behavior change, a determination to change, and repetitive practice.

With all exercises, the leader must elicit the thoughts of the group regarding their reactions and observations while the exercises were being enacted. Experiential insights of group or family members, whether positive or negative, are valuable for the entire group to hear, consider, and discuss. When exercises and/or techniques are used, the length of time, purpose, and appropriateness must always be carefully planned by the leader. Group or family discussions can be directed sensitively toward learnings intended to be attained by the use of the exercise. Often a group or family will bring out the points desired without specific intervention of the leader. Insights gained by individual members through experiential exercises are not perceptible or known to exist unless the member shares his or her thoughts with the group. The leader must accept that insights occur differently with individuals—some are spontaneous and some germinate, waiting for the right time to sprout.

ASSERTIVENESS TRAINING

Enrolling for assertiveness training in a class or group has been an activity which many individuals have considered essential in recent years. The incorporation of the principles of assertiveness training in the content of classroom lectures for nursing students has been received enthusiastically by many of the students. The quiet passive-type students have responded, knowing that they need the training, but are frequently frightened to try it.

As stated by Bakker, all people need a territory, a place to live, a field of action, a stage on which to act out the story of their life. In the daily practice of everyone's life from birth until death, all persons' borders are disputed in one way or another. To maintain territory which they regard as their own, individuals have to exert steady outward pressure. In daily human affairs the territorial boundaries of individuals are continually under stress; borders can move outward or inward, and the pressure on each side can be increased or decreased. Persons attempting to expand their territory and consequently move in on another person's territory are labeled as exhibiting aggressive behavior. In the context of territoriality, *aggression* means any act which results in the extension of the territory that a person holds.[26] *Assertiveness* is an act of independence whereby people maintain control over all parts of their territory. In other words, the defense of one's territory is assertive when it is direct and specific to the area under attack. Assertive persons rely on feelings of adequacy and strength. Defensive persons give the appearance of weakness because they are unsure of their borders or of their ability to defend them. Consequently, they do not convey self-assurance to others.[27]

In learning how an individual defends or acquires territory, the word "weapon" is used to signify the means that is used for aggressive or

[26]Cornelis B. Bakker and Marianne K. Bakker-Rabdau, *No Trespassing: Explorations in Human Territoriality,* Chandler & Sharp Publishers, Inc., San Francisco, 1973, pp. 49–52.
[27]Ibid., pp. 59–62.

assertive purposes. Every person uses weapons, uses the ones best known and which have been effective on previous occasions. For example, to resolve an interpersonal conflict, there must be a clear understanding of the issue involved. Whose territory has been invaded? What weapons were used by the aggressor? There are a great variety of weapons used to take over another's territory, and frequently, they are not obvious ones, are not recognized as weapons, and are successful in distracting the defender from the primary issue.

Assertiveness training classes deal with the concepts of human territoriality, assertive behavior, and ways to handle selected situations assertively. Recognition of subtle fighting techniques or weapons and learning to defend one's territory consciously, honestly, and successfully has value in achieving the objectives that one desires. Also, a keen insight into techniques used in interpersonal conflicts leads one to evaluate the consequences of any selected behavior. On occasion, an individual may choose to consciously acquiesce to an aggressive behavior because of the secondary undesirable consequences of assertiveness. Consciousness of one's own behavior and weapons, and another's behavior and weapons when an issue is at stake—whether assertive or aggressive—whether overt or very subtle—is the desired goal.[28]

When nurses have studied, practiced, and feel well-acquainted with the concepts of human territoriality, assertive behavior, and weaponry, they can teach assertiveness training to groups of citizens desiring to learn. Lists of weapons and how they are used and successfully counteracted can be role-played and practiced in a variety of practical situational contexts.

COMMUNITY ACTION GROUPS

There are times when nursing students come into contact with citizens who are dissatisfied with their immediate conditions and want to do something about them. It is helpful to assess where the citizens are, listen to the issues that bother them, elicit all the facts of the situation, inquire regarding obstacles that may interfere, and investigate if participation from "outsiders" will be accepted. If the citizen group is willing to incorporate the various skills of nursing students, a number of valuable activities can be implemented. Students can act as informal leaders, consultants, data-gatherers, active participants, facilitators, advocates, investigators, instructors, or in capacities where action and/or knowledge are required. Many of the activities are opportunities for experiential learning and prepare students for future citizen and/or professional leadership activities.

[28]Ibid., pp. 169–172.

The principles of community organization practices must be remembered and reviewed with the citizen group if necessary and appropriate. After the issue for which action is deemed essential is decided and objectives determined, other factors bearing consideration by community action groups include recruiting additional interested citizens, gaining support from recognized power structures, fund raising, informing through publicity, and campaigning through legislative or political channels.

Recruiting   To recruit additional interested citizens, it is necessary to talk to various individuals in the community informally. The ideas and opinions of those who may be interested in the issue should be elicited in one-to-one informal conversations. Whenever a citizen seems to have a conviction about an issue, an invitation should be extended to attend a planned meeting which will convene at a well-known and easily accessible location in the local community. The suggestions of various citizens should be integrated and implemented as feasible. Personal invitations to attend meetings which fit the schedules of citizens get best results. If transportation or baby-sitting facilities are needed in order to persuade citizens to attend, arrangements should be made for these resources. Citizens should be reminded before scheduled meetings by telephoning, sending postcards, or canvassing door-to-door. When the meeting is held, the chairperson should be a recognized and well-liked leader of the local community. After the purpose for the meeting has been explained, all persons attending the meeting should have the opportunity to speak and participate in formulating plans. Assignments or short-term action projects can be designated and divided among group members so that each is involved and feels a part of the group. A meeting that is well-paced and purposeful is the responsibility of the leader. If all participants feel they have contributed in some way, the meeting is generally considered successful, and additional citizens are recruited.

Support from power structures   Support of an identified issue from certain key leaders or recognized establishments in the community is always helpful. To determine which leaders are sympathetic to an identified issue requires initiative and risk-taking behavior of citizen-participants. Visiting recognized influential citizens or talking to representatives of the news media, government, schools, professional organizations, labor unions, and other recognized establishments takes preparation. The organizational structure of each establishment should be requested in advance so that preparation for entering the bureaucratic system with a formal hierarchy of authority can be made. Desired results are best attained when correct procedures for entering a system are followed and the appropriate persons representing the chain of command of the bureaucratic institution are approached. Facts, logic, and straight-forward arguments about the identified issue should be well-formulated in the mind and easily articulated. It is good strategy to listen to the position of the community leader first, agree on points when there is agreement, and be ready to question or answer points with which there is disagreement. It is always wise to be objective, friendly, and respectful in manner. When support from a community leader is obviously unavailable, the visit should be terminated and other leaders consulted from whom to request support. When a community leader is sympathetic to an identified issue, the form of support which he or she is able to give should be requested directly. This may be a signature, request for money, use of a building, equipment, an advertisement, or active membership in the citizen group.

Fund raising Solicitation for funds can be done through mailings, advertisements, pledge groups, parties, garage sales, bake sales, dinners, dances, special events, fairs, canvassing, or by writing a grant proposal. For the citizen participants who are involved with planning for and raising money, the method decided upon for soliciting funds requires knowledge about details ensuring successful implementation. Small fund raising can be fun, such as organizing a raffle, garage sale, dinner-dance, and similar functions. If the citizen group decides that a grant proposal has distinct possibilities for procuring the needed funds, a committee can be assigned the task of writing and submitting a proposal. Organizations from whom funds can be solicited, should be identified and the required explanatory documents obtained regarding correct procedures to follow. Usually guidelines are available for writing a formal application for funds. The guidelines must be read carefully and followed exactly. The written proposal must make use of clear, succinct language, contain documentation of facts, objectives, evaluative methods, a bibliography, and a reasonable budget. Writing a grant proposal is an excellent learning experience for citizen participants since the process consolidates the purpose, objectives, planning, implemention, and evaluation of a project into a complete whole. The act of writing a proposal tends to increase the commitment and conviction of participants.

Informing through publicity Communicating about an identified issue to the general public can be achieved by various means. Whatever method is selected, it is necessary initially to catch the public's attention, be explicit about the content of a message, have all necessary details included in a message. If the message addresses itself to immediate concrete problems that citizens are experiencing, attention will be easily secured. Pictures, cartoons, phrases, and colors are noticed if they show humor, emotion of some type, or timeliness. It is advisable to know the selected target population—what they are thinking and feeling—and address the content of the message within a context that has meaning for the target population.

The means for informing the public include leaflets, newsletters, newspapers, posters, television media, slide shows, films, exhibits, and letters to the editor. Organizing a speaker's bureau is another way of informing community groups. The choice of the publicity method must be carefully planned. Learning to prepare an attractive poster, leaflet, or newsletter may require consultation from local community artists and publicity experts. Knowing the strategy for approaching a local news-paper or writing an acceptable article has advantages toward getting desired results. Slide shows can be created by citizens committees and be "right on target." If films are used, they must be previewed and carefully selected in terms of the intended message. Canvassing on a door-to-door basis is a grass roots method which can be done for some projects. It tends to broaden one's perspective of human behavior and is best done in selected neighborhoods. (See Chap. 4.)

Campaigning through legislative or political channels   A knowledge about the legislative and political process locally, statewide, and national-ly is increasingly essential for community groups (and nurses) to compre-hend. When a community action group supports a health issue requiring a change in the law, sophistication regarding the mechanics of changing the law has definite advantages.

A referendum can be drawn up which brings a selected health issue to a public vote. To prepare a referendum, it is advisable to consult an attorney about the mechanics of writing a referendum and any other local requirements which should be known. The number of signatures to be gathered and the correct procedures for soliciting signatures should be elicited. When the proposed referendum is written and ready for signa-tures, as many workers and supporters of the health issue that can be mustered must be gathered so that they will distribute the referendum, publicize it, and ensure ample support of voters at the polls during the election period.[29]

Lobbying is the direct personal presentation of citizen views to government representatives. It is best done by an organized constituency aroused over a specific issue, such as the League for Women Voters or the American Nurses' Association. It is important to know the local state legislators' records regarding positions on various issues. The legislators should be supplied with facts about identified health issues for which

---

[29]The O.M. Collective, *The Organizer's Manual,* Bantam Books, Inc., New York, 1971, pp. 169–170.

support is desired. All studies, articles, statistics, data, and research with which to persuade legislators should be made available to them. The best arguments are individualized personalized ones whether delivered in person or in a brief, yet convincing, letter.[30] It is important to learn how legislative bills are processed. When hearings are held by legislators on identified health issues important to a citizen's group, as many supporters as possible should be gathered to attend the hearing and speak in support of the bill. Evidence of enthusiasm, conviction, and commitment from an organized group of citizen participants has an influential impact on legislators.

Knowledge about campaign tactics and political strategies generally are not well known by nurses in general. As reported by Livingston and Dodd, who collected campaign contributions for a nurse running for city office in a Northwest city, contributions were received from approximately one-third of the nurses contacted. They stated that naïvety exists among nurses regarding sums of money to give, the process and organization of campaigning, the role of a candidate and her campaign manager.[31] For political clout and increasing visibility in public and professional affairs, nurses must study and participate in the political process if they wish to have a voice regarding the future delivery of health-care services.

EVALUATING GROUP MEETINGS

In a study done by Chopra which evaluated the ingredients contributing to successful groups, the primary characteristic was found to be their high degree of motivation. Concurrent with the motivation are the attributes of enthusiasm, a high level of interest, and commitment. He found that the nature of the group task is not as significant in motivating as the fact that members of such groups are *motivated to work with each other.* He concluded that the factor which is critical to the success of a group is the way members interact with each other and treat each other's ideas. In successfully motivated groups, when an idea is disclosed by one member, other group members will spend a lot of time and energy trying to fully understand the idea, exploring its implications, and suggesting ways to overcome its limitations. In other words, members of a motivated group work *with* the person who offered the idea and try to help him or her to strengthen it. All too often, this kind of strengthening behavior is not common in community groups. The reversal is more apt to be practiced—that of immediately raising objections and reasons for why an

[30]Ibid., pp. 170–172.
[31]Carolyn A. Livingston and Marylin J. Dodd, "Neophytes in the Campaign Process," *Washington State Journal of Nursing,* **47**(4):13–14, Fall 1975.

idea will not work. As a consequence, the person who suggested the idea, regardless of his overt reaction and behavior, feels "put down," and the meeting goes on and on.[32]

When evaluating group meetings, factors to consider for analysis include the following:

1 Goals. Were the goals explicit? Were the group members interested and involved in attaining the group goals? Was the interaction goal-directed?

2 Leadership. What were the interpersonal influences of the leader? Was leadership distributed and participatory in nature or was it obviously controlled by one or two individuals? Was there evidence of a coalition of power?

3 Psychosocial environment. Was the psychosocial climate warm, friendly, spontaneous, formal, informal, cold, threatening, etc.? Were group members generally responsive and considerate of each other?

4 Physical environment. Were the arrangements (seating, chairs, table, blackboard, equipment) suitable? Were the temperature of the room, lighting, acoustics satisfactory?

5 Mechanics of meeting. Was the meeting well-paced? Was the agenda followed? Were all reports included? If a group decision was made, was this managed satisfactorily?

6 Skills of group members. Which members attended to the task functions of initiating, seeking information or opinions, giving information or opinions, clarifying and elaborating, summarizing, and checking for consensus? Which members performed the maintenance functions of harmonizing, gatekeeping, encouraging, compromising, and setting standards? Did all group members interact and/or participate? Were communication skills used such as paraphrasing, perception checking, giving "I" messages? Was there evidence that nonverbal behavior was noted?

7 Problem-Solving skills. Were all group members cognizant of the issues? Was the group productive? Did they listen to each one's ideas in a constructive fashion?

8 Other factors. Were there other factors that were generally helpful or upsetting in terms of the group's behavior and productivity?[33]

Evaluation is a necessary ongoing process and, when done conscientiously, assists in improving future meetings. In every community, group meetings are convened with little thought directed toward evaluation. One such community council meeting which met regularly was observed by a nursing student and described as follows: "Group dynamics showed a

[32]Amarjit Chopra, "Motivation in Task-Oriented Groups," *Journal of Nursing Administration,* **3**(1):55–60, January–February 1973.
[33]Jack R. Gibb, Grace N. Platts, and Lorraine F. Miller, *Dynamics of Participative Groups,* National Training Laboratories, Washington, D. C., 1951.

loosely knit group purposelessly meandering toward a vague goal. There were poor habits of communication, little verbal expression of feelings, and an underlying atmosphere of tension. There was little cooperative effort, give and take, and limited efficiency."

The above description occurs all too frequently in community meetings. Group participants do little to change or improve meetings, and general deterioration and dissatisfaction occurs. For groups convened by nurses, evaluation must always be considered essential if success and goal attainment is the desired end product.

COORDINATION OF INTERDISCIPLINARY PERSONNEL

Nursing is a highly diversified occupation and there are some tasks which nurses undertake that are not noted to be their function exclusively. One such task for community health nurses is that of *coordination* of patient care. When working intensively with families, community health nurses learn of a variety of agencies or personnel who are communicating with one or more members of the family constellation and often arrange for a conference of all interested personnel or call the representative of each discipline individually in an effort to coordinate the services given to the family. This particular task is essential and must be *stressed* as an important, vital attribute of community health nurses.

When people are drawn together to combine their efforts for a given purpose, this is coordination. *Coordination* is the orderly arrangement of group effort to provide unity of action in the pursuit of a common purpose.[34] In community health nursing, the common purpose that is focused upon by the various health representatives is the integration of community health services to the patient or family. Communication among personnel of all community health facilities is essential to share information and discuss what is involved in sustaining or improving the health status of the given patient and family. All too often coordination of health personnel is not initiated spontaneously and duplication or overlapping of services to a family occurs. By assuming the task of coordination with responsibility, the community health nurse contributes to the assurance that continuity of patient care will be achieved.

Health Teams

In community health nursing the composition of health teams varies according to the purpose for gathering the group and the nature of the personnel attending. Community health teams can consist of professional

---

[34]James Mooney, "The Coordinative Principle," in Joseph A. Litterer (ed.), *Organizations: Structure and Behavior,* John Wiley & Sons, Inc., New York, 1963, p. 39.

persons or a combination of lay and professional persons. Some examples of health teams include: (1) a group of community health nurses working in an agency; (2) a group of community health nurses, licensed practical nurses, home health aides, and community aides working in an agency; (3) a community health nurse representing a health department, a social worker representing the department of public assistance, a physician, a school principal, a school nurse, an individual representing the housing authority, etc.; (4) a community health nurse and paraprofessional personnel representing a clinic service such as family planning; (5) a community health nurse, a medical nurse representing the hospital, a family member, a family counselor, a school teacher, and other involved personnel; (6) a community health nurse and a group of lay volunteers getting ready to execute a screening test for vision, hearing, or a related health measure.

When the nurse is a member of any health team, she must know her purpose for being included as a participant and must be willing to assume responsibility for leadership when it is needed or implicit. The preceding discussion about "Working with Groups" is applicable to developing effective health teams, particularly if the team meets on a regular basis. The emphasis of health teams should always be focused on their mutual purpose, action directed toward agreed-upon goals, and effort expended toward maintaining working relationships which facilitate satisfactory progress. Sharing of information in a noncompetitive fashion enables all team members to function in a responsible, satisfying manner and expedites the purpose for which the group was brought together.

Multidisciplinary Conferences

When the community health nurse initiates a plan for a conference of professional persons representing several community agencies to discuss a care plan for a specified family, she must call all the professionals serving the family and invite them to a stated place at a specific time for the purpose of pooling their information about the family. All too often representatives of the various community agencies working with a given family are not called together to unify their purposes and goals in giving assistance. If the conference is to be one in which confidential information is disclosed, the nurse should clear the exchange of such information with the patient by asking him to sign a release-of-information form. In so doing, the patient is made aware that such a conference is in the planning stages and realizes the purpose is to facilitate the integration of health services in his or her behalf. When talking to the professionals who are being invited to the conference, the nurse should state that the patient has signed a release slip, indicating that it is permissible to bring confidential records and reports. She should also state her expectation of the contribution the professional person will make to the conference, and if he or she wishes to bring printed materials that will aid in the group's understanding, this would be desirable. If it seems expedient to invite the professional worker's supervisor to the conference, the procedure for doing so correctly should be requested. By being knowledgeable about the organizational structure of allied community agencies and complying to their modus operandi, coordination is facilitated.

A review of the four points in the discussion of "Leading or Facilitating a Group" will give the nurse ideas regarding her plan of procedure for the conference. It is important to remember that all group members should be introduced. Too often in professional groups, the assumption is made that everyone knows each other, and this is not necessarily so. Another essential point to realize is that the initiator of the conference must act as the leader or facilitator. When the group is composed of community professional leaders, it is often tempting for the nurse to transfer the leadership of the conference to another person who holds a more imposing position. However, when the nurse is the initiator, she *must* perform responsibly as the leader or facilitator. If she thinks refreshments will serve the function of relaxing the group members, she should plan for and offer coffee and cookies early in the conference. If a blackboard is available and the listing of issues coming out in the discussion seems indicated, the leader should feel comfortable about writing the ideas on the blackboard herself or asking someone else to do so. Regardless of the composition of the group, whether it is made up of eminently more important persons professionally than herself, the nurse leader should perform the tasks of facilitation with confidence and responsibility.

Coordination with Other Community Professionals

It is essential that the community health nurse keep open lines of communication with the family physician at all times. This may require several telephone calls or a visit to the physician's office. When the nurse interprets her function with the family to the physician, she can emphasize the nature of her role as a coordinator. She can explain how she was referred to the family, and the contract agreed upon by the family and herself for continued service. She can describe her assessment of the family situation and identify her need for validation of specific information given or activities prescribed by the physician. By bringing out omissions, misperceptions, or incompletions of the family's health knowledge or practices in the home, the nurse can demonstrate the efficacy of her role as a coordinator. By working *with* the physician, making him or her knowledgeable about the obstacles which are hindering the family's implementation of stated recommendations, and the goals toward which she is working, the nurse communicates the essentiality of her function with the family.

It is equally important for the nurse to keep open lines of communication with all allied professionals representing different community facilities who are serving commonly known families. For example, if the family receiving public assistance is on the active roster of the housing authorities and family counseling service, those workers representing allied disciplines should be made aware that the nurse is also serving the family. The main objective for keeping open lines of communication is to work toward common, unified goals in serving a family. Otherwise, families are given the opportunity to exploit the services of several community facilities in a number of ways or become confused about the multiplicity of professionals who are communicating varying suggestions. When the nurse starts working with a family, she should inquire about the possibility of other community facilities to whom the family is known. She should make a point of requesting the names of other workers who are serving the family currently and explain that she wishes to talk to them. If it is necessary for the family member to sign a release-of-information slip, the form should be made available and signed at the time of the visit. The nurse can then arrange for a multidisciplinary conference or talk to each professional individually. It is vital that all community workers, professional and nonprofessional, discuss their contact with the family so that common goals are determined and methods of working toward goals are synchronized. Attitudes toward a given family are concomitantly revealed, discussed, and adjusted toward the purpose of accomplishing the mutually accepted goals. To reiterate, the community health nurse is in the best position to initiate and implement coordination of community health services to the patient and family whenever several professionals are involved.

Coordination with Other Community Nonprofessionals

The utilization of nonprofessionals or paraprofessionals in the medical and nursing ranks is increasing rapidly in our society. With the advent of a wide selection of trained and untrained community workers, it is essential that all community professionals relate in a manner that enhances and enriches the capabilities of these people. The term *nonprofessional* refers to those persons whose tasks are mainly of a technical nature, i.e., licensed practical nurses, nurse's aides. Paraprofessionals refer to those persons within the community who are unskilled, have little formal education but are being trained successfully as assistants in some capacity to professionals, i.e., home health aides, community aides, nutritional aides. Studies have shown that locally selected trainees or paraprofessionals living in impoverished neighborhoods have a strong desire to work and earn a decent living. When they have received on-the-job training, they contribute effectively to a given program because they know a great deal about the persons living in the "hard to reach" neighborhoods who have need for health services. The paraprofessionals can be genuinely open, empathic, supportive, and persuasive of people they serve because they have lived through very similar circumstances. They can overcome barriers of cultural differences, communication difficulties, lack of motivation, and understanding which have often interfered when professionals have dealt with the disadvantaged groups.[35]

Because nonprofessionals and paraprofessionals are demonstrating their effectiveness in the health field, it is essential that professionals recognize and utilize their services to a maximum degree, promote the idea of teamwork, and take advantage of the extra time to perform professional functions which they alone can best fulfill, i.e., managerial tasks or research studies. Relating effectively to nonprofessionals is no different from relating to any other group of people. Nonprofessionals want to be seen and heard, deemed worthy, and considered a part of the team. They generally know their assets and limitations, appreciate recognition of their strengths, and are honest about their limits. They appreciate and want supervision when their competencies are uncertain. Even though they are not so well educated academically as professionals, they have knowledge and attitudes about the local community which are valuable for the professional to know. Often they have an intuition and compelling warmth for the consumer which the professional may not possess. In team meetings, the skilled, effective nurse is one who provides a comfortable environment and encourages all members to contribute their ideas whether they have a professional, nonprofessional, or paraprofessional status. It behooves the nurse leader to recognize all her team members, regardless of their professional standing, as worthy of her respect and interest. By working *with* the nonprofessionals and paraprofessionals and not *over* them, the performance of the team as a whole is enhanced and satisfying.

It is not unusual for professionals to demonstrate lack of enthusiasm toward the skills of nonprofessionals. When a negative reaction of professionals is perceived, it often results from a lack of understanding and acceptance of paraprofessionals in any field of nursing. One way to counteract negative attitudes is to provide the opportunity for professionals to talk openly about their feelings and attitudes in a series of closed sessions. When it is appropriate and timely, their special strengths and capabilities as professionals should be pointed out in conjunction with the

[35]Wilbur Hoff, M.D., "Older Poor Adults Trained as Home Health Aides," *Public Health Reports,* 83(3):184–185, March 1968.

paraprofessional's requirement for competent supervision, and a new relationship which is reality-based and very much needed may be started. Emphasis on the responsibility for directing or supervising other personnel to give skilled health services to consumers is highly important and demanding. When done well, the professionals can take pride in the fact that they played an essential role in facilitating expert care to the patient, which restored the patient's dignity, worth, and health.

Interdisciplinary Teams

Interdisciplinary coordination implies team-centered leadership which is based on the nature of tasks to be completed and usually connotes an extended period of time. An interdisciplinary team is made up of several persons, each representing a specific discipline, who agree to work as a group toward a common purpose with mutually acceptable goals. The interdisciplinary team differs from the multidisciplinary team in its commitment, mode of operation, and shared responsibilities.

Working as a member of an interdisciplinary team requires an understanding of the goals, roles, tasks, and communication processes of the group. Each member must have respect for and accept all other members of the group. A team composed of several persons representing different disciplines and professions does not always exemplify what is commonly considered "team spirit." For the group who has consented to be a team, effort, commitment toward common goals, understanding of the role boundaries of each discipline, willingness to learn each other's language and viewpoints in problem-solving and decision-making sessions, patience, and persistence must be realized.

Initially when an interdisciplinary team comes together, they have limited knowledge about each other. They must assess the level of education each member possesses in terms of each one's discipline; interpret and clarify the capacities, territories, and roles of each discipline, including functions which seem to overlap or duplicate; and feel comfortable about communicating openly so that viewpoints and assumptions can be questioned and criticized. In getting acquainted, sometimes members show deference to particular individuals—a reaction representative of the caste system in each profession. Or relationships with persons of the opposite sex are such that a characteristic superior-subordinate manner is apparent. If this happens, the behavior must be consciously changed before a true team-centered leadership can evolve. It takes time and patience to understand about the territories, limitations, and extensions of roles of other disciplines. When there is role ambiguity or role conflict, negotiations must be made eventually about who will do what. It helps to develop ground rules for governing the communication processes and operation of the team. As necessary, the rules can be cited when contradictions or stalemates take place. The process of solving problems and making decisions as a team is a shared responsibility which, practically speaking, differs considerably from practicing independently, an activity which each individual is accustomed to doing. Learning to share, coordinate, and integrate with others takes time, patience, and persistence but can be rewarding, eventually, when the many inevitable obstacles have been arduously overcome and the goals of the endeavor have been attained. Experimentation with interdisciplinary teamwork is on the increase and when the demonstration of collaborative relationships has shown that the provision of health care is superior in terms of efficiency, efficacy, quality, and satisfaction to all concerned, these new interdisciplinary models may well be accepted and emulated.[36]

USE OF CONSULTATION

There are many times when a community health nurse needs consultation. Because she is a generalist, consultation in specialized fields of nursing and closely allied disciplines such as nutrition, social work, psychology, community development, and others is essential and edifying in improving the quality of services given to the consumer. Consultation can be gained from many sources, such as nursing supervisors, clinical specialists, physicians, social workers, nutritionists, specialists for specific disease categories or social conditions, and others.

The consultation process involves the following three features: (1) the consultee, an individual who has defined a need—something she wishes to know; (2) the consultant, the person with the expertise to fulfill the need; and (3) the problem area with which the consultee wants help. The problem can be a health need of a patient or a community activity in which the consultee is involved. The assumption is made by the consultee that the consultant can fulfill her need, and the consultant assumes that the consultee will be prepared with all the data relevant to the problem.

When the consultee desires help in regard to a problem, she requests an appointment with the appropriate consultant and gathers all data she believes will be pertinent to the consultation. This may involve making a summary of all essential information from the family record and forwarding a copy of the summary to the consultant prior to the appointed time. Or, it may involve reading more-inclusive references pertinent to the problem to enable the consultation to be on a sharing, knowledgeable basis between two professionals.

The success of the consultation is dependent on several factors listed

[36]Robert A. Hoekelman, "Nurse-Physician Relationships," *American Journal of Nursing,* 75(7):1150–1152, July 1975.

as follows: whether the consultee (1) has correctly diagnosed her needs, (2) is adequately prepared with all essential data, (3) has adequately communicated her needs to the consultant, (4) has selected the appropriate consultant, and (5) has thought through the consequences of implementing ideas or changes that may be recommended by the consultant.[37] The conversation between consultant and consultee should be two-way, not in one direction only. Ideas suggested by the consultant should be thoroughly explored by both parties as to their feasibility in relation to the specific problem area being studied. Since the consultee is personally acquainted with the problem area, its idiosyncracies and complications, she alone can suspect if an idea will work. When the consultee is helped to see a problem area more comprehensively and is actively involved in reaching realistic conclusions regarding her next steps, she is more likely to feel satisfied with the consultation process and will demonstrate subsequent activities which reveal successful learning. Rather than expecting the consultant to provide answers, the consultee should anticipate the problem-solving approach to be used, during which the consultant aids in sharpening the diagnosis of the problem area and suggests ideas or alternatives that have not already occurred to the consultee. It is up to the consultee to make the ultimate decision as to what action to take, since she is fully acquainted with the uniqueness of the problem. Inherent in the consultation process is the requirement for openness in discussion, a comfortable, sharing environment, and a bond of mutual respect which facilitates a helping relationship between the two participants.

As the community health nurse learns to make use of a wide selection of available consultants within the community, she develops her own expertise in becoming an exceptional generalist who is recognized by all community specialists. She is the individual who has a grasp of the wholeness of health practices occurring within her particular community.

SUMMARY

Community health nurses have started utilizing group work as an efficient means for reaching out and facilitating growth of consumers with whom they come in contact. In conducting group work they must know the problems of entering a new group—how to focus on the content of meetings, how to utilize the communication process, how to lead or facilitate, and how to evaluate group growth.

Some community groups with whom community health nurses should be knowledgeable were identified as therapeutic groups, self-help

[37]Schein, op. cit., p. 5.

groups, growth groups, reference groups, assertiveness training groups, and community action groups. Nurses must seek out opportunities to act as leaders, co-leaders, consultants, data-gatherers, facilitators, advocates, instructors or in any capacity where action and/or knowledge is required. Group work provides excellent experiential learning for professional leadership roles and activities.

The coordination role of the community health nurse is vital to ensure that health services to a family are integrated and purposeful. Someone must bring into a common focus all of the elements of the health-care system which are directly or indirectly involved in giving services to individuals, families, or groups. This means teamwork with professionals, nonprofessionals, and paraprofessionals who are working in the various health facilities in a community. Because the community health nurse is a generalist, she must be prepared to use consultation, which will result in increased expertise for herself and beneficial activities for consumers.

SUGGESTED READING

Bakker, Cornelis B., and Marianne K. Bakker-Rabdau: *No Trespassing: Explorations in Human Territoriality,* Chandler & Sharp Publishers, Inc., San Francisco, 1973.

Beckhard, Richard: *Organization Development: Strategies and Models,* Addison-Wesley Publishing Company, Inc., Reading, Mass., 1969.

Beier, Ernst G.: *The Silent Language of Psychotherapy,* Aldine Publishing Company, Chicago, 1966.

Berne, Eric: *Principles of Group Treatment,* Grove Press, Inc., New York, 1966.

Bradford, Leland P., Jack R. Gibb, and Kenneth D. Benne: *T-Group Theory and Laboratory Method,* John Wiley & Sons, Inc., New York, 1964.

Bumbalo, Judith A., and Delores E. Young: "The Self-Help Phenomenon," *American Journal of Nursing,* **73**(9):1588–1591, September 1973.

Cartwright, D., and A. Zander: *Group Dynamics,* 3rd ed., Row, Peterson & Company, Evanston, Ill., 1968.

Eichhorn, Suzanne Finn: *Becoming,* Institute for Health Team Development, Montefiore Hospital and Medical Center, Bronx, New York, 1973.

Horwitz, John: *Team Practice and the Specialist: An Introduction to Interdisciplinary Teamwork,* Charles C. Thomas, Publisher, Springfield, Ill., 1970.

Jacobson, Sylvia R.: "A Study of Interprofessional Collaboration," *Nursing Outlook,* **22**(12):751–755, December 1974.

Janis, Irving L.: "Groupthink," *Psychology Today,* **5**(6):43–46, November 1971.

Johnson, David W.: *Reaching Out,* Prentice-Hall, Inc., Englewood Cliffs, N.J., 1972.

Knowles, M., and H. Knowles: *Introduction to Group Dynamics,* Association Press, New York, 1969.

Lewis, Howard R, and Harold S. Streitfeld: *Growth Games,* Harcourt Brace Jovanovich, Inc., New York, 1970.

Lippitt, Ronald, Jeanne Watson, and Bruce Westley: *The Dynamics of Planned Change,* Harcourt Brace Jovanovich, Inc., New York, 1958.

Marram, Gwen D.: *The Group Approach in Nursing Practice,* The C.V. Mosby Company, Saint Louis, 1973.

Maslow, Abraham: *Toward a Psychology of Being,* D. Van Nostrand Company, Inc., Princeton, N.J., 1962.

Nirenberg, Jesse S.: *Getting Through To People,* Prentice-Hall, Inc., Englewood Cliffs, N.J., 1963.

The O. M. Collective: *The Organizer's Manual,* Bantam Books, Inc., New York, 1971.

Perls, Fritz: *The Gestalt Therapy,* Julian Press, Inc., New York, 1956.

Redman, Eric: *The Dance of Legislation,* Simon and Schuster, New York, 1973.

Rogers, Carl: *On Becoming a Person,* Houghton Mifflin Company, Boston, 1961.

Satir, Virginia: *Peoplemaking,* Science and Behavior Books, Inc., Palo Alto, Calif., 1972.

Schaefer, Marguerite J.: "The Political and Economic Scene in the Future of Nursing," *American Journal of Public Health,* 63(10):887–889, October 1973.

Schein, Edgar H.: *Process Consultation: Its Role in Organization Development,* Addison-Wesley Publishing Company, Inc., Reading, Mass., 1969.

Schmidt, Cheryl Klouzal: "Five Become a Team in Appalachia," *American Journal of Nursing,* 75(8):1314–1315, August 1975.

Sedgwick, Rae: "The Role of the Process Consultant," *Nursing Outlook,* 21(12):773–775, December 1973.

Sherif, Muzafer, and Carolyn Sherif: *Interdisciplinary Relationships in the Social Sciences,* Aldine Publishing Company, Chicago, 1969.

Sullivan, Harry Stack: *The Psychiatric Interview,* W. W. Norton & Company, Inc., New York, 1954.

Thomstad, Beatrice, Nicholas Cunningham, and Barbara H. Kaplan: "Changing the Rules of the Doctor-Nurse Game," *Nursing Outlook,* 23(7):422–427, July 1975.

Veninga, Robert, and Delphie J. Fredlund: "Teaching the Group Approach," *Nursing Outlook,* 22(6):373–376, June 1974.

Watzlawick, P., J. Beavin, and D. Jackson: *Pragmatics of Human Communication,* W. W. Norton & Company, Inc., New York, 1967.

Chapter 8

Developing a Prevention Package

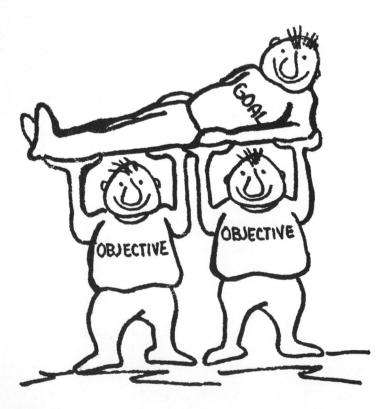

Health is the third largest industry in the United States. Health spending today is eight times the spending of twenty years ago.[1] Knowing this and considering ways to divert the process leads one to the concept of prevention.

In newspapers and magazines written for public consumption, articles are appearing increasingly which have to do with prevention measures. Titles such as "Keeping Cool at Gimbels: Controlling Hypertension," "The Mormons' Secrets for Their Low Cancer Rate and Fewer Heart Attacks," or "Keeping Young with Yoga" are samples of catchy phrases designed to intrigue readers' interest. The current trend toward focusing on factors of prevention and influencing greater numbers of consumers to change unhealthy health habits is gaining in momentum and encompasses the human being's whole life-style.

All health professionals are familiar with the three levels of prevention which are classified as primary, secondary, and tertiary. Primary prevention connotes health promotion, which involves activities directed toward promoting general well-being and is not focused on a particular disease. Primary prevention also includes specific protection for selected diseases, such as immunizations for diptheria, whooping cough, tetanus, and smallpox. Secondary prevention focuses on early diagnosis and instigating measures to stop progression of disease processes or handicapping disabilities. Tertiary prevention deals with rehabilitation activities for disabled patients in an effort to return the person to a level of maximum usefulness.[2] In our present era, health promotion or the primary level of prevention is receiving more emphasis than ever before and consumers are reading persuasive messages about dieting, exercising, relaxing, meditating, and similar activities.

The statement was made in Chap. 10 that infection is not synonymous with disease. A person can have an infection but not be overtly ill or aware of any untoward activities going on internally. Whether an individual experiences illness or wellness at any given point in time is dependent upon both personal and situational factors.[3] A person can be well and feel ill or vice versa—can be ill and feel well. The state of health at a given moment in time is indeterminate. Of the vast majority of people who are actively and productively functioning on a day-to-day basis, most believe themselves to be well and healthy. To appeal to this population to maintain optimal health and become interested in preventive measures is a challenging task for community health nurses.

[1] National Health Insurance Resource Book, op. cit., pp. 2–6.
[2] Hugh R. Leavell and R. Gurney Clark, *Preventive Medicine for the Doctor in His Community: An Epidemiologic Approach*, 3rd ed., McGraw-Hill Book Company, New York, 1965, pp. 19–28.
[3] Ruth Wu, *Behavior and Illness*, Prentice-Hall, Inc., Englewood Cliffs, N.J., 1973, p. 83.

It is accepted practice that when consumers enter a hospital as patients, they receive a gamut of professional services, all of which are included in the package, whether requested directly by the patient or not. If the American public can be aroused to expect or anticipate optimal health or "feeling good" as part of a prevention package, promoted as a fringe benefit of employment or normal health-care services, new directions for community health nursing activities can be instituted.

It is well known that excellent health in and of itself has no attractive appeal to the average citizen who takes health for granted. Therefore, the traditional methods used by health professionals for changing undesirable health habits must be studied, analyzed, and, for the most part, discarded. New ways for reaching citizens, causing them to consider changing a life-style must be devised and tried. Nursing students are innovative and eager to try new ideas when given the opportunity to do so. Selling a prevention package to selected consumer populations can be experimented with in a variety of settings. In place of insidiously and unintentionally suggesting that catastrophic illnesses may be end results of stressful and competitive lives, emphasizing the joys and satisfactions of day-to-day living in terms of sensory awareness, intrinsic energy, "feeling good," can be dangled as a carrot for those individuals who want to live an active life, productive until death. The task entails knowledge of marketing and motivational strategies. If the basic need for physiological stability as identified by Maslow can be translated into a conscious expectation by the citizen, then the potential demand for prevention services has a start. Many potential consumers of health-care services are currently questioning the quality, efficiency, and costs of health care. Perhaps, a turnaround can be effected whereas instead of protestingly accepting health-care delivery services and costs, preventive health services can be "sold as a bargain," the fringe benefits including less pain, little cost, less boredom, less fatigue, and more fun, more energy, and more satisfaction.

A model of preventive health action proposed by Suchman advises that individuals and groups be assessed according to factors of personal readiness, social control, and situations or actions.[4] This means that in addition to studying motivational factors designed to change the behavior of individuals, the nature of the environment or social pressures must be critically examined in terms of influences on individuals. A change of behavior, if it gives pleasure, does not entail a great amount of effort, seems socially acceptable, and is presented in an attractive package, may have a chance for success. An example illustrating the factors identified

[4]Edward A. Suchman, "Preventive Health Behavior: A Model for Research on Community Health Campaigns," *Journal of Health and Social Behavior,* **8**(3):197–209, September 1967.

by Suchman is given for purposes of reflection. For citizens who are now middle-aged and smoke or have smoked, it is interesting to reflect what motivated each person to begin smoking at the age they did. For many, when they were teenagers and young adults, the social pressures or appearance of social acceptability attracted their desire and readiness to smoke. Today the social pressures have changed, and the segregation of smokers in identified smoking areas, the denial of smoking during meetings, and the social acceptability of nonsmoking behavior has had curious effects. Many middle-aged citizens who were avid smokers at one time no longer smoke. The factors that strongly influenced these individuals to successfully stop the habit perhaps were related to social control and specific situations. The means they utilized to effect the change of behavior and the factors that contributed to their readiness to stop would provide useful data for studies in motivation.

Initiation of preventive projects or programs requires a knowledge of risk factors and curiosity about new data which are being published continuously. For the purpose of stimulating nursing students to be possibility thinkers—persons who perceptively probe every problem, proposal, and opportunity to discover the positive aspects present in almost every human situation[5]—and to investigate and experiment with primary preventive health measures which will impress consumers, the subsequent sections will deal with risk factors, exercise, relaxation or stress reduction, nutrition, and ecology or environment.

Risk Factors

Heart disease, cancer, and stroke now cause nearly seven-tenths of all U.S. deaths.[6] Disease takes a long time to develop and symptoms appear a long time before a clinical disease is manifested. The problem with many early symptoms is that they can be associated with temporary ailments which are not taken seriously, such as indigestion, heartburn, chronic fatigue, and chest pain. As stated by McCamy and Presley, risk factors that are known to lead to heart disease are smoking; being overweight; having no regular exercise; feeling tense a great deal of the time; having a familial history of heart disease; consuming refined sugars and starches, junk foods, saturated animal fats, and coffee; having an elevated blood cholesterol level; and an elevated blood pressure. For strokes, cerebral vascular accidents, the risk factors are similar in many respects to those for heart disease. McCamy and Presley report that for cancer, data are being published suggesting a correlation between sexual life-style and

[5]Robert H. Schuller, *Move Ahead with Possibility Thinking,* Doubleday & Company, Inc., Garden City, N.Y., 1967, p. 2.
[6]National Health Insurance Resource Book, op. cit., p. 82.

cervical or uterine cancer; the risk factors of smoking, drinking alcoholic beverages, having a long-term nutritional deficiency, and feeling esophageal irritation (drinking beverages or eating food too hot) with cancer of the esophagus; obesity, constipation, and consumption of nitrates (chemical additives used as preservatives) with cancer of the colon. For the person who exercises properly and regularly, a top resistance factor for warding off cancer seems to have been found.[7]

It is of interest that in a study published in the medical journal *Cancer,* September 1975, Enstrom found that citizens of the state of Utah (nearly three-fourths Mormon) have the lowest cancer death rate of any state in the Union. In view of his findings, the life-style of Mormons is worthy of examination because they abstain from alcohol, tobacco, coffee, tea, eat a diet based on wholesome grains, fruits, vegetables, and exercise regularly.[8] Whether an individual accepts the implication that a life-style contributes to the risk of having heart disease, cancer, or stroke or not, a curiosity about and an investigation of this kind of data must be pursued. In experimenting with and preparing primary preventive health projects or programs, community health nurses can appeal to target populations of consumers who are interested in avoiding catastrophic diseases.

A community-based project for controlling hypertension was done at Gimbels in New York City by doctors and nurses at Cornell University Medical College and the United Storeworkers Union. Following an educational campaign, 84 percent of the employees were screened for high blood pressure. Of the 186 with hypertension, two-thirds accepted free treatment for the next year, which included medication and checkups by nurses and paraprofessionals. The union participated by sending reminders and telephoning employees who missed their appointments. After a year of treatment, 81 percent of the employees had a satisfactory reduction in blood pressure. This project demonstrated that the place of work is an effective setting for conducting preventive programs, particularly when all persons in the community-based approach work together as a team. Incidentally there was no loss of work time for the employees![9]

The National Heart and Lung Institute reported that a substantial number of Americans are becoming aware that they have high blood pressure and are in a position to seek treatment. It was estimated that twenty-three million American adults have high blood pressure. Surveys

[7]John C. McCamy and James Presley, *Human Life Styling,* Harper & Row Publishers, Incorporated, New York, 1975, pp. 17–31.

[8]James E. Enstrom, "Cancer Mortality Among Mormons," *Cancer,* **36**(3):825–841, September 1975.

[9]Jody Gaylin, "Keeping Cool at Gimbels: Controlling Hypertension," *Psychology Today* Magazine Newsline, October 1975, p. 27.

in 1971 indicated that nearly half of those who had high blood pressure did not know it. Results of a 1974 survey showed that the percentage of people unaware of their high blood pressure dropped 19 percent. This suggested that in three years, four million Americans became aware that they had high blood pressure.[10]

Preventive health programs are being conducted with demonstrable success. Community health nurses have the opportunity to reach diverse target populations with the same chance for success. However, it must be remembered that although prevention is the goal of a planned project, additional considerations must always include plans for effective advertising, campaigning, educating, reminding, and reinforcing consumer participation.

EXERCISE

Exercise is the means to an alert, vigorous, and lengthy life. Inactivity can kill you.[11] Physical activity can and should be fun, not a chore, and it should be done *daily*. Body tissues and functions are improved by physical activity.[12]

Many citizens are responsive to the idea of exercise and enjoy participating in a program of active sports such as tennis, golf, swimming, bicycling, regular visits to a gymnasium or spa, jogging, attending yoga or body conditioning classes, and similar activities. For citizens who are generally inactive, depressed, listless, and bored, and such people can be found, the challenge for the community health nurse is to entice or persuade these people to start exercising daily—a little at a time, yet increasing the tempo and complexity of movements as their physical fitness progresses. Projects can be tried such as introducing classes or groups to yoga, aerobics, Air Force exercises, walking clubs, or bicycling clubs. Getting a group started takes energy, enthusiasm, and persistence. It may require the utilization of many persuasive techniques including bribery or coercion. However, if consumers become conscious of feeling better and realize that their capacity level to do the activities they enjoy doing has increased, then it is possible to assume that they may continue their exercise regime on their own. A good example of a person who exercises conscientiously every day is an active self-supporting elderly woman of 89 years who swings her arms and legs religiously every morning for a self-prescribed period of time and number of movements.

---

[10]Al Rossiter, Jr., "More Becoming Aware of High Blood Pressure, Seek Treatment," *Seattle Post-Intelligencer,* December 25, 1975.

[11]Laurence E. Morehouse and Leonard Gross, *Total Fitness in 30 Minutes a Week,* Simon & Schuster, Inc., New York, 1975, p. 20.

[12]Ibid., p. 75.

Even when she feels pain on movement, she exercises because "I feel better and walk better after I exercise. If I didn't exercise, I wouldn't be doing the activities that I do today." This lady lives alone, drives her own car, and maintains her own garden.

RELAXATION

No one quarrels with the fact that life today is stressful for most Americans. The tensions of everyday life—transporting oneself to work or school, coping with behavior of others in the immediate environment, meeting one's self-requirements in terms of performance, returning home—all contribute to variable stress-responses. Many persons associate relaxation with sleeping, exercising in a pleasurable activity, or being temporarily inactive. However, for those individuals who engage in meditation or complete relaxation states, they become conscious for the first time of the true meaning of relaxation. Relaxation means the complete absence of holding any part of your body rigid. By relaxation of muscles is meant the complete absence of all contractions. Limp and motionless, the muscle offers no resistance to stretching. It is physically impossible to be nervous in any part of your body, if in that part you are completely relaxed.[13]

Rest is nature's remedy for tension. Learning to relax or control tensions leads to more efficient living through conservation of human energy. By conserving human energy, freedom to accomplish those things a person wants to do is increased because fatigue states are avoided. Jacobson states that a course in scientific relaxation or tension control teaches an individual to run his or her own organism successfully. Advantages concurrent with this accomplishment may be increased job productivity, longer daily working ability, clearer thinking, lessened self-consciousness, harmonious staff meetings and relations, diminished sensitivity to criticism, lessened friction, lessened anxiety, decreased fatigue, decreased absenteeism, better working attitudes.[14] In a course of scientific relaxation, students are taught to become familiar with the sensation, location, and degree of tensions, to note the control sensation which is the sensation from muscular contraction. As students progressively learn tension control, they utilize a self-discipline which leads to relaxation, self-operation, and improved general health. An instructor's text written by Jacobson contains the essential information required for teaching scientific relaxation.[15]

[13]Edmund Jacobson, *You Must Relax,* McGraw-Hill Book Company, Inc., New York, 1962, pp. 84–85.

[14]Edmund Jacobson, *How to Teach Scientific Relaxation: Instructor's Text,* Auspices, Foundation for Scientific Relaxation: Inc., Chicago, 1958, p. 17.

[15]Ibid., pp. 1–147.

Bernstein and Borkovec have written an informative training manual which describes progressive relaxation training in terms of its history, current status, research findings, clientele who can benefit, the rationale for relaxation training, basic procedures, and possible problems with suggested solutions. The manual is concise, is in paperback, and is available for health professionals who wish to teach relaxation training to prospective clients. As cautioned by Bernstein and Borkovec, relaxation training is not a panacea for all clients; it is a technique which must be used with discrimination and judgment. It has been found to have considerable value for persons with high tension levels[16] and can be initiated with clients who are responsive and consenting to preventive measures as suggested by health professionals.

In an article written for business executives, Benson described the "relaxation response" as a simple way for individuals to alleviate stress and thus moderate or control many of its undesirable effects—effects which may range from simple anxiety to heart disease. The "relaxation response" is an innate integrated set of physiologic changes which appear to counteract the harmful physiologic effects of stress.[17] The relaxation response elicits changes similar to those described by persons promoting the regular practice of meditation. It cannot be denied that conscious relaxation, meditation, or temporary withdrawal from the busy activities of the day, when done regularly and for brief time periods, will have beneficial effects for all individuals engaged in the practice. However, for persons with high tension levels and showing physiological damage, such as elevated blood pressure, learning progressive relaxation and practicing it daily diminishes the amount of work required of the heart; and general health, a sense of well-being and renewal, is the result.

As explained by Jacobson, taking a rest or nap each day is beneficial, yet is not as effective in lowering blood pressure as the employment of scientific relaxation. Until an individual has acquired habits of muscular relaxation when resting, the arms and other parts of the body can continue to be in a tense state. Training to relax is an easy treatment and produces lasting results.[18]

Persons of all occupational levels and ages exhibit varying degrees of tension levels and are potential candidates for progressive relaxation training. A project of four relaxation classes was conducted by two senior nursing students with a population of elderly citizens living in a retirement facility. Preceding each class, blood pressure readings were taken, then a thirty-minute tape was played giving instructions for eliciting the relaxa-

---

[16]Douglas A. Bernstein and Thomas D. Borkovec, *Progressive Relaxation Training,* Research Press, 1612 North Mattis Ave., Champaign, Ill., 61820, 1973, p. 11.

[17]Herbert Benson, "Your Innate Asset for Combating Stress," *Harvard Business Review,* 49–60, July–August 1974.

[18]Jacobson, *You Must Relax,* op. cit., p. 231.

tion response. Following the tape, blood pressure readings were taken again. Since the attendance of the class was voluntary, participation of the residents dropped gradually, possibly due to a variety of extraneous factors. However, the data collected at each session showed a reduction in blood pressure following the elicitation of the relaxation response. The average drop in blood pressure per session for each group varied from −3.9 mmHg drop to −16.6 mm. It was found that the particular individuals who attended the four classes regularly had a consistent progressive decline in blood pressure readings which implied the benefits of regularly applying the technique.

For community health nurses who wish to teach progressive relaxation training, thorough knowledge of the technique, personal experience with it, attention to the physical setting, knowledge of muscle groups and familiarity with the sequence for training, and evaluative forms and devices are all requisite before initiating any teaching sessions. Training classes can be utilized in a variety of settings with a diverse range of citizens who consent to participate. Information can be given about stress, consequences of stress, process of relaxation, tension control, physiologic changes, body awareness, significance of breathing, and related subjects. The need for citizens to learn techniques of relaxation and its benefits is an opportunity which is a "natural" for community health nurses and should not be overlooked, particularly when practicing primary prevention.

NUTRITION

Obesity is one of the serious nutritional health problems in the United States. Contributing to the problem is the sedentary nature of our culture which indulges in excessive TV watching and eating "garbage" foods. Income is not necessarily a single important factor that contributes to obesity, as much as eating high caloric foods, junk foods, sweets, habitually eating as a conditioned response, having a daily cocktail, inactivity, eating at all social gatherings or coffee breaks, snacking at all hours of the day or night, eating too fast, and cleaning up your plate. The affluent have a problem with nutrition as do the poor. Selected groups of consumers are demonstrating an avid interest in nutrition as evidenced by the proliferation of natural food and health food stores, soup and salad restaurants, recipe and diet books.

Studies are showing that nutrition has a great deal to do with our daily capacity to perform. Findings of a study done by Viteri demonstrated that when a group of respondents received a diet supplemented with high quality protein and calories, they spent 33 percent of their time in rest or sleep and 67 percent of their time being active at work or after work. In comparison, a nonsupplemented group of subjects who were studied at the same time spent 49 percent of their time at rest or sleep and 51 percent of their time being active at work or after work. The study stated that the nonsupplemented subjects were extremely tired and almost exhausted during the work period whereas the supplemented respondents were not.[19] This study suggests that people who are receiving inadequate nutrition (by scarcity, lack of income, ignorance, or choice) are being robbed of a percentage of their potential active life, their vitality, their sense of well-being, and their freedom from excess fatigue.

In another study done by Cabak and Najdanvic, it was reported that children who were hospitalized for severe malnutrition at less than twelve months of age had a reduced IQ in the later school years as compared to children who had not been malnourished.[20] This study suggests that nutrition not only affects physical energy and vitality, but also intellectual development. In view of the suggested associations which these studies bring out regarding the effect of nutrition on physical and mental performance, it seems imperative for community health nurses to evince a deep interest and curiosity about the diet patterns of the families they visit.

FAMILY NUTRITION

Nutrition, or the lack of it, has played an important part in the long history of human beings. It has been an instrument of government and politics and often a cause of war and conquest. It has led to exploration, discovery, and colonization and has participated in the fate of whole populations. In recent history it has been closely allied with industry through agriculture, transportation, and trade and plays a part in all aspects of modern living. The ultimate aim of nutrition is to provide for the health of the individual and the prevention and treatment of, and recovery from, diseases.

The community health nurse needs an appreciation and knowledge of the culture and background of the families she serves and to use this understanding in developing her nutrition teaching, utilizing the current diets of the families as far as possible, but urging changes as necessary. People and animals have always sought food to satisfy their hunger, but the science of nutrition has shown that not only quantity but *quality* is necessary for health and that an adequate diet is essential to strengthen the body's general resistance to disease.

[19]Milton Terris, "Approaches to an Epidemiology of Health," *American Journal of Public Health,* **65**(10):1037–1045, October 1975.

[20]Herbert G. Birch, "Malnutrition, Learning, and Intelligence," *American Journal of Public Health,* **62**(6):773–784, June 1972.

The prevalence of malnutrition and hunger is a problem and concern of nearly every country, not just the so-called "developing countries." Hunger and malnutrition can only be attacked successfully by a combination of several means. Economics and money, education, food production and distribution, and the recognition of the nutritional value of certain foods are all necessary in meeting the problem. There is no single way of overcoming hunger and malnutrition, for its control is closely associated with the need for adequate shelter and clothing, for fresh water, sanitation, requisite cooking facilities and equipment, and on occasion, the overcoming of communication and language barriers. Home visits often take place in the kitchen, and the nurse can utilize the opportunity to observe the conditions under which the homemaker must prepare meals.

Many families, both rich and poor, lack adequate nutrition despite the availability of food. This is caused by lack of knowledge of nutrition, by faulty traditional food habits, by religious beliefs and taboos, food dislikes, and food fads based on pseudo-science.

Families as well as persons living alone need to learn more about foods that provide normal nutrition and how to spend their money wisely and economically. A report relating to the 1969 White House Conference on Food, Nutrition, and Health in Washington, D.C., considered that previous efforts in nutrition education have been to a large degree ineffective and concluded:

> Most Americans today are abysmally ignorant about the most elementary principles of applied nutrition. This ignorance makes the middle and upper classes ideal targets for food faddists and the poor suffer because their limited food budget allows them no room for mistakes. Although food habits are difficult to change, a national nutritional policy will only become a working reality if we are able to find new effective ways to educate the population in the basics of food and nutrition.[21]

This evaluation of the situation offers a challenge to the nutritionist and the community health nurse working in the home, health center, school, and place of employment. Regardless of adequate money for food, knowledge and understanding of food values, and the availability of food, there can be little success in combatting hunger and malnutrition unless people are *motivated* to eat the nutritious foods their bodies need. This is partly a matter of nutrition teaching, although more than teaching is involved. Learning must take place and be implemented by change, motivation, and new patterns of food use. Acting as a nutrition counselor, the nurse needs to be flexible and develop ways to apply nutrition values

[21]"Message from the White House," Editorial, *The Journal of Nursing Education,* 8(4):5, McGraw-Hill Publications, New York, 1969. By permission of the publisher.

to families' eating habits. She works to bring about needed change when necessary, but the motivation to change must be present for it to last. In seeking to bring about change, she must guard against imposing her own values, standards, and enthusiasm on others. She also needs to recognize that there is no standardized cultural patterns even among people of the same nationality. Although every family on the block may be of the same national origin, there will be wide variations in familial customs and values. They may come from different regions of a country, speak different dialects, and have different standards of living.

Counseling About Nutrition

It is extremely difficult to persuade people to change food habits and can rarely be done based on a "It's good for you" approach. It is always advisable to elicit the families' opinions about food before introducing any of your own ideas. However, before the nurse engages a family in discussion about nutritional ideas and habits, it is good preparation for the nurse to browse through local grocery stores and look at food displays and prices in the neighborhood. In view of her findings, she may want to assist low-income families to set up buying clubs or food cooperatives or at least inform them where food cooperative stores are located. She may want to try cooking some recipes which avoid preprocessed preprepared foods and see if the end result is tasty or not. A good recipe book to experiment with is "Diet for a Small Planet" by Lappé.[22]

The purposes of adequate nutrition are to provide for body growth and development, to maintain general health and resistance to disease, to provide for activity, and to maintain a desirable weight. Margaret Mead has said, "Food affects not only man's dignity, but the capacity of children to reach their full potential, and the capacity of adults to act from day to day."[23]

Every nurse learns that a normal, adequate diet includes a balance of proteins, carbohydrates, and fats in combination with vitamins, especially A, B complex, C, and D, minerals, especially calcium and iron, and an adequate amount of fluids. The problem, and at the same time the challenge, in teaching is to interpret to the homemaker in the family or the person living alone what this means in terms of economics, availability of food, attractive food combinations, preferences of family members, and what contributes to growth and development and to general health and well-being.

Many changes in family organization and living patterns have taken

[22]Frances Moore Lappé, *Diet for a Small Planet*, Friends of the Earth, Ballantine Books, New York, 1971.
[23]Margaret Mead, "Changing Significance of Food," *Journal of Nutrition*, 2(1):17–18, Summer 1970.

place in recent years that affect family nutrition and eating habits. The movement of families from rural to urban areas, varying work shifts at factories and plants of different family members, the increase in the number of homemakers working outside the home, and the many interests and social activities that family members have, such as scouting, clubs, unions, and church meetings, make it increasingly difficult to plan and serve nutritious meals to the family as a group. The extensive advertising of foods and food supplements such as vitamins and iron compounds and some of the "fear" advertising regarding the value of low-calorie foods are responsible in part for a considerable lack of accurate knowledge and understanding of nutrition by many people. It has been said that more Americans are malnourished because of nutritional ignorance and misinformation than because of poverty. In teaching, the nurse should consider some barriers to learning she may encounter, such as apathy, ignorance, and lack of understanding of basic principles of nutrition, long-established family food habits, personal tastes, and lack of money.

Homemakers should be encouraged to include in their meal planning foods selected from the four major food groups: milk and milk products; meat, fish, poultry, eggs, nuts, and vegetables high in protein, e.g., dried beans and peas; fruits and vegetables, especially citrus fruits, tomatoes, and carrots; and enriched or whole grain bread and cereals.

Many homemakers do not always find it possible to provide a completely balanced diet in each meal, but the homemaker or person living alone might think of the meals eaten within a twenty-four-hour period as a unit of meal planning, since meals are affected by modes of modern living and individual needs and preferences. Usually the body has been at rest and has had little food intake for the ten to twelve hours preceding breakfast. For many persons breakfast is an important meal and requires more nutritive elements than are supplied by a sweet roll or doughnut and a cup of coffee. Consideration should be given particularly to children's growth and energy needs and also to those family members engaged in physical activity. Protein should be an important part of breakfast, such as milk, fish, meat, or eggs. In some European countries, cheese is frequently eaten for breakfast. Bread, toast, and cereals, hot and cold, help to provide energy for the coming day. Many families include fruit or fruit juices for breakfast. This may or may not help to provide the daily requirements for vitamins. It depends on the source of the fruit and the juices, how long the fruit has been in storage in the market and the home, and how it has been treated in preparation, for freshness is essential to the vitamin content. Some vitamins may be destroyed by prolonged cooking, also.

A carefully planned and prepared breakfast is a necessity in our urban society, as lunch is often a sketchy meal, eaten away from home and usually in a short time period. This is in contrast to many foreign countries, where the midday meal is an important family activity, with one to one-and-a-half hours allowed for the meal and a rest or relaxation period. When family members carry their lunch to work or school, it is wise to include some fresh fruit, such as oranges, bananas, or apples, and raw vegetables, such as carrot sticks. Mothers should be warned that if they send their children to school with carefully planned and balanced lunches, children have been observed exchanging their lunches for those that contain dill pickles and other interesting but nonnutritive foods.

The evening meal is important to the family's nutrition and should be carefully planned to include adequate servings of protein foods, such as meat, fish, cheese, eggs, or vegetable protein dishes with leafy and root vegetables, milk for children, and a simple dessert—fruit, fresh or cooked, gelatins, or various milk and egg puddings. The dinner should be eaten under as pleasant surroundings as possible.

These are some of the points to be considered in relation to normal diets of an average family without special food needs beyond that of growing, active children and active adults whose health maintenance must be met.

In nutrition teaching and working for change in dietary habits, the nurse should help the homemaker or person living alone to build whenever possible on the accustomed diet. A "meat and potato" diet meets many nutritional requirements and with the addition of such leafy vegetables as spinach, broccoli, or a salad and some fruit could be made a satisfactory one. Low-income families tend to use a diet high in "starchy" foods, because it is less expensive, is temporarily filling, and gives quick energy. However, it does not meet the body's requirements for growth and development of muscles, bones, and teeth or for general well-being.

There are many approaches to teaching nutrition for the alert nurse that will enable her to help the homemaker or the person living alone. There are times when a visit is made before the remains of breakfast or lunch have been cleared away and by observing unobtrusively, the nurse can learn something about the family's eating patterns. In discussing diet and foods, the nurse needs to ask questions that will provide more information than just a "yes" or "no" response.

A review of a record of the family's menus for two or three days will provide insight into some of the nutrition problems. In one instance, the sixth-grade daughter of a family had a severe problem of overweight. By reviewing the family menus, including snacks the girl had at school, for three days, it was discovered that the snacks alone—candy bars, ice cream, and doughnuts—came to more than 600 calories a day. This brought out several psychological problems of which the family was not aware.

The nurse needs to be nonthreatening in her teaching, recognizing that the homemaker may be doing the best she can under the circumstances and in the face of such problems as meal preparation on a low income and meal planning with foods available from "surplus foods" and "food stamps." Some nurses have recipes they can share or exchange with homemakers for casseroles, the cooking of cheap cuts of meat, and simple desserts. On occasion, a productive way to teach is to accompany the homemaker to the market to give assistance in economy buying, showing her how to read the labels and compare sizes and prices of cans and packages.

Not only are the nutritionists in health centers, health departments, and hospitals available to the nurse for consultation, but also many private health organizations, such as the local heart association, employ nutritionists who can be most helpful. Nutritionists associated with some of the commercial businesses such as food processing plants and dairies often help. They are interested in the nutrition problems the nurse encounters in her work with families. In one "company" town suffering from a severe economic depression, the nutritionist from the local gas and electric company worked with the nurse to present some cooking demonstrations of low-cost menus and provided copies of the recipes demonstrated.

When certain dietary restrictions conform to religious beliefs or cultural practices regarding the eating of meat or other foods, substitutions can be worked out. Assistance for this can be secured from a local nutritionist.

NUTRITIONAL NEEDS OF SPECIAL GROUPS

Pregnant and Lactating Mothers

Every expectant mother needs dietary supervision throughout her pregnancy. When carefully planned, meals for *both* the mother and her family can provide for all those nutrients needed for growth and development, energy, and general well-being. Many foods are sources for more than one nutritional requirement. In planning for her diet with the pregnant and lactating mother, consideration should be given to her age. Is she a teen-ager? or does she belong to a later age group? If she is a single teen-ager, she faces difficult problems—personal, emotional, familial, and health, with all their complications. Furthermore, these problems can have a direct effect on her baby.

Most teen-age pregnant mothers are still in their own growth period. Studies have shown that the nutritional status of many adolescents is unfavorable for an early pregnancy. The unfortunate outcome of many teen-age pregnancies, including maternal morbidity and mortality and infant morbidity and mortality, reflects this. Attention should be given to the nutritional status of this group, based on individual needs determined by careful physical examination to discover the presence of nutritional anemias and poor dietary habits. The pregnant woman who has passed through adolescence and who spaces her pregnancies so that her body has the opportunity to rebuild its nutritional well-being can expect a much more favorable outcome of her pregnancy and a healthier infant.

Calcium   With the growth of the fetus and accessory tissues during pregnancy, a significant need for calcium and iron occurs in the mother's body. This becomes more pronounced in the second and third trimesters and even more so during the lactation period. Pregnant women should understand the importance of calcium in their diet and its contribution to the growth and development of the infant's tooth and bone structure. Milk and milk products are good sources of calcium. Turnip and mustard greens, broccoli, and cooked dry beans are considered fair sources, and oranges are also a fair source.

Iron   Iron is an essential in the prenatal diet and in the second and third trimesters there is an increasing need to include it in the diet in order to:

1   Maintain the mother's hemoglobin level
2   Maintain her body stores of iron
3   Provide iron for fetal development
4   Furnish the infant with iron stores needed for blood formation during the neonatal period before iron-rich foods are added to the diet

It requires careful planning to include sufficient iron in the mother's daily diet. Good sources of iron include liver (both pork and beef), kidneys, oysters and clams, heart, lean pork and beef, raisins, cooked dried beans, canned peas, dried peaches, apricots, and prunes. Fair sources include spinach, mustard greens, eggs, and whole wheat bread and cereals.

Vitamins   The pregnant mother has an increased need for vitamins, especially in the last six months, and also during the lactating period.

Vitamin A   A fat-soluble vitamin, vitamin A is an essential factor in cell development, in normal bone formation and tooth development, and for a healthy skin. Good sources include liver, kidneys, egg yolk, whole milk, cream and butter, dark green and deep yellow vegetables such as broccoli and carrots, and such fruits as peaches, apricots, and canta-loupes. If buttermilk or nonfat milk is used in place of whole milk, being cheaper, other sources of vitamin A should be added to the diet. Such foods as salad dressing made with mineral oil are not advised because mineral oil interferes with the body's ability to absorb carotene (vitamin A) and other fat-soluble vitamins and also affects calcium and phosphorus absorption.

Thiamine (B-1)   This vitamin helps to keep both the appetite and digestion normal. It is necessary for completion of carbohydrate metabolism and is a factor in the maintenance of a healthy nervous system. It occurs widely, but in small amounts in many foods; thus, it points up the value of a varied diet. Again the second and third trimesters of pregnancy require additional intake of thiamine, as does the lactation period. Good sources include liver, heart and kidney, lean pork, dried beans and peas, whole grains, nuts, peanut butter, white potatoes, and oranges. Fair sources include fish, poultry, other meats, eggs, milk, and many fruits and vegetables.

Riboflavin (B-2)   Riboflavin assists in the metabolism of carbohydrates and amino acids. It has an increasing importance in the second and third trimesters of pregnancy. Milk is a good source, also liver, heart, and kidney. Fair sources include lean meat, poultry, cheese, eggs, dark green leafy vegetables, and whole wheat bread and cereals.

Niacin (B-3)   This vitamin aids the body in translating sources of energy into usable form. When the protein in the diet is of good quality and of sufficient amount, the body's niacin intake will be adequate. Good sources include fish, heart, liver, kidney, poultry, and peanuts. Fair sources are found in milk, whole grain bread and cereals, and white potatoes.

Ascorbic acid (vitamin C)   Vitamin C is an essential element in the diet of the entire family, but especially for the pregnant mother. During the second and third trimesters and lactation period, it is recommended that her diet include a minimum of one serving a day from a good source and one from a fair source. Vitamin C increases the body's ability to absorb iron and is necessary for the development and maintenance for normal connective tissue in bones, cartilage, and muscle. Good sources are to be found in fresh fruits, including oranges, strawberries, cantaloupe, and grapefruit, and in such vegetables as cooked greens (turnip, mustard, and spinach), brussel sprouts, and red and green peppers. Fair sources include fresh tomatoes, cooked cauliflower, sweet or white potatoes, raw cabbage, and liver. The body does not store vitamin C as it does vitamin A, so it should be included in the daily diet.

Vitamin D   Sources of vitamin D, a fat-soluble vitamin, include not only certain foods, but also sunshine. The pregnant mother requires an additional amount of vitamin D in her diet during the second and third trimesters and in the lactation period. This vitamin promotes the absorption and retention of calcium and phosphorus in the body and is necessary during the fetal growth period for the formation of teeth and bones. Frequently the physician orders supplementary vitamin D for the pregnant woman, especially during dark winter months, when there is little sunshine. The mother should be warned against the dangers of overdosing of vitamin D. Food sources include fortified milk, butter, fish oils, egg yolk, and liver.

Special Health Problems

Pregnant and nursing mothers with special diet problems for underweight or obesity should have continuous medical supervision throughout pregnancy and the lactation period. Efforts to reduce during pregnancy should not be made, except under physician's orders and close supervision. The weight of current medical opinion is to the effect that "severe caloric restriction is potentially harmful to the developing fetus and to the mother and almost inevitably restricts other nutrients essential for the growth process."[24] The need for this medical supervision applies also to mothers with chronic diseases of the heart, nephritis, or diabetes, all of which would require dietary restrictions of certain foods.

Folk Medicine: Use of Herbs

Folk medicine practice is the curative and maintenance behavior used by individuals to solve health problems. The response of many consumers to the ideas of folk medicine and herbalism (the knowledge and study of herbs) is growing. Visits to health food stores, natural or organic food stores, spice or herbal shops will reveal a wide selection of foods, supplements, and herbs at variable prices. Consumer advocates can always be found in these stores who are knowledgeable, firm, and persuasive about particular products recommended for purchasing. Some people buy herbs for medicinal reasons, some like to try different herbal teas experimentally, and some buy for healing purposes. An intellectual curiosity and a willingness to listen to persuasive arguments about the use of herbs and folk remedies is enlightening. Many of the folk remedies and folklore of different ethnic groups which are handed down from generation to generation have merit and bear investigation before discrediting them altogether. It is good practice never to laugh at or ridicule a belief no matter how wierd it sounds. The wise nurse will listen and learn about home remedies and practices the family is carrying out and will suggest complementary health measures as necessary or advisable.

In their study of food taboos, Bartholomew and Poston concluded there was a "need for further investigation and study of the background,

---

[24]National Academy of Sciences, *Maternal Nutrition and the Course of Pregnancy: Summary Report*, Washington, D. C., 1970, p. 13.

beliefs and customs of an individual before determining his or her nutritional status and giving constructive guidance. Every effort should be made to explore new avenues and approaches in motivation, education and guidance in this area."[25]

NUTRITIONAL NEEDS OF INFANTS, PRESCHOOL, AND SCHOOL CHILDREN

Infants

Breast feeding is the natural way to feed a new baby. Human breast milk is suited to the digestive system of the normal baby and provides the nourishment needed in the first few months of life. When breast feeding is not feasible for the new baby for reasons such as the mother's health or allergies, unusual food needs of the baby, or because of social or economic conditions, the baby should be under close medical supervision and a suitable formula prescribed, with semisolid foods added gradually upon the doctor's recommendation.

Babies develop at different rates of speed even within the same family. Some have teeth at five or six months, while others get teeth months later. Some infants are walking by their first birthday, while others begin later. It is the same with foods; all children are different, but usually by their first birthday they should be having some soft foods, such as pureed fruits, vegetables, and meats, eggs, bread, rice, and other cereals. Children begin new foods slowly, and it is better not to urge them to eat foods which at first taste they appear to dislike, but rather to wait and reintroduce the food again a few weeks later with one they do like.

Until they are about three years old, children are in a rapid growth period in relation to their size. If their mothers have eaten wisely and carefully during their pregnancy, the children will have good head starts nutritionally. Their diet for the first three years of life is important to future growth and development and for their general health. They need protein body-building foods and calories for energy. Their stomachs are small and they will not be able to eat much at a time. Usually they will need food more often than the family's three-meals-a-day pattern.

Preschool Children

At about three years of age, the rate of growth tends to slow down and appetites may decrease. Parents should not be unduly concerned unless there are other symptoms. A basic menu pattern for preschool children is suggested (Table 8-1) that can be adapted to meal planning for the entire family.

[25]Mary Jo Bartholomew and Frances E. Poston, "Effect of Food Taboos on Prenatal Nutrition," *Journal of Nutrition Education,* 2(1)15–17, Summer 1970.

Table 8-1

Breakfast	Lunch	Dinner
Fruit or juice	Meat or substitute	Meat or substitute
Meat or substitute	Vegetable or salad	Vegetable or salad
Bread and/or cereal	Bread or substitute	Bread or substitute
Butter and milk	Butter and milk	Butter and milk
	Dessert: fruit,	Dessert: fruit,
	jello, or ice cream	jello, or ice cream

Children often need between-meal snacks. These can be fruit, fruit juices, milk, celery or carrot sticks, bread and peanut butter, or a *small* serving of a sweet—cookies or ice cream. The between-meal snack contributes to the child's total nutrition intake.

School-Age Children

Children who have formed good eating habits in early childhood will have few diet problems at this age period. As they grow older, their energy needs increase. They need larger servings, and some sweets added to their diet. It should be emphasized to parents that all growing children need *protein*—meat, milk and milk products, fish, and eggs; *carbohydrates*— bread, cereals, fruits, vegetables, and simple desserts; *fats*—butter, peanut butter, cream; and *vitamins* and *minerals* from fruits and vegetables.

Teen-Agers

Boys In this age period, boys are in a time of rapid growth and energy needs. They need foods richer in nutrients than perhaps at any other time of their lives. Many need snacks that have nutrition value, not just a cola or a candy bar, but foods selected from the four major food groups.

Girls The teen years are an important period of physical and psychological development for girls. They also need more essential nutrients than at any other time of their lives, except perhaps during the later months of their pregnancy and lactation periods. Yet, according to dietary studies, teen-age girls often have the poorest eating practices of any age group. They tend to become figure conscious and inclined to cut down on amounts of food without respect to the quality and nutritive content.

Breakfast is often neglected in order to allow more time for sleeping or for dressing. In these times of fashion awareness, many girls of normal weight consider themselves to be too fat and try for a more slender figure by "crash" or "fad" diets of calorie counting at the expense of essential nutritious foods, especially those needed for tissue development and for body reserves. It should be stressed that in attempting to reduce weight it is the quantity of food that should be restricted and not the nutritive *quality.*

Iron intake is frequently lessened in these diets with resulting nutritional anemias and susceptibility to colds and other infections, even tuberculosis. Teen-age girls with anemias are inclined to be apathetic, irritable, or fatigued and to lose interest in school achievement. Motivating this group to eat the foods they need is often difficult, but the nurse must try to be original and innovative in making suggestions. A good breakfast decreases the hunger and energy needs at lunch time, when it is so easy to consume high-calorie foods, such as potato chips, pie, and candy bars. Participation in such physical activities as swimming, hiking, tennis, or skating should be encouraged. Finally, giving the girl some responsibility for the planning, purchasing, and preparation of family meals stimulates interest in nutrition. With the increasing number of teen-age marriages and pregnancies, the nutritional status of the teen-age girl has a high priority, not only for her family but for society as well, since many teen-agers will be mothers before they are twenty.

Teen-age girls and boys with serious overweight problems should be seen by their physician for several reasons before commencing a weight-reduction regime. To date, the etiology of adolescent obesity is not clearly defined, and certain physiologic factors may be operating that are not understood. Some cases of obesity might possibly be associated with certain diseases, such as diabetes or heart and kidney difficulties, and this should be ruled out before undertaking a reducing program. In some instances, the obesity might result from genetic traits, which would involve several approaches to the problem. A large proportion of obesity cases, however, appear to result from physical inactivity coupled with the availability of the ample and varied food supplies in our society. A psychological approach may be the most effective one, an approach in which there is no nagging or teasing, but a sense of support, cooperation, and encouragement by other members of the family. The content of the diet should be carefully watched to ensure that the foods so necessary to the growing adolescent are included.

In some cultures, children and other family members are urged to overeat, with the idea that the resulting obesity indicates that the parents, especially the father, have sufficient money to feed the family "well." The nurse and the nutritionist need to approach such a situation with extreme caution and delicacy, as this is a matter of family pride, and careful teaching is involved or the results could be destructive.

Appearances for girls and physical prowess for boys are the activating forces for good nutrition and the underlying relationships of sound nutrition to these forces should be demonstrated to all teen-agers. Nutrition affects appearance and is related not only to weight but to posture, as good posture is determined by strong muscles and bones. Skin, hair, and eyes will also reflect the teen-ager's nutritional state. It is important to teach, but not to preach, nutrition to teen-agers. There is no magic formula that will persuade them to eat the foods they really need. The challenge lies in presenting nutrition information in such a way that it will motivate them to think and voluntarily select wisely from the variety of available foods.

The Middle-Aged (Over Thirty-five Years)

The need for protective foods remain as high for this age group as for young adults. Adequate nutrition will help to lengthen the period of maximum enjoyment and vitality as well as the life span. Milk, meat or substitutes, fruits and vegetables, and bread and cereals are as necessary as in earlier years to maintain general good health and replace tissue. Many people of this age group are not as active as they were in former years. They need to watch their food intake, cutting down on quantity but not on quality, for there is still the need for food of nutritive value. General outdoor exercise such as walking, golf, and swimming should be encouraged and "crash" or "fad" diets discouraged.

In this age group, some of the chronic diseases may appear, such as diabetes or cardiac disturbances, that require diet restrictions. This will provide opportunities for teaching nutrition to the patient and the homemaker. When obesity is a problem, reducing should be undertaken on the physician's advice and the nurse can offer assistance and support. Obesity might have a psychological basis, with compulsive eating resulting from feelings of frustration or of not having a sense of being necessary now that the children are grown and have assumed their own responsibilities. Helping the individual to build new interests and diversions might aid in overcoming the obesity. In general, middle-aged persons need a well-rounded diet, still high in quality, but lower in quantity, and with sufficient outdoor exercise and interests.

The Elderly

During their working years, most people invest their money with the hope and anticipation of adequate financial resources upon retirement. During this time they should also be making an investment in good health for their retirement years through sound dietary practices. Difficulties can result when there are not habits of good nutrition for retirement, when living patterns will be different. Preparation for retirement is more than just financial, for sound nutrition patterns will be important.

Faulty diets in the aged are commonly results of loneliness and financial worry, which can lead to a malnutrition so severe that life cannot be enjoyed. Loneliness tends to increase poor eating habits, such as overeating of starchy, unbalanced meals and nibbling sweets, eating too little food at irregular times, or foods that contain slight nutritional value, at times a "tea and toast" diet. Some elderly people excuse themselves for this by a "what's the use?" attitude.

The nurse's challenge is to encourage an interest in all aspects of the meal: the planning, shopping, cooking, and eating. People should be encouraged to have their meals in as pleasant a situation as possible, to eat slowly and savor the food. For some, listening to the radio, watching television, or reading while eating can contribute to the pleasure of the meal.

Many retired men and women living alone have never learned to plan, buy, or cook a meal, and they need help to undertake such a program for themselves. There are some community resources to help them, such as senior citizens center classes and clubs. They particularly need help with shopping when the food budget is limited, for it may be a problem in relation to small buying and cooking. Emphasis should be on the importance of a varied diet selected from the four major food groups. A home economist has offered the following suggestions for planning and shopping under these situations for this group.

1 Keep up-to-date on food prices by watching advertisements.
2 Buy no more food at one time than can be used easily; a big economy-sized package is not a bargain if it grows stale or spoils or the person tires of it.
3 Buy dry mixes for breads, cakes, and puddings; a portion can be used and the remainder will keep in a cool place.
4 Cook small amounts when possible; half a cup of shelled peas or cut string beans makes a normal serving.

The elderly need one or more servings a day of meat, fish, eggs, or other protein foods, also milk and milk products, cereal or bread, fruit, or fruit juices, and vegetables. Some elderly people may be unable to tolerate certain foods, such as raw fruits and vegetables. Vitamins and minerals play an important part in the individual's health and can be supplied through careful selection of foods. Although these persons may not be as active as formerly, a varied diet with plenty of fluids is still essential for good health.

Chronic diseases requiring diet restrictions occur frequently in this age group, including diabetes and cardiac disturbances, also degenerative diseases such as cancer and paralysis agitans. The physician will prescribe diets for these conditions, but the nurse will need to explain—more than once—why it is important to avoid salt or sugar and why soft foods may sometimes be necessary. Salt and sugar substitutes are available at pharmacies and grocery stores; they can make meals more palatable. Often patients must experiment with them to find the one they like best, as their flavors differ.

When older persons live in a household with younger people their diet regime can be adapted to the regular family meal, with the omission of raw fruits and vegetables as necessary and the avoidance of certain foods that are too rich or highly seasoned.

It is important to point out to the elderly, especially those living alone, the close relationship of nourishing food to good health and a sense of well-being in order to enjoy life.

DIET IN DISEASE

Nutrition is not only essential in maintaining good health, but it is also an important factor in restoring the patient to health or at least enabling him or her to function to as normal a degree as possible. A discussion of the implications of nutrition in diseases frequently encountered by the community health nurse in the home is included here.

Diabetes

Known to man for centuries, diabetes is a disease of nutritional interest and is encountered frequently by the community health nurse in her work. It is widespread, found in every economic and age group, but most often in women above forty years of age. There are indications that it might have an inherited tendency, although there are other causes.

When diabetes occurs in children and young adults, it is of a more serious nature. These young patients usually require insulin treatment and a special diet planned for their nutritional needs by the physician. Usually the patient or a family member is taught insulin administration at the health center, the physician's office, or during a hospital stay. The nutritionist confers with the patient and family members regarding the prescribed diet and ways of following it. She teaches the use of scales and other measures as needed and advises on menu planning and meal preparation. The community health nurse's responsibility is to follow up the teaching in the home by: (1) supervising the insulin administration until she is satisfied that either the patient or a family member understands and can carry out the procedure satisfactorily; (2) advising and assisting with diet problems as they arise in the home; and (3) watching for any unusual condition.

When diabetes occurs in patients over forty years of age, it usually has a milder course and can frequently be controlled by diet, sometimes a strict one. Obesity aggravates diabetes and often is a complicating factor and must be considered in the patient's entire treatment program in relation to diet, calorie intake, and exercise.

Diet Obviously, any form of sugar, such as candy, cake, jam, cookies, pie, syrup, or honey, must be omitted from the diabetics' diets, yet they must have adequate nutrition for energy, body-building tissues, maintenance of good health, and resistance to infection. Their food should have a psychological appeal and be attractively served. When patients are placed on diabetic diets they usually will have some resistance to the restrictions, and this is normal. In introducing patients to their new diet, the nurse's objective is to change or adjust their behavior and former patterns of eating. It is important to teach them about the new diet slowly, as learners must progress from one new idea to the next until they understand the restrictions the disease has put on their choice of foods. At first, some patients will place too much reliance on the effect of the insulin and tend to cheat a little in eating. The nurse should direct her teaching to activating these patients to accept the diet for its positive outcomes, e.g., lessening the chances of cataracts or foot circulation difficulties. It is important to help patients recognize and accept their disease as a way of life. Listen to their accounts of frustration with the prescribed diet, the food substitutes, elimination from the diet of favorite foods, and change of eating habits. The nurse needs to amplify and reinforce what they have learned and assist them in translating it into their own changed dietary behavior.

The exchange Diabetics, like other people, must have some carbohydrates, protein, and fat each day in their diet. It is essential for all but those with a very mild diabetic condition to eat the exact amount of the foods planned for their daily intake—no more, no less—especially if they are taking insulin. To facilitate planning for the patient's dietary needs, foods necessary to the diabetic's health were classified and divided into six "exchanges": (1) milk, (2) vegetables, (3) fruits, (4) bread and cereals, (5) meats, and (6) fats. These are considered to be "protective" foods.

Most diabetic lists are made out in definite terms, indicating carefully weighed or measured amounts of carbohydrate, protein, and fats by grams—such as one cup of whole milk is carbohydrate, 12 grams; protein, 8 grams; and fat, 10 grams. One slice of baker's bread is carbohydrate, 15 grams; protein, 2 grams; and fat, 0 grams. Three ounces of cooked ground beef contains carbohydrate, 0; protein, 21 grams; and fat, 15 grams. The diet list and menus are made out for a twenty-four-hour period. An "exchange" system provides for wider choice in the diet and at the same time keeps the diet within the limitations of the patient's required grams of carbohydrate, protein, and fat for the twenty-four-hour period. A simple example would be that if a patient wanted a soft boiled egg for dinner in place of a meat serving, the egg would be considered equivalent to a meat allowance of 1 ounce in an exchange. A more involved exchange would be an apricot, cottage cheese, and lettuce salad for lunch, which would provide exchanges for one fruit, one meat, and one vegetable from the "A" list.

Vegetables on the "A" list include those that contain 3 grams or less of carbohydrates per one-half-cup serving; examples are lettuce, broccoli, young string beans, or greens. Usually they are allowed "as desired." Group "B" vegetables contain 7 percent or more carbohydrates per 100 grams and must be considered in the carbohydrate allowance for the twenty-four hours. They include green peas, winter squash, and such root vegetables as carrots, onions, beets, and turnips.[26]

Until diabetics have full appreciation of the need for strict compliance to their required diet and are completely motivated to follow it, they will need the support of family and close friends to protect them from well-meaning people who will say, "This cake is very simple, it can't possibly hurt you." Or "Just one little piece of candy isn't anything."

Many patients have a diabetic condition so mild that medication is not indicated and treatment is based on a low carbohydrate intake. High blood sugar or sugar in the urine usually appears in this group only after a high carbohydrate intake including such sugar-rich foods as candy or cake. These patients need to be highly motivated to keep on their diet. The nurse can be of assistance to both patient and family in teaching the value of the diet and by her understanding and appreciation of the frustrations at not being able to have some of the "favorite" foods and foods that others are eating.

Together the nurse and patient and/or the family can plan a nutritious, satisfying diet that will maintain health and well-being. This should be a normal diet, but low in carbohydrate, and include meat and meat substitutes, some fats, and adequate vitamins and minerals. Fresh fruits can be used for dessert. Some bread and cereals are needed as a source of vitamin B complex. Families are always looking for new flavoring products which will mitigate the feeling of restriction regarding the patient's diet. Sugar and salt substitutes are available, which will enable the patient to have some favorite dishes. The addition of lemon juice or herbs and spices will often increase the tastiness of food that was lacking with the use of sugar substitute alone. When recipes can be devised which will satisfy patients' tastes, they are happier and the cook's work is made easier.

Patients should be alerted to the recognition and care of diabetic symptoms and conditions. The nurse should help them to learn the importance of following their diet and maintaining their personal care,

[26]Linnea Anderson and John H. Browe, *Nutrition and Family Health Service,* W. B. Saunders Company, Philadelphia, 1961, pp. 47–58.

e.g., care of the feet and daily exercise, so that their health and well-being can be sustained.

Because of improved diagnostic techniques, this mild type of diabetes is being discovered more frequently than in the past and provides the nurse with many opportunities for health teaching to patient and family regarding the disease and its care.

Heart Disease and Stroke

There are multiple causes for a person's suffering a heart attack or a stroke. Among them are obesity and a faulty diet extending over a period of years, lack of sufficient physical activity, emotionally stressful situations at home or at work, environmental factors, family history of such attacks, habitual cigarette smoking, and certain diseases such as diabetes. Usually an attack follows a combination of two or more of these causes or situations.

Many Americans have a diet high in cholesterol and animal (saturated) fats, such as eggs and meat, and dairy products such as butter, cream, and whole milk. Other foods of high caloric value such as ice cream and rich cakes and pies are common in the American diet. These foods tend to increase the cholesterol in the blood of many individuals, which in turn contributes to the development of atherosclerosis, a disease that underlies most heart attacks and strokes.

Diet The diets of patients convalescing from a heart attack or a stroke are of major importance in their return to health. They should understand that in all likelihood they will follow it fairly closely for the remainder of their lives. In most cases, the physician orders a low-sodium diet, based on 1,200 to 1,800 calories per day. It is important that the patients and homemaker understand the major objectives of this diet, which are to provide for low calories, low-sodium intake, and low roughage and yet at the same time to supply sufficient amounts of vital nutrients. The patients' food likes and dislikes should be determined and respected in diet planning as far as possible. Sodium is an essential mineral for all human beings, animals, and plant life and a diet too low in sodium could prove harmful, but since sodium appears in practically all foods and drinking water, this is not of unusual concern. It is believed that the average person ingests between 5,000 and 8,000 milligrams of sodium in the daily diet. One level teaspoon of table salt contains approximately 2,300 milligrams of sodium. There are many sources of sodium in the average diet that the patient and the family might overlook in diet planning. In addition to table salt, foods may contain baking soda, baking powder, and often monosodium glutamate, the latter used for flavor accent. It is important to read food labels carefully on packaged, canned, or frozen foods to determine the amount of sodium included. Many frozen vegetables are processed with table salt, such as frozen lima beans, so patients and families should be alerted to the salt content of these foods.

A low-sodium diet is often flat and uninteresting to the taste, but care must be exercised in the use of seasonings. Table salt is to be avoided, also prepared mustard, meat sauces, celery and parsley flakes, and garlic, onion, and celery salts. Other herbs and spices, such as pepper, oregano, and paprika, may be added in small amounts unless limited by the physician. Fresh lemon and lime juice may be used for enhancing flavors. These juices could add to the vitamin C content of the diet, as well. Here, too, the family often needs help in finding substitutes for salt which will satisfy the patient's taste and increase variety in the diet. The nurse should show the patient or family how to appraise the content of the salt substitute so that they are aware of the meaning of the symbols on the label. Often the doctor will recommend a specific substitute.

The physician's diet list will include the foods the patient may have. This will be influenced by the severity of the attack and the resulting condition. Foods most patients should avoid include baked beans, bacon and ham, canned meats, canned soups, bread, crackers, and some cereals. Exchanges can provide flexibility in the diet, and with the physician's approval can be used by the heart patient as they are by the diabetic patient.

In planning a low-sodium diet to meet heart patients' dietary needs, the homemaker or the patients themselves must bear in mind the requirements for protein, carbohydrate, and fat as well as vitamins and minerals needed for general good health. It is important not to lose sight of these patients' general nutritional needs, while at the same time meeting those special dietary needs required by their heart condition. In other words, do not overlook the forest for the trees.

Prevention As a preventive measure, the community health nurse should be alert while working with families to situations or health problems in the home that could lead to heart attacks in later years, such as emotionally stressful situations, heavy cigarette smoking, obesity, and diets apparently high in those foods conducive to heart disease. Helping families to face these situations objectively and before they become too serious provides opportunities that could be productive for teaching prevention of faulty heart conditions that could result in invalidism in later years.

Helpful material may be secured from the American Heart Association, and its local or state associations that the nurse can use in her teaching and the patient and family can have for reference.

Phenylketonuria

There are other diseases of a chronic nature that require strict adherence to a specific diet if the patient is to live a normal, productive life. Our knowledge of biochemistry, genetics, and other sciences is increasing at a rapid rate. This knowledge has implications for the health and care of many people with diseases about which little is known currently. The disease phenylketonuria, frequently referred to as PKU, is an example. The only treatment to date is severe dietary restrictions of certain proteins and a substitute formula, beginning at birth if possible and probably continuing throughout life. The physician prescribes a special diet which provides little variation, although as more knowledge is acquired about the disease it may be possible to widen the content of the diet. Research in this disease is still in the experimental stages. The nurse's function is to work closely with the physician and the parents, teaching the parents the reasons for the diet and for carrying it out to the letter. Some recent studies have pointed to the value of the mother following the diet, if indicated, during her pregnancy.

Parents need considerable emotional support because of the rigorous food restrictions that must be imposed on the infant and child and the frequent blood samples to be taken. Many parents and grandparents have some guilt feelings also, since this is a disease linked with heredity. Some members of the medical profession estimate that control of this disease eventually could result in the reduction of patient population in institutions if the disease is discovered immediately after birth and treatment is instituted.

ECOLOGY AND ENVIRONMENT

A person's involvement with the natural environment is inescapable. How you live and what you do has an impact, either directly or indirectly, on the world around you. Whether you are overtly concerned or not, social actions related to pollution (air, noise, water), recycling, disposables, solid wastes, conservation of energy and natural resources, population control—all affect you.

Historically, as humanity has evolved, the sociocultural system has been able to protect and insulate us increasingly from certain injurious effects of our environments. In other words, over time the human population has adapted to its native environment and maintained a dynamic equilibrium with processes of environmental change.[27]

[27]Solomon H. Katz and Anthony F. C. Wallace, "An Anthropological Perspective on Behavior and Disease," *American Journal of Public Health*, **64**(11):1050–1052, November 1974.

In our current era, there is a great deal of concern about the encroachment of undesirable problems such as pollution, overcrowding, and limited natural resources due to technology and carelessness. Where there is high population density (urban environment) there is increasing worry about the environmental problems of noise, accumulating garbage, occasional power outages. In addition, metropolitan areas tend to manifest disordered relationships due to crowding, stress, deprivation, and lack of territorial control.[28]

Many people believe our present quality of life is endangered unless steps are taken to safeguard and protect our environment. This means that actions must be directed toward reducing air, water, noise pollutions, saving or conserving our natural resources, and adopting life-styles which assure a reasonable expectation of the necessities of life for everyone. Even though it seems fashionable today to be pessimistic and forecast crises of many different types, the purpose is served of alerting the general population to possible environmental catastrophes.

What can be done about environmental problems? As possible from a community action standpoint, a pathological pattern of behavior (individual or social) can be changed, or a protective behavior pattern can be introduced. A familiarity with social epidemiology can lead a student to investigate cultural situations, social situations, and personality situations as they interrelate with the host and agent, so as to provide knowledge about intervention points toward which prevention can be directed. As stated by Graham, there is much epidemiological knowledge about the agent, vector, and host, and what should be done to effect prevention; however, behavioral changes that are necessary and the sociological knowledge regarding how this behavior can be successfully altered to effect prevention is lacking.[29] When scientific inquiry becomes more devoted to studying social factors within the environment which are of a preventive nature, perhaps incidences of diseases and environmental wastages or pollutions will be reduced markedly.

On a small scale, local citizens and nurses can become active in ecological organizations such as the Audubon Society, the Wilderness Society, Common Cause, or any antipollution group. Campaigning for legislation which provides for cleaner air or water measures in the local community is an activity which can gain constructive results. In addition, individually, each committed person can reduce the amount of electric energy used daily, may organize car pools, save all materials which can be recycled, avoid use of disposable products, plant a garden, and recruit

[28]John Cassel, "An Epidemiological Perspective of Psychosocial Factors in Disease Etiology," *American Journal of Public Health,* 64(11):1040–1043, November 1974.

[29]Saxon Graham, "The Sociological Approach to Epidemiology," *American Journal of Public Health,* 64(11):1046–1049, November 1974.

friends into the ecological movement. Every nurse should maintain an active interest and concern regarding ecological and environmental issues. When problems become apparent within local communities, community health nurses should be knowledgeable about the environmental issues under discussion and be able to inform citizens about recommended actions.

SUMMARY

Emphasizing the concept of primary prevention persuasively to citizens in an effort to gain their attention and interest in maintaining optimal health was the message of the chapter. Preventive health projects already have been implemented with satisfactory results. Many innovative projects can be initiated by community health nurses which are primarily preventive in nature. These programs can be related to exercise, relaxation or stress reduction, nutrition, or ecology and environment.

In all these fields of study the nurse must keep abreast of current findings and studies, work closely with or seek consultation from the professionals who have the expertise and knowledge, and grasp opportunities to teach creatively or advocate preventive health measures for individuals, families, and groups. By being visible and articulate, the community health nurse will be contributing her own expertise and knowledge of human behavior toward the actualization of citizen health in local communities.

SUGGESTED READING

Birch, Herbert G., and Joan Dye Gussow: *Disadvantaged Children: Health, Nutrition and School Failure,* Harcourt Brace Jovanovich, Inc., New York, 1970, and Grune & Stratton, Inc., 1970.

Boston Women's Health Book Collective: *Our Bodies, Ourselves,* Simon and Schuster, New York, 1973.

Callahan, Catherine L.: "The White House Conference on Food, Nutrition and Health," *Nursing Outlook,* **18**:58–60, January 1970.

Christakis, George: "Nutritional Assessment in Health Programs," *American Journal of Public Health,* Supplement, **63**:1–73, November 1973.

Cooper, Kenneth H.: *The New Aerobics,* M. Evans & Co., Inc., New York, 1970.

Crim, Sarah R.: "Nutritional Problems of the Poor," *Nursing Outlook,* **17**:65–67, September 1969.

Devi, Indra: *Yoga For Americans,* Prentice-Hall, Inc., Englewood Cliffs, N.J., 1959.

Dong, Collin H., and Jane Banks: *The Arthritic's Cookbook,* Thomas Y. Crowell Company, New York, 1973.

Echeveste, Dolores W., and John L. Schlacter: "Marketing: A Strategic Framework for Health Care," *Nursing Outlook,* **22**(6):377–381, June 1974.

Elting, L. Melvin, and Seymour Isenberg: *You Can Be Fat-Free Forever,* Penguin Books, Inc., New York, 1974.

Jacobson, Edmund: *How to Teach Scientific Relaxation.* Instructor's Text, Auspices, Foundation for Scientific Relaxation, Inc., Chicago, 1958.

Jacobson, Edmund: *You Must Relax,* McGraw-Hill Book Company, Inc., New York, 1962.

Jarvis, D. C.: *Folk Medicine,* Fawcett Publications, Inc., Greenwich, Conn., 1958.

Krause, Marie V., and Martha A. Hunscher: *Food, Nutrition and Diet Therapy,* 5th ed., W. B. Saunders Company, Philadelphia, 1972.

Lappe, Frances Moore: *Diet for a Small Planet,* Friends of the Earth, Ballantine Books, 1971.

Lerza, Catherine, and Michael Jacobson, (eds.): *Food for People, Not for Profit,* Ballantine Books, Inc., New York, 1975.

Lust, John B.: *The Herb Book,* A Bantam Book, Benedict Lust Publications, Sini Valley, Calif., 1974.

"Making Health Education Work," *American Journal of Public Health,* Supplement, **65**:1–44, October 1975.

Martin, E. A.: *Nutrition In Action,* 3rd ed., Holt, Rinehart and Winston, Inc., New York, 1971.

McCamy, John C., and James Presley: *Human Life Styling,* Harper & Row, Publishers, Incorporated, New York, 1975.

Morehouse, Laurence E., and Leonard Gross: *Total Fitness in 30 Minutes a Week,* Simon & Schuster, Inc., New York, 1975.

National Research Council Report: *Recommended Dietary Allowances,* 7th rev. ed., National Academy of Science, Washington, D.C., 1968.

Royal Canadian Air Force: *Exercise Plans for Physical Fitness,* Pocket Books, 1962.

Samuels, Mike, and Hal Bennett: *The Well-Body Book,* Random House/ Bookworks, 1973.

Terris, Milton, "Approaches to an Epidemiology of Health," *American Journal of Public Health,* **65**(10):1037–1045, October 1975.

Toffler, Alvin: *The Eco-Spasm Report,* Bantam Books, Inc., 1975.

Chapter 9

Aging

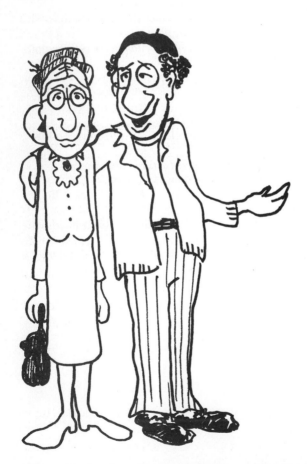

"First—it's lunch at the senior center . . . then bowling with the neighborhood oldsters, exercise class at 4:30—and then dinner and dancing with the Grey Panthers."

Aging is a process that can be viewed from several perspectives. The positive view is analogous to the aging of wine—the more years that it ages, the more priceless and exquisite it becomes—a veritable treasure to possess! The natural view accepts the normal sequence of aging as when the hardy crocus withers; the beautiful rose loses its bloom and gradually drops its petals; the apple becomes dry, wizened, or wrinkled; the leaves of the vine maple become brilliant before fading and becoming brown and dry. The negative view is analogous to fashion. When an item is no longer in style, it is considered old, useless, and generally discarded. All these views of the aging process are existent in our society, and are transferred to our aging citizens for assimilation as they see fit.

Gerontological and geriatric nursing has emerged as a popular, special field and has provided valuable content for community health nurses. Insights relative to the processes of aging and how it affects persons in our society have provided nurses with a basis for understanding physical and behavioral changes. With this increased understanding, nurses are able to support healthful living practices among the aging and to more readily identify symptoms and signs of incipient disease. Interpretations by nurses enable elderly patients and their families to better utilize medical, social, and personal resources in planning for more healthful and satisfying living in the later years.[1]

DESCRIPTIVE DATA ABOUT THE AGED

As defined by the lawmakers, sixty-five years of age is the legal time for people to retire with social security benefits, and this influences the attitudes and expectations of many citizens regarding the transition to becoming old. The 1970 census disclosed that people over sixty-five years of age constitute approximately 10 percent of the total population.[2] In 1971 the average length of life in the United States was estimated to be 71.1 years.[3] The life expectancy for women is nearly five years longer than that of men. Most older people live in a family setting, usually in their own households. Of every 100 older people, 28 live alone or with nonrelatives. Only 5 percent of old people live in institutions. Most elderly people live in the central city; approximately 35 percent live in small towns, and 5 percent live on farms.[4]

[1]Myrtle Irene Brown, "Nursing of the Aging and Aged," *Working with Older People: Clinical Aspects of Aging,* Austin B. Chinn (ed.), vol. 4, U. S. Department of Health, Education, and Welfare, July 1971, p. 354.

[2]Jack Botwinick, "Who Are the Aged?" Reprinted from *Geriatrics,* © 1974 by the New York Times Media Company, Inc. 29(7):124–129, July 1974.

[3]Committee on Ways and Means, *National Health Insurance Resource Book,* U. S. Government Printing Office, Washington, D. C., 1974, p. 242.

[4]Botwinick, op. cit., pp. 124–129.

Ninety percent of senior citizens have some income from retirement payments; others work, but a great majority are categorized as poor economically. The elderly have chronic diseases and have medical expenditures $3^1/_2$ times those of people under sixty-five years of age.[5] In personality and behavior, senior citizens are people as various and as individual as any younger group; possibly, they are more so.[6]

In a longitudinal study done by Maas and Kuypers, the life-styles and personality orientation of 142 respondents were examined over a forty-year time period.[7] Most of the subjects were economically well-off and very few had below average incomes. All the respondents were parents of children when originally selected for study.

A conclusion of this study, based on the accumulated data, shows that there are innumerable potentials for variety in life-style in old age. The findings brought out that fathers characteristically had a continuity of life-style from young adulthood into old age, due to relatively few changes in their environment, other than retirement. For mothers, life-style changes were more apparent, sometimes radical, due to pressures of marital, parental, occupational, and environmental factors that forced adaptation to a greater or lesser degree. It was found that qualities of life in old age are highly associated, in complex ways, to qualities of life forty years earlier. Mothers revealed continuities in personality, from early adulthood to old age, more so than fathers, and this finding was most evident for those mothers whose late-adult personality was characterized by anxiety and ego disorganization. The only suggested explanation for this finding was the presence, both in old age and in early adulthood, of depressive tendencies, low self-worth, tension, and high self-doubt.

Conclusions from these findings suggest that old age, to be properly understood, should be viewed as an integral part of the life cycle and not as a terminal period apart from the earlier years of life. Wives and mothers should expand their interests and involvement beyond the circle of the family if their later years are not to become problematic ones. Health is a crucial correlate of total personal functioning in old age. Health problems in old age are likely to be clearly foreshadowed in the early-adult years.[8]

For community health nurses, whether talking about housing, retirement, economic factors, leisure-time experiences, or health services, it must be remembered that aging persons have a wide diversity of interests, capacities and needs and should be provided with a wide diversity of

[5]Ibid., p. 126.
[6]Ibid., p. 129.
[7]Henry S. Maas and Joseph A. Kuypers, *From Thirty to Seventy,* Jossey-Bass Publishers, San Francisco, 1974, pp. 1–215.
[8]Ibid., pp. 1–215.

opportunities and provisions. As pointed out in the Maas and Kuypers study, most parents in their old age are not traveling a downhill course; they are involved in rewarding and diversely patterned lives. They demonstrated that different ways of living can be developed as social environments change with time. For some, old age provided a second and better chance at life.[9]

PROBLEMS OF THE AGED

Some of the crises which must be met by the elderly include the following: completion of the parental role; withdrawal from active community and organizational leadership; termination of marriage through death of one's mate; loss of an independent household; loss of interest in distant goals and plans; the necessity of depending on others or on society for support, advice, and management of funds; physical disabilities, such as arthritis and cataracts; assumption of a subordinate position to adult persons; taking up membership in groups made up largely of old people.[10] Other crises which are often unanticipated are loss of mobility due to failing sight or inability to walk any distances, the potential for robberies or muggings, nutritional deficiencies due to limited mobility, depressed affect, inadequate funds, change in living situation, and possibility of falls, fractures, and fires.[11] The manner in which the elderly person copes with and adjusts to these crises as they occur in life depends on the individual's personality, attitude, and past experiences, which may have been negative or positive. In order for aging to occur satisfactorily, it is essential that flexibility in adjustment to new situations be developed. Frequently, clients are not aware of crisis potential and may need to be alerted to preventive practices or improved coping mechanisms which will serve as precautionary measures.

Community health nurses can play an important role in assisting the elderly to strengthen their coping abilities, as the nurses interact with the aged in their home situations. In some cases, clients do not seek help actively because of a variety of factors, such as pride of independence, a stoic acceptance of difficulties, a sense of helplessness, a fear of the unknown, or unawareness of available resources.[12] When these particular clients come to the attention of the nurse, she must take the initiative to become thoroughly aware of the home situation, assess the health status

[9]Ibid., p. 215.

[10]Paul L. Niebanck, *The Elderly in Older Urban Areas*, Institute for Environmental Studies, University of Pennsylvania, Philadelphia, 1965, pp. 96–97.

[11]Priscilla Pierre Ebersole, "Crisis Intervention with the Aged," *Nursing and the Aged*, Irene Mortenson Burnside (ed.), McGraw-Hill Book Company, New York, 1976, pp. 272–273.

[12]Ibid., p. 280.

and capabilities of the client, elicit the concerns of the client, and introduce preventive measures which will support optimal, satisfying living conditions. In so doing, she must have a relationship with the client which is trusting and understanding of the basis for all actions taken.

Retirement

Retirement has a definite effect on the elderly, because it forces them to change many of their basic relationships and habits. Some of the expectations directed toward retired persons is that they will assume responsibility for managing their own lives; they will live within their income regardless of its adequacy; they will avoid becoming dependent on their families or on the community; they will engage in leisure time or volunteer roles.[13] Whether retirement is anticipated as desirable, inevitable, or dreadful, the complexity of this social role becomes gradually apparent as specific privileges, expectations, and relationships evolve. A new framework of activity and interests have to be developed. Since a basic psychological hunger of people is for time structure, the retired person must find new purposeful and satisfactory ways of structuring the day. A variety of tasks, activities, or hobbies can be undertaken, dependent upon the energy, enthusiasm, and interest of the person. Sometimes a reduction of income affects the manner in which the retired person lives. Or the income may be ample but a decline in health changes the living pattern so that some former activities can no longer be enjoyed. When widowhood occurs, this often means a severance of a fundamental relationship that has given stability and meaning to life. The process of readjustment is a lengthy one, and often important decisions have to be made during this critical period which affect the remainder of the person's life.[14]

Loneliness

The elderly often experience a deep sense of loneliness and isolation as they try to reaffirm meaning to their lives. Conti described several elderly persons who had individually adapted to life-styles that were unsatisfactory because of their loneliness. She described how the community health nurse visited these persons who initially denied their loneliness, but consented to receiving the attention of a "caring" person and eventually made adjustments to more satisfactory coping patterns. For some, this meant attendance of senior citizen groups for socialization or participation in a range of activities. The work of the nurse with these elderly people meant communicating her value of them as human beings and

[13]Robert C. Atchley, "Retirement," ibid., p. 532.
[14]Niebanck, op. cit., pp. 97–102.

showing acceptance, understanding, and patience with them before they were ready to reveal their feelings or willingness to make a change in adjustment.[15] Pets are very important to some elderly persons. For those clients who have difficulty with the English language, bringing persons to visit who speak their native tongue gives pleasure. Certain times of the day or night are lonely periods for some clients. By arranging a telephone call or social visit at these particular times, the loneliness may be assuaged.[16]

Nurses should be particularly observant of symptoms of depression in the elderly. Because the aged have difficulty tolerating the loss of physical health, special attention should be focused on impairments of vision, hearing, or ambulation. When a client complains of anxiety, nervousness, insomnia, loss of energy, loss of appetite, the nurse should become alerted to feelings of depression. The therapy of hope is one of the best strategies to use as opportunities are devised for social contacts and the strengthening of self-esteem. In as many creative ways as the nurse can discover, efforts should be directed toward increasing the sense of usefulness of the client. Simple rewards are satisfying and appreciated when given in recognition of even a small gain.[17] By caring and being sensitively supportive of the client's concerns, the nurse strengthens the client to face each day.

Elderly persons sometimes move slowly and think slowly, but they are very responsive to the enthusiasm and warmth of young people and delight in any kind of exchange with young people. They also are very responsive to sensory stimulation and should be touched or stroked whenever a practical opportunity arises. Sensory experiences are important for psychological well-being. For example, the nurse should always feel the pulse, whether she needs to know it or not, comb the hair, press the ankle for edema, or give a reassuring body squeeze whenever she wants to communicate approval or acceptance. In many ways, elderly persons are like little children and do not mind being treated with warmth, fun, or simple games. If encouraged to attend small group discussions where a subject of interest is being explored, participants can find this to be a stimulating way of sharing ideas or receiving recognition, particularly when they have an able nurse leader or facilitator.

MYTHS ABOUT AGING

Some myths about the elderly which must be checked out in terms of the acquaintance of the nurse with any aged patient include the following:

---

[15]Mary Louise Conti, "The Loneliness of Old Age," *Nursing Outlook,* 18(8):28–30, August 1970.

[16]Irene Mortenson Burnside, "Mental Health in the Aged," op. cit., p. 143.

[17]Irene Mortenson Burnside, "Depression and Suicide in the Aged," op. cit., p. 172.

(1) the expected passive behavior pattern of the person in retirement. The right to "take it easy" has been earned, and the patient now can rest. Does the patient conform to this myth? Is the patient content? What is his or her philosophy of life? Is satisfaction with resting evident? (2) Dependence on others for advice and assistance is a natural and inevitable consequence of advancing age. Does the patient accept dependence graciously or seem to be fiercely independent? Who are the acceptable persons from whom advice and assistance will be taken? (3) Custodial care in institutions is the answer to chronic illness, invalidity, and mental disturbances. How does the patient feel about institutional care? Has he or she personally visited any nursing or retirement homes? If custodial care is needed, what does this mean to the individual? (4) Withdrawal from social participation tends to accompany departure from employment. Is the patient active socially? Has the patient withdrawn from former social groups voluntarily? Is he or she lonely? Is encouragement needed to join new groups, such as a senior activity center? (5) No preparation for retirement is required or expected. How is the patient adjusting to retirement? Were most of the changes anticipated? How would he or she advise others to prepare for retirement? (6) Older persons are unable to learn new skills.[18] Since cognitive processes do not decline with age, what generally happens in learning a new skill is the necessity for unlearning a well-established way of doing things. This means willingness to change. For most individuals, the initial response to a new idea is resistance which is more a function of intelligence, cultural, and experiential factors than one of age.[19] Will the patient be willing to try out a new skill? Is the patient a *possibility* thinker—a person who perceptively probes every problem proposal, and opportunity to discover the positive aspects present in almost every human situation? Or is the patient an *impossibility* thinker—a person who makes swift, sweeping passes over a proposed idea, scanning it with a sharp, negative eye, looking only for reasons why something will not work instead of visualizing ways in which it could work?[20]

WORKING WITH THE AGED

For nurses visiting the elderly in their homes, it is a delight to witness the uncovering of each personality as the history of each person is evoked. The pictures, belongings, and other memorabilia in the home provide the nurse with clues regarding the client's interests and sources of comfort.

[18]Ernest W. Burgess, *Aging in Western Societies,* The University of Chicago Press, Chicago, 1960, p. 20.
[19]Kathy Gribbin, "Cognitive Processes in Aging," *Nursing and the Aged, op. cit., p. 49.*
[20]Robert H. Schuller, *Move Ahead with Possibility Thinking,* Doubleday & Company, Inc., Garden City, N. Y., 1967, pp. 2–3.

Elderly persons love to talk with animated young nurses who are client-centered and willing to draw out their thoughts about past events, present concerns, and future desires. Whenever special interests, skills, and hobbies are discovered that had meaning for them in the past, they might respond to persuasion to resume the favored activities, if feasible. Sometimes a modification of procedures must be devised because of physical impairments or economic factors.

A firm, persistent, persuasive, encouraging approach works well with elderly clients. The "laying on of hands" is advisable whenever an opportunity presents itself, i.e., taking a pulse, checking for edema of extremities, or reaching out with a friendly touch.

As pointed out by a nursing student:

> . . . even if health care is readily accessible to the elderly patient, the formal technological care they receive is not the care they want. Frequently they are lonely. A patient may dutifully take medications for hypertension, cardiac or respiratory diseases every day and have monthly checkups, but he may not be healthy if he does not feel someone is definitely concerned about him—not his blood pressure or urine, but himself as a total human being. Affection is a primary element in caring for the elderly, and many of our older citizens are environmentally isolated in our modern life. If an older person lives alone, he may not see or talk with another person for a week or more. As his isolation develops, he may not bother with reading a paper or using other communication media. With the decrease in sensory stimulation, apathy and/or mental deterioration becomes an inevitable eventuality.

To maintain the health status of elderly citizens, community health nurses must:

1 Be warm, caring, person-centered nurses.
2 Do a health assessment of each referred client.
   a Check vital signs, take blood pressure, height, weight, listen to heart and lungs, check condition of feet and nails. Has the patient had a recent physical examination? If he or she uses a corrective device (hearing aid, glasses, dentures), are they in good working order?
   b Examine all medications taken, frequency, method of administration, purpose of medications, patient's understanding about the importance of each medication and possible side effects, reminder system for taking medications as prescribed by the physician. "Elderly patients frequently have multiple chronic disease states that require long-term multiple drug therapy."[21] Errors of omission, erratic dosage, and overdosage when medications are self-administered are not uncommon.

---

[21]Ronald C. Kayne, "Drugs and the Aged," *Nursing and the Aged,* op. cit., p. 438.

    c Do a nutritional assessment or diet history, determine the adequacy of nutrients (minerals, vitamins) in the diet, assess the patient's knowledge about essential foods, foods to avoid, regularity of meals, practice of snacking, recommended supplemental foods, food likes and dislikes, fluid intake. "The person who eats alone should be suspected of marginal nutrition and this fact should lead to observation and inspection for further signs."[22]

    d Ascertain ADL (activity of daily living) of each client, ability to give self-care, mobility, housekeeping ability, amount of exercise done on a daily basis, patient's receptivity to learning simple exercises, avocational interests.

    e Determine client's ability to relax or method of reducing stress, client's receptivity to learning relaxation measures.

3 Examine the home for environmental hazards, need for minor repairs, recommended safety measures.

4 Find out who are the significant family members or neighbors in case of emergency.

5 Ascertain the client's knowledge of available community resources according to personal needs, such as senior citizen centers, meals on wheels, transportation resources, recreational facilities, volunteer opportunities, mobile library, home health services, and educational facilities.

6 Assess the life-style of the client, friends, frequency of socialization with others, recreational interests, hobbies, crafts, ability to reach out and join others, client's willingness to learn new occupational skills.

When all essential data has been gathered, the nurse has knowledge of most of the client's needs, and can make a contract with the client which fulfills the need with highest priority. Often, the need as determined by the nurse is not the one having highest priority with the client. When this happens, it is generally advisable to work with the need the client has identified.

For example, a nursing student described the home of an elderly male client as being a "tumbled down, dark, damp hovel." She went on to say, "When I first saw the conditions in which Mr. C. was living, my first thought was to get him out of there and tear down the house. I then assumed that if he would not leave the place, he would *certainly* want to clean it up. But Mr. C's perspective of his needs differed greatly from mine. His greatest concerns were to insure the continued satisfaction of his physical needs; mine were for his safety needs. His need priority included refilling needed prescriptions, getting new glasses so he could

---

[22]Mary Opal Wolanin, "Nursing Assessment," ibid., p. 406.

read again, and cleaning out the driveway so that 'you and the meal lady can get in.'

For another student working with an arthritic, hypertensive elderly lady who had been advised by family and friends to move into a retirement facility and who had numerous reasons for delaying such a move, discussion of the client's situation led to the realization that the elderly lady hoped to die in her home. So, as a temporary but necessary and immediate measure, the student negotiated with the client to fulfill two goals: (1) order a bedside telephone to replace the telephone on the wall in case of emergency and (2) visit her physician whom she had not seen for a year and secure a current assessment of her physical condition. By working with the client to fulfill immediate needs, compliance with future advisable medical and nursing measures becomes more assured as changes in health status occur.

While actively engaged in working with elderly clients, the community health nurse may be calling and coordinating with professionals of many related disciplines, such as the physician, nurse practitioner, physical therapist, occupational therapist, nutritionist, social worker, consumer advocate for senior citizens, homemaker, housekeeper, or environmental health specialist. By freely consulting with members of the related disciplines, services are individualized, clarified, and facilitated for elderly clients. At all times, family members and significant others should be kept informed and approving of all developments and decisions.

RESOURCES FOR THE ELDERLY

In every community, resources for the elderly are multiplying and services are available which provide a wide variety of programs designed to meet the physical, emotional, social, recreational, economic, and environmental needs of senior citizens. To become knowledgeable about the services in each local community, the nurse or citizen must locate the information and referral center for senior citizens. This can be done by securing a people's yellow pages book, or looking in the yellow pages of the local telephone book for the headings: aging, senior citizen services, social service organizations, or social and health services. The mayor's office in every community, the welfare department, or social security office should also be able to direct telephone inquiries to the proper local resources.

Services that are available through senior service centers or departments of aging cover a gamut of needs. A visit to these agencies is very illuminating and frequently engenders enthusiasm to reach out and inform more aging citizens about the opportunities they might be missing.

Questions are answered or directions given about the many resources available, such as health-care facilities, medicare, medicaid, housing, employment, transportation, volunteer opportunities, social security, supplemental security income, food stamps, leisure-time activities, educational opportunities, and senior services activities and events.

Volunteer Opportunities

A program with which to be familiar is RSVP (Retired Senior Volunteer Program) which is sponsored by ACTION, Washington, D.C. It offers senior citizens, sixty years of age and older, the opportunity to volunteer for a variety of interesting and vital jobs. The volunteer chooses the activity in which he or she has expertise or an interest and, subsequently, gives real services or teaches important skills needed by the clientele with whom he or she is working (school children, disadvantaged persons, handicapped individuals, other senior citizens, etc.). Activities from which the volunteer can select are inclusive of occupations, such as recreational and craft interests, newspaper or newsletter abilities, employment services, office or food preparation skills, handyperson skills, musical or entertainment abilities, or friendly visiting. In-service, on-the-job training sometimes is given in community agencies receiving volunteer aid if it seems necessary. While giving service, volunteers are covered by an insurance plan which gives protection for accidents on the job or travel to and from a station. Sometimes, mileage compensation is given, if desired. Periodically, social events are planned to provide recognition, honor, and awards to volunteers. RSVP not only gives senior citizens the opportunity to volunteer services, it also serves as an excellent resource for the disabled and homebound elderly who need some kind of assistance in the home.

Health Care

Health-care facilities, such as local health departments, visiting nurse associations, and home-care agencies, are cognizant of the needs of the elderly and occasionally offer free programs screening citizens for early symptoms of diabetes, glaucoma, tuberculosis, and hypertension. Or, foot-care clinics are maintained on a regular basis so that senior citizens can have their nails clipped, corns and calluses examined for infection, receive preventive protective remedies, counseling, and referral.

Many home-care agencies provide health-care and supportive services to sick and disabled persons in their places of residence. This includes medical, nursing, dental, physical therapy, occupational therapy, homemaking, and housekeeping services as recommended. Day-care centers provide supervision for elderly persons who cannot be left alone for extended periods of time. The goal of the day-care center is to keep citizens residing in their own homes as long as possible yet provide them with a protective daytime therapeutic environment according to their needs. Day-care centers are particularly valuable resources for family members who want their aging member to be in a protective environment while they work during the day.

On an increasing scale, nurse practitioners are making their services available in retirement homes, low-income housing projects, and senior citizen centers. They do health assessments, foot care, screen for hypertension, diabetes, glaucoma, counsel about preventive health measures, refer special problems to physicians or to appropriate community resources as necessary. When residents become acquainted and familiar with the services of the nurse practitioner, they respond very positively to her ministrations and suggestions for improved daily living.

Protective and Advocacy Services

Familiarity with legal services for citizens is becoming essential for nurses to know. In every community there are legal resources which will advise or give information about what to do when a problem is causing concern. People's yellow pages maintains a list of legal resources, and local telephone books have listings of numbers to call for information, such as the mayor's office or community information and referral services. Legal knowledge and direction frequently needed by nurses and family members are ways for securing common legal protection of persons and property, such as power of attorney, guardianship, trusts. Explanations and requirements for acquiring specific protection can be secured from any legal aid or legal referral agency.

Helping elderly citizens or family members to protect their money and property is a preventive measure that can always be encouraged by nurses. Making a will, the appointment of an executor of the will, joint ownership of bank accounts and trusts, and after-death arrangements should be suggested as important preventive functions to have clarified among family members.[23]

The Gray Panther Movement suggests that people in their later years need not remain passive and impotent when faced with unacceptable conditions. With increasing assertiveness and organization, the senior citizens are mandating appropriate responses from all sectors of society as to appropriate provision of their needs. Elderly citizens should be encouraged to request that their names be put on the mailing list of state and local committees for aging. In this way, they are kept informed of all legislation pertaining to their interests.[24] Through organizations which

[23]Bernita M. Steffl, "Prevention Measures and Safety Factors for the Aged," ibid., pp. 483–485.
[24]Marie A. Fasano, "Community Resources," ibid., p. 515.

present a united front, senior citizens secure publicity, public concern, and remedial action for many problems which are of particular concern to them.

Financial Resource

Supplemental security income (SSI) is a minimum income for older people with limited financial resources who are sixty-five years or older and people under sixty-five who are blind or severely disabled. The monthly checks take the place of basic cash payments which were once paid by state and local public assistance offices to the aged, blind, and disabled. People who are eligible for SSI may be earning a small amount of money or have no income, or have minimal assets which can be turned into cash. To determine if qualifications of senior citizens meet expected criteria, it is advisable to call a social security office to obtain the most recent essentialities for eligibility. The amount of payment to each citizen is variable according to the income and assets each individual or couple has. Even though the Social Security Administration runs the program, supplemental security income is not the same as social security. People who get social security can get supplemental security income also if they are eligible for both sources of payment.

Aged, blind, and disabled people receiving SSI checks also are eligible for medical assistance and social services from the state public assistance office. To determine the extent of specific services available for these clients, the local welfare office should be contacted.

Nutrition Resources

The food stamp program is funded by the United States Department of Agriculture and enables low-income households to buy more food of greater variety to improve their diets. Food stamps are coupons that can be used similarly as cash at authorized food stores to buy food, seeds, and plants for growing food. They cannot be used to buy tobacco, alcoholic beverages, paper products, soap, or anything inedible. To purchase food stamps, participants pay a sum of money based on their family size and net monthly income. Households with a low net income are eligible for food stamps. A *household* is a group of people living together who buy and cook their food together. They pool their income and share expenses. While most households are families, other groups of people who are not related to each other can also be a household.

Application for the food stamp program is made by requesting an interview with a representative of the state agency (welfare office). It is advisable for all applicants to have documents showing: where the household is; how many are in the family; the proof of income; paid bills and receipts showing expenses, such as rent, medical bills, child care, education; a savings account passbook; and the most recent checking account statement. If a household is eligible, an authorization to purchase (ATP card) is issued. The amount each household is required to pay for food stamps each month is determined in the eligibility interview.

A requirement of the program is that all able-bodied individuals in the household between eighteen and sixty-five years of age must register for work and accept suitable employment. When registered, they report to the state employment service, and are referred to employers when suitable employment is found. For food stamp recipients who are over sixty years of age, are physically handicapped, feeble, or cannot prepare all their meals, meals on wheels will accept food stamps. In the event of a disaster, such as a fire, hurricane, tornado, flood, storm, or other severe catastrophes, the food stamp program can be converted into an emergency plan which issues free food stamps to all adversely affected households. To apply for emergency assistance, disaster relief agencies or the welfare office must be contacted. It is the responsibility of each household to report an increase or decrease of household size, change of income, or other alterations of household status within ten days of the change. Misuse of food stamps and ATP cards is illegal and subject to penalty.

Other Resources

Senior citizen centers or information and referral centers are the best sources of knowledge about all available services provided in the community. They can answer inquiries about transportation resources, bus schedules, and services. They know if mobile libraries are available for individuals who are homebound. They can provide information about meals on wheels or locations of hot meals in neighborhood settings. They have a listing of all adult education classes held in local community settings and dealing with a variety of subjects—theoretical, vocational, or recreational. For citizens who want to focus on pure enjoyment, information is available about dances, bingo games, card games, field trips, and other activities that represent some of the amusements planned for senior citizens. A wide variety of special services are constantly in the process of development, so inquiries regarding special needs should always be made in the event that services are obtainable or that ideas for new services will culminate into special projects.

Avocational counseling is a free professional service which helps disabled and retired citizens to discover their interests and potentials and then finds activities in their communities best suited to their needs. Avocational activities include a range of interests, such as games, sports, nature, collecting, art, music, education and culture, volunteer work, and organizations.[25] When a citizen is desirous of learning more about a

[25]"Health Professionals Told of Avocational Counseling," *Geriatrics*, **29**(5):43, May 1974.

special interest, inquiries should be directed toward senior citizen centers or information and referral centers.

For community health nurses who have never visited local community facilities giving special services to specific clientele, it is advisable to become acquainted with these resources. Many community facilities give service to all ages of clientele; however, when a certain portion of senior citizens are actively interested in a particular service, it is helpful to study the basis for the magnetism of the service, the facility, or the promised results. Suggested places to visit with an open mind, observe, and make use of all the senses are health food stores, nutrition and vitamin centers in supermarkets, low-income housing authority offices, missions on skid road, centers serving hot lunches, herb stores, natural food stores, and health clinics in inner cities.

CHRONIC DISEASE STATES AND DEATH

For those individuals and family members who must learn to adjust to the changes evoked by the symptoms of chronic and degenerative diseases, such as multiple sclerosis, arthritis, emphysema, terminal carcinoma, cerebral vascular accident (stroke), and similar debilitating diseases, special attention must be given. Not only the patient but all family members are affected in some way or other by the required adaptation to the existence and concurrent dependencies produced by chronic diseases. All patients and families adjust in their own individualistic ways and many need assistance in learning to accommodate with essential changes necessitated by the disruption of roles and tasks in the home. Many professional references deal with the stages of adaptation or coping mechanisms undergone by patients when chronic diseases are diagnosed or terminal prognoses are given. However, few authors as yet take heed of the distinct adjustments expected of family members who are directly affected by the change of status of the patient, a family member with a one-time vital role in the family structure. Kubler-Ross discussed the physical and emotional adjustments undergone by family members of patients who were dying and recognized that family members also went through emotional stages of adjustment very similar to those described for dying patients. She pointed out the importance of someone to befriend family members, allow them to work through their rational or irrational feelings about a pending death, and ease the movement of feelings toward acceptance without guilt.[26] The family-centered community health nurse is the qualified person for the role of comforting and assisting family members when chronic degenerative diseases are diagnosed and terminal prognoses are anticipated.

[26]Elisabeth Kubler-Ross, *On Death and Dying*, The Macmillan Company, New York, 1969, pp. 157–180.

The stages of adaptation or coping mechanisms undergone by patients and family members when they realize the necessity for accepting a change in their lives have been identified by various authors as sequential and progressive in nature for most people. According to Crate, who studied stages of adaptation for the diagnosis of multiple sclerosis, the first stage is one of *denial* and *disbelief,* which is manifested in a variety of ways, depending upon the individual's life-style of coping with crisis or conflict. Denial can be exhibited for a short period or it can be long-lasting. The nurse should listen to all expressions of feeling noncritically and help the individual to articulate with clarity. By drawing out existing feelings of resentment and bitterness, she facilitates the adjustment process. The second stage consists of a *developing awareness,* which is commonly manifested as anger. By being empathic, the nurse can listen to arguments, criticisms, and attacks without responding as a singled-out target. She must be aware that anger is a realistic defense when a person's life is capriciously changed without consent. The nurse must consciously not argue with the patient or moralize about any issue. The third stage is one of *reorganization,* in which relationships with family members are adjusted and accommodations are made in the activities of daily living. At this time the nurse must continue to listen to the expressions of feelings of the patient and family members, suggest suitable practical rehabilitative methods for readjusting their household routines, encourage the use of appropriate self-help devices, and give verbal support for accomplishments successfully attained by the persons assuming new roles and duties. The fourth stage consists of *resolution* or *identity change,* in which the patient acknowledges the reality changes he sees in himself. He begins to identify that he is similar to other patients with the same diagnosis. Dependent upon the diagnosis and the home situation, the nurse at this point must consider releasing the patient, encouraging him to become self-directive within his limits, and to seek out relationships with others.[27]

For patients and families who are concerned about the time when admission to an institution becomes eminent, the nurse must elicit the perceptions of the patient regarding the meaning of institutionalization. Acute care hospitals are generally viewed differently from nursing homes, convalescent homes, or retirement homes. Family members must be alerted to the advantages and disadvantages of particular institutions in terms of the patient's viewpoint, physical condition, recommended treatments, and home situation. A problem-solving approach can be used with the patient and family members as all alternatives for care are carefully considered. Visits to the institutions to view their assets and limitations can be encouraged. An assessment and recommendation from the attend-

[27]Marjorie Crate, "Nursing Functions in Adaptation to Chronic Illness," *American Journal of Nursing,* **65:**72–76, October 1965.

ing physician always is valuable at this critical moment of decision making for patients and families. For the most part, if the patient voluntarily decides to enter a selected facility, the transition from home to institution is greatly eased for all concerned.

When the diagnosis is a terminal one, the early stages of denial and anger precede the latter stages of adaptation, which are aptly described by Kubler-Ross as those of bargaining, depression, and acceptance. *Bargaining* is a period when the patient makes a bargain with God in the hope that his death will be postponed. *Depression* is the natural state during which a patient is filled with sorrow that he will soon lose everything and everyone he loves. If he is allowed to express his sorrow, he becomes emotionally prepared for the final stage of *acceptance*. During the final stage, effective communications are predominantly nonverbal rather than verbal.[28] For a nursing student who did not know how to say what she wanted to say to a young mother dying of cancer, she chose to sit with the patient for a period of time in quietness and empathy. This nonverbal expression seemed to give comfort and peace to the patient.

The concept of hope was graphically described by Kubler-Ross as an essential ingredient in all people. They are nourished by it and appreciate any small fragment of hope that is offered on a realistic basis. The hope may not necessarily be directed toward total cure, but a remission of the illness or an anticipation about the next life.[29] Until the patient gives some cue that he is ready to talk, the nurse is in a position where asking direct questions may seem awkward. If she has a knowledge of the patient's religion, values, and beliefs, she is better able to speak words of comfort and strength that prepare the patient for the final task. Communicating a genuine individualized concern to the patient, accepting his health status realistically in a verbal or nonverbal manner, and incorporating hope in such a way that the patient finds it believable is the most supportive behavior the nurse can give.

SUMMARY

An overview of some of the problems, concerns and resources for aging as commonly encountered by community health nurses was given. Nurses can be supportive of aging as a process which leads to more healthful and satisfying living in the later years. In working with the aged, the nurse must be a warm, caring, person-centered nurse who carefully applies and individualizes the nursing process with each client. Knowledge and familiarity with the ever-growing community resources and services available for all senior citizens is essential, as well as illuminating.

[28]Kubler-Ross, op. cit., pp. 82–136.
[29]Ibid., pp. 138–156.

SUGGESTED READING

Becker, Ernest: *The Denial of Death,* The Free Press, New York, 1973.

Birren, J. E., R. N. Butler, S. W. Greenhouse, L. Sokoloff, and M. Yarrow: *Human Aging,* Public Health Service Publication no. 986, Washington, D. C., 1963.

Bonner, Charles D.: *Homburger and Bonner's Medical Care and Rehabilitation of the Aged and Chronically Ill,* 3d ed., Little, Brown and Company, Boston, 1974.

Botwinick, Jack: *Aging and Behavior: A Comprehensive Integration of Research Findings,* Springer Publishing Co., Inc., New York, 1973.

Burnside, Irene Mortenson: *Nursing and the Aged,* McGraw-Hill Book Company, New York, 1976.

Chinn, Austin B. (ed.): *Working with Older People: Clinical Aspects of Aging,* vol. 4, U. S. Department of Health, Education, and Welfare, July 1971.

Griffin, Jerry J.: "Family Decision," *American Journal of Nursing,* 75(5):795–796, May 1975.

"Hypertension: A Special Feature," *American Journal of Nursing,* 76(5):765–780, May 1976.

Krieger, Dolores: "Therapeutic Touch: The Imprimatur of Nursing," *American Journal of Nursing,* 75(5):784–787, May 1975.

Kubler-Ross, Elisabeth: *On Death and Dying,* The Macmillan Company, New York, 1969.

Maas, Henry S., and Joseph A. Kuypers: *From Thirty to Seventy,* Jossey-Bass Publishers, San Francisco, 1974.

"Middle Years—A Special Supplement," *American Journal of Nursing,* 75(6):993–1024, June 1975.

Miles, Helen S., Dorothea R. Hays: "Widowhood," *American Journal of Nursing,* 75(2):280–282, February 1975.

McIntyre, H. Mildred: *Heart Disease: New Dimensions of Nursing Care,* Trainex Press, Garden Grove, Calif., 1974.

Moustakas, Clark: *Loneliness,* Prentice-Hall, Inc., Englewood Cliffs, N.J., 1961.

"Options for the Aging," *American Journal of Nursing,* 75(10:1799–1822, October 1975.

Ten State Nutrition Survey, 1968–1970, Department of Health, Education, and Welfare Publication No. (HSM) 72-8134, Atlanta, Ga., 1972.

Wolff, Ilse S.: "Retirement: A Different Season," *Nursing Outlook,* 21(12): 763–765, December 1973.

Chapter 10

Applying Epidemiology, Statistics, and Research

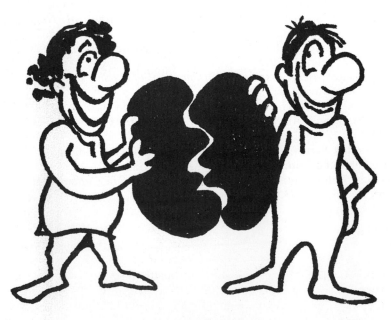

Problem-solving

The emphasis on clinical, laboratory, and epidemiologic research in the past decade dictates that the nurse have an understanding and appreciation of research methods and statistics. The Community Health Nursing Section of the American Nurses' Association requires the nurse to have knowledge of the research method within the broad categories of evaluating, studying, and research. Also, an understanding of epidemiology and statistics is necessary for continuing appraisal and evaluation of health situations which concern patients, families, and communities.

STUDY AND RESEARCH

Searching for increased knowledge in a systematic way requires curiosity, self-discipline, and familiarity with research methods. Nursing students who wish to promote the advancement of improved patient care must have a beginning acquaintance with basic principles and methods in order to study any aspect of the health-illness continuum which concerns them. For the nurse who is sufficiently curious about an intriguing health problem, a beginning step into research activities can be initiated by doing a ministudy. By investigating the variety of methods for doing studies, getting an idea from readings whether any other nurse has done a similar study, and determining exactly what she wants to find out, the neophyte nurse can start investigative activities which may bring exciting discoveries to light. Some problems that might be interesting to study include identification of consumers' attitudes and opinions regarding specific health issues or advertised products, the coexistence of specific stress factors with specific chronic diseases, and the investigation of factors that promote wellness in families—why some families rarely if ever have upper respiratory illnesses while others seem to have them constantly. Other areas of interest are only limited by the concerns of the nurse, and the demands of her position. They could include learning about the skin care routines followed by adolescents with acne, or how families react if one of the children has enuresis. What factors influence the utilization of health-care facilities in the community?

Nurses working in the community, wanting to improve the health status of its residents, need to become better acquainted with research methods, evaluation, and interpretation of results. They need knowledge of the principles and methods of epidemiology because their patient is the community. *Epidemiology,* and its research techniques, describes and explains the distribution and determinants of disease in population groups, with the ultimate goal of promoting health and furthering preventive measures. This is in contrast to clinical research, which pertains to the individual patient who usually already has sought health care, and the efficacy of diagnostic tests or therapeutic regimens. The community

· health nurse often is trying to prevent the need to seek curative health services.

The purpose of presenting an elementary discussion of epidemiologic and statistical concepts is to enable the nurse to participate in or to conduct studies of her own. Familiarity with these concepts will be of value in presenting and analyzing quantitative data, such as showing how great a problem hypertension is in her community. Also, it will help the nurse be more critical of the validity of the proliferating new knowledge in the health sciences area. Terms such as variation, population, sample, data, observations, and central tendency, which may be familiar to the nurse in other contexts, are explained from the point of view of epidemiology and statistics. The authors present this limited discussion knowing that the material is too elementary for some readers, that it will be a review for others, and that it will be helpful for some; it is in no way intended to bring about mastery in the sciences of epidemiology and statistics. (The student is directed to references in the bibliography at the end of the chapter for a detailed discussion of both subjects.)

DEFINITIONS

Epidemiology has been defined above. Basically, its purpose is to learn why some people get sick and others do not and then apply the knowledge to prevent other people from getting sick. Another way of saying this is that epidemiology tries to identify "risk factors"—those elements or variables in an individual's life or environment which give him or her a greater than average risk of developing a particular disease—and then developing a strategy to counteract those factors and thus reduce the risk.

The term *statistics* is defined in various ways. For the purpose of this presentation, statistics refers to a systematic approach for obtaining, organizing, and analyzing numerical facts so that scientific conclusions can be drawn from them. Statistics allow for description and for inferences. The rather specialized techniques that are used for biological data are often called biostatistics. They present fact rather than an assumption or hunch.

Vital statistics in the broad sense refers to births, deaths, populations, illnesses, marriages, and divorces. In the narrow sense the term refers to births, deaths, and populations. Illnesses in the population are classified as morbidity statistics, deaths as mortality statistics. Generally marriage and divorce statistics are used more frequently by social agencies than by health agencies. Since the disciplines of public health and community health nursing are concerned with people, vital statistics are an important tool in their fields.

SOURCES OF DATA

The family record is an excellent source for such statistical information as age, sex, ethnic background, and specific disease or condition. Information from the records facilitates program planning and is useful in evaluating the services given to the family. Study of the records should also give the interested and curious nurse ideas as to some of the problems that need to be researched in order to learn more about them. Roberts and Hudson developed a method of studying the patient's progress through his or her record. Their study method gives direction for collecting, presenting, and analyzing data concerning the following:

1 The scope of needs identified in patients and families by the community health nurse (Does the patient or family also recognize these needs?)

2 The progress made by families in meeting their own needs for nursing care (What factors seem to influence how successfully this is done?)

3 The proportion of persons who obtain needed immunizations and diagnostic tests (Which families do, and which do not, get their children immunized, and why?)

4 The number and kinds of conditions which are brought to medical attention for diagnosis, periodic medical evaluation, and treatment (Are the preventive programs in the community really aimed at the most important targets?)

5 The extent to which patients with chronic illness and disability attain self-care[1] (Again, why are some successful in doing this, and others not?)

The questions in parentheses were added to indicate possible questions that an alert nurse might have, and which she may wish to research for answers.

Information from records is used in compiling monthly and annual reports required by the agency. Such information is used by the local community health agency as well as by state and federal health agencies, grant-in-aid programs, voluntary and contracting agencies—insurance companies, schools, or industrial firms that pay for services—and by sponsoring or coordinating groups, such as the community chest or the united funds. The information is used to make comparisons with previous years, to predict and to determine needs for ensuing years, and to interpret to the community in order to obtain better understanding and support for community health nursing services.

[1]Doris E. Roberts and Helen H. Hudson, *How to Study Patient Progress,* Public Health Service Publication 1169, April 1964, p. 1.

The staff nurse rarely is responsible for compiling the agency's monthly or annual reports, but she is responsible for knowing the information contained in them. Her responsibility includes knowledge and understanding of the major accomplishments of the year, such as quantitative and qualitative attainments, concerns and plans for change, trends in activities and service needs, and the relation of service given to the estimated needs for such services.

Staff nurses may be involved in compiling statistics for special investigations of such topics as well-child care, child abuse, premature births, epidemiologic problems, home-care programs, school health, congenital defects, rehabilitation, mental retardation, migratory workers, and many more. The individual nurse may be interested in conducting a study within her district. The opportunities are unlimited and will vary according to the nurse's interest and the policies of the agency.

PRINCIPLES OF EPIDEMIOLOGY

Epidemiology, in the strict sense of the word, is a branch of medical science and centers on distribution and causation of disease in populations with the goal of discovering means of disease prevention. The methods used to determine disease causation can be adapted to many other areas of concern. At first it was concerned with the epidemic diseases, as the word indicates, but now it is being applied to all diseases, including trauma. It is more a system of methods than a body of knowledge, and uses knowledge from many areas such as biostatistics, microbiology, and clinical medicine.

One of the underlying principles is that no disease occurs by chance alone, because each follows its own recognizable pattern of occurrence. The pattern may not be seen when looking at one sick person, but when information is collected on many people with the same disease, some common elements in their total life experience may begin to emerge. Compiling a list of these common elements helps to delineate the group in the community that has a high risk of developing that specific disease. Currently this is well-illustrated by the fact that cigarette smokers have a much higher risk of developing lung cancer than people who do not smoke. The "profile" of the group at high risk for coronary heart disease is fairly well-known. It includes such risk factors as being male, overweight, underactive, a smoker, high blood cholesterol level, high blood pressure, and certain personality characteristics. Knowledge of the risk factors provides a basis for preventive programs. Today, preventive efforts against the major diseases are not as simple as producing a vaccine and administering it. The efforts to prevent disease may affect a person's life-style.

Health is a state of equilibrium, a delicate balance of many factors. When this balance is lost, disease results. These factors can be grouped as those related to the host, the agent, and the environment. The host is the human being at risk of acquiring a disease. Some of the factors which determine whether or not the host will do so include age, sex, genetic background, general health status, immunologic status, personal health habits, and more. The agent is the factor which is essential to disease causation, such as microorganisms, physical forces, chemicals, or even food. Environmental factors are all those things external to the particular host, including other people. Disease prevention depends, in large part, on what we know about these factors and their interrelationships. As an example, we have learned how to prevent some infectious diseases by giving vaccines. We have protective clothing and heating devices to protect us from harm by extreme cold weather.

Disease causation is complex. Some diseases, such as coronary heart disease, may be the outcome of several interacting factors rather than of a single specific factor. Even when a specific infectious agent is known, there may be contributing factors that influence whether or not exposure to that agent will produce disease. Many common colds are caused by rhinoviruses, but a rhinovirus infection often fails to cause illness. Contributing factors here could include the person's general level of health or previous experience with that particular agent. When investigating the cause of a disease, it is necessary to pay attention to contributing causes as well as the primary agent.

Another important concept is that infection is not synonymous with disease. Sources of infection in a community are not limited to ill people. The term "infection" means that an infectious agent has invaded the host and started to multiply, in intimate relation to host tissues. There are at least four possible outcomes of this invasion. First, there may be overt clinical illness. Second, an inapparent, or subclinical, infection may occur in which the person shows no symptoms but is shedding the agent. In a study of family illnesses, rhinoviruses were recovered sometimes from healthy people. Another outcome is that the infected person may become a carrier. After recovery from clinical illness, he or she may shed the agent, continuously or at intervals, for a long period of time. With typhoid fever, the ex-patient sometimes excreted the agent at intervals for the rest of a lifetime, and so was still infected. Fourth, whether or not disease occurred, the agent may persist quietly in the host's tissue for long periods of time. Periodically it may produce symptoms, The best known example of this is probably herpes simplex, the cold sore. This is called a latent infection.

Knowledge of the distribution of disease over time is very valuable to the nurse in the community. Many diseases, such as hepatitis type A, are

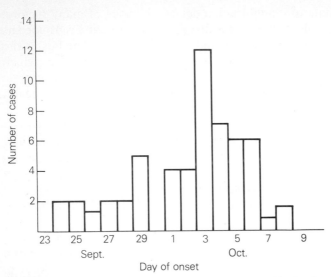

Figure 10-1 Symptomatic cases of infectious hepatitis, by day of onset.

often present at a low level of incidence. This is the endemic, or background, level of incidence. When a significant increase in the number of new cases occurs, it is called an epidemic. That term originally referred to communicable diseases but more recently is being applied to chronic diseases as well, such as the "epidemic of coronary heart disease." Occasionally a disease occurs in large numbers in many countries, such as pandemics of influenza that affect most of the world.

An epidemic curve is merely a graphic display of disease onsets over time, be it hours, days, or weeks. It can give insight into the source of the disease. If a school nurse observes that several students develop hepatitis within a brief period (a few days to two weeks) and none after that, she will consider the possibility of a common-source, or "point" outbreak. Fig. 10-1 presents such an epidemic. A group of students drank water contaminated with hepatitis virus on only one day. Illness onsets began after a reasonable incubation period, and continued over a two-week period, then stopped. The nurse would focus her investigation on events in the period consistent with the usual incubation period, i.e., fifteen days before the first case to thirty-five days before the last one. This pattern of the epidemic curve strongly suggests that all the patients were exposed at the same time and probably at the same place.

If an unusual number of new cases keeps occurring over months, it indicates that the source of the infection is continuing in the community, and exposure is occurring intermittently. Figure 10-2 illustrates a typical continuing-source epidemic curve. It displays the onset dates of infec-

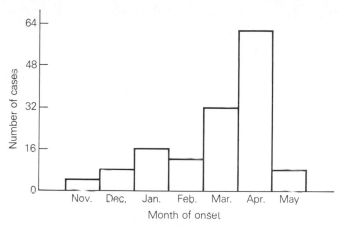

Figure 10-2 Symptomatic cases of infectious hepatitis, by month of onset.

tious hepatitis in a cottage-type institution over more than a five-month period and indicates that exposure was occurring over a much longer time than the usual incubation period.

EPIDEMIOLOGIC INVESTIGATIONS

A nurse working with school children observed that some of them were having an unusual type of eye infection. In her concern for the health of her school, she learned how many students had this disease by observing those present and learning if any were absent because of it. She wanted to prevent a major epidemic. She phoned the family physicians of the sick children to learn if each one really had the same infection. Careful inspection of the list of children with the eye infection led her to recognize that they were all members of the swimming team. When she questioned them about this, she learned that they were on the team which practiced after school. Checking farther, she found that no members of the team that practiced early in the morning were sick. The school custodian told her that chlorine was added to the pool very early in the morning. Careful tests showed that by late afternoon the chlorine level in the well-used pool was low. From then on, chlorine was added at noon also. No new cases of eye infection occurred.

What had the nurse done? Most importantly, she had promoted the health of the pupils by stopping an epidemic. She had accomplished this by using two types of epidemiologic studies. First, she did a survey to find out precisely how many pupils in her "community" had the particular disease, and verified the diagnosis so that she knew it was indeed the same disease. It is necessary to learn how much disease occurs and who gets it before any efforts can be started to learn what causes it. The diagnosis must be reasonably accurate. The survey that determines this is a *descriptive observational study.*

Next, she had done a case-control study. She had gathered information about common exposures and experiences that the children with the infection had had—that all were members of the swimming team that practiced in the afternoon. This led her to the hypothesis that it could be caused by faulty chlorination, and the fact that no one on the morning-practice team (the control group) had an eye infection strengthened the possibility. The cooperation of the custodian and proper tests proved the hypothesis and resulted in preventing more eye infections.

The example illustrates some important features of case-control studies. They are designed to discover what possible causative factor is more often associated with people with infection than in otherwise similar healthy people. Factors to be studied may have been suggested by careful observation, extensive reading, or even by a hunch. Then to learn which factor(s) more frequently affects diseased people, the study must include a comparison or control group of unaffected people. They should be as much like the patients as possible except for presence of the disease. Selecting the right control group is one of the most important parts of the study. In conducting any study, the assistance of people with other areas of knowledge is usually needed. This the nurse got from the custodian. Probably the statistician is the one most frequently consulted in order to select the control group, analyze findings correctly, and draw proper conclusions.

Another type of epidemiologic investigation is called the *cohort study.* Once a factor has been shown to more often affect people with the disease, we need to estimate the risk associated with it. This type of investigation starts with a group of people, or cohort, exposed to the factor and observes them over a period of time to determine the frequency with which the disease develops. Again, a comparison group is needed, as similar as possible but not exposed to the factor. Studies of lung cancer used cigarette smoking as the suspect factor and observed smokers and nonsmokers over years for the development of lung cancer.

The major difference in study design is easy to recognize. The case-control study starts with the disease, while the cohort study starts with a possible causal factor. The former design will give you an estimate of relative risk or an answer to the question: How much greater are my chances of getting lung cancer if I smoke than if I do not? The cohort design will give you a direct estimate of risk: What are my chances of getting lung cancer if I smoke?

The study designs described so far are all observational designs, used to describe the pattern of disease occurrence in a community or to determine and analyze the importance of suspected causal factors. Another design is that of the *experimental study,* in which the investigator actually manipulates the experience of one group under study, but not that of the comparison group. For ethical reasons, these are usually limited to clinical trials or to evaluating the effectiveness of a vaccine.

STATISTICAL CONCEPTS AND TECHNIQUES

To aid the nurse in developing a systematic approach in classifying and analyzing data, certain statistical concepts and techniques are necessary. Those to be described are variation, qualitative and quantitative data, population and sample in collecting data, tables and graphs in presenting data, and analyzing the data.

First and foremost is the concept that any particular subject or subject area is characterized by variation. The field of nursing is an example, since nurses may work in a hospital, office, community health agency, clinic, school, or industry. Another example is provided by people. Some people are young, others are old; some are thin, others are obese; some are males, others are females; some have a specific disease, others do not. Human behavior differs, for no two persons are alike, and all respond to the environment in different ways. The variables or factors are the characteristics which have more than one value to be studied.

TYPES OF DATA

There are two types of data; qualitative and quantitative. *Qualitative data* refer to those variables that describe a quality or attribute observed in the people or subject being studied. The variables in qualitative data are referred to as enumerations, classifications, and discrete or counting data. Qualitative data are developed by counting the number of persons who possess or do not possess a quality or attribute, e.g., the number of persons who are male or not male, who wear dentures or do not wear dentures, who have chickenpox or do not have chickenpox. The number of children in a family or the number in a group is a discrete value, as one does not have a proportion or one-half of a child or person. Qualitative attributes are easy to classify since there is only a definite number of possibilities, such as sex, race, presence or absence of a disease. Caution must be taken in categorizing subjective judgments of such matters as severity of a disease, appearance, or behavior. Personal bias may affect the classification when it is made by other persons, even though specific criteria are set up. Also, counting data can be misleading when they are based on small numbers of cases.

Quantitative data or variables are those having measurable values,

Table 10-1 Frequency distribution of weight in pounds of 65 senior nursing students at school X

Weight, lb	Number of Students
100–104.99	1
105–109.99	1
110–114.99	5
115–119.99	11
120–124.99	12
125–129.99	19
130–134.99	10
135–139.99	4
140–144.99	1
145–149.99	1
Total	65

instead of counts or enumerations as in qualitative data. Quantitative variables allow for measurement by recording the amount of a variable possessed by each person (or thing) studied. Age in years is measured by subtracting the birth date from the present date. Incubation period for a disease is the time interval in hours or days between the infection of a susceptible person or animal and the appearance of signs or symptoms of the disease in question. Variables in quantitative data are called continuous data, in the sense that they are capable of assuming any value of measurement, as seen in measuring heights, weights, temperatures, and blood pressure.

Grouping of quantitative data in which the measurements are made in a continuous scale should be done with care to avoid loss of detail. For example, classifying sixty-five nursing students weighing 100 to 150 pounds would not tell how many students weighed 110, 120, 125, or up to 150 pounds. Generally, to determine groupings, one divides the range into equal size intervals from five to twenty and makes each group nonoverlapping with the succeeding one. The range is the difference between the largest and smallest observations. For instance, if class intervals of five were used for weight, you would count the number of people falling into the class interval from 100 to 104.99; 105 to 109.99; or 110 to 114.99; and so on, through 149.99 The distribution is summarized in Table 10-1. Such characteristics as heights, temperatures, pulses, blood pressures, or specific laboratory findings also could be shown in a frequency distribution table.

COLLECTING THE DATA

The kind of data to be collected, the way in which they are collected and from whom or where, depend on the hypothesis or purpose of the study.

Two concepts important to data collection are those of population and sample. Population refers to the full group, the universe, all the people in the community. In practice, access to the total population may be impossible or even undesirable. Epidemiologically, a population can be defined as all the people who meet a prescribed definition, such as the same sex, or age, or engaged in the same activity. Sometimes the word "population" is used in reference to the group on whom observations are to be made, e.g., the study population. The observations made are measurements of characteristics of people, such as cholesterol levels or height.

A sample is a portion or a fraction of the population or the universe which is to be investigated. Sampling is a method of selecting a smaller subgroup from the total population, which will be as representative of the entire group as possible. This helps you to generalize the results of your observations to the entire group. If you could assume that the sixty-five senior nursing students previously mentioned were truly representative of all such students you would generalize that the weight range for senior nursing students is from 100 to 150 pounds. It is impossible to select a truly representative subgroup or sample, so any generalizations to the larger group must be made with caution. However, samples are used—in part because of the tremendous saving of time and money that is accomplished by studying only a small portion of the whole population.

There are many types of samples, but only the simple random sample will be mentioned here. This is a sample selected from a population in some random way so that every individual in that population has the same probability of being included in the sample. This helps eliminate bias. Another advantage of the random sample is that there are mathematical techniques which allow for drawing conclusions about the population on the basis of the sample.

When dealing with small numbers, a way of selecting a sample would be to copy the name or measurement on a piece of paper, place the pieces of paper in a hat or box, mix them up, and draw without looking into the hat or box, so that the sample is drawn by chance alone. For larger samples, one technique is to assign consecutive numbers to the entire population and then use a table of random numbers to select the sample. Tables of random numbers are found in most statistics books.

The method of collecting data depends on the hypothesis, the size of the sample, and the variables being studied. A few sources for data are records from the community health nursing agency, clinic, school, or industry; employment records, birth and death certificates, United States census reports; morbidity and mortality reports from local, state, national, or international agencies.

There are many ways of developing a form for recording the variables, or the information. The form may be a simple listing of facts,

Table 10-2 Source of referral for nursing service

Nursing service	Source					
	Private physician	Patient or family	Hospital or out-patient department	Health department clinic	Community health nurse	School	Total
Newborn.						
Infant.						
Preschool.						
School.						
Adult.						
Maternity.						
Tuberculosis						
Communicable disease. . . .						
Noncommunicable disease.						
Chronic disease						
Orthopedic disease						
Mental health						
Total.						

such as age and sex; a complex form may contain age, sex, race, housing, income, occupation, education, immunizations, behavior, attitudes and beliefs, and work history. The form may be a checklist used for entering a few items, or a punch card for many items, up to the limit of the card. Use of punch cards or large cards with a number of items makes tabulation more difficult unless mechanical means are employed.

TABULATING THE DATA

Tables are the most common way of presenting observations in a systematic arrangement, as they show the interrelationship among the variables. The simplest form of a table is a two-column frequency table, which may be used for quantitative or qualitative data. The first column gives the classes into which data are grouped, and the second column lists the frequencies for each classification or group. Table 10-1 is an example of a two-column frequency table.

Since tables show the interrelationship between variables, the form may be arranged showing several variables. This type of table presents data in relation to the specific variable and in relation to any combination of the variables. For example, to determine the source of referrals to a district during a certain period of time, the data would be tabulated as shown in Table 10-2. In this example the total number of referrals from all sources can be determined. In addition, the table gives information concerning the interrelationship between the source of referral and the service given, as well as the combination of sources referring persons to a particular service.

A table should be self-explanatory, and the title should tell exactly what the table shows. All columns should be specifically labeled. Do not put more data in one table than the eye can readily comprehend. Lined columns can be distracting to the reader, so do not use them unless it is necessary to separate data.

GRAPHICAL PRESENTATION OF DATA

A graph is a pictorial way of showing quantitative data. It allows a rapid overview of the material presented. There are many types of graphs; a few of the most common, such as the bar graph, histogram, and polygon, will be presented. There are some guidelines that apply to all graphs. The simplest type that will show the data is the best to use. Any graph should be self-explanatory; the title should tell precisely what the graph shows; scales should be marked and labeled; and any symbols used should be explained. The data on a graph usually proceed from left to right, from bottom to top, with frequency of the event on the vertical scale and the

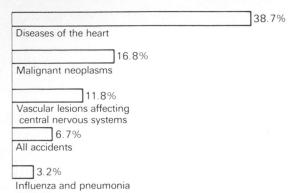

Figure 10-3 Five leading causes of death in the state of Washington in 1969.

method of classifying the data on the horizontal scale. (See Fig. 10-3.) Finally, when an arithmetic scale is used, the same distance on the scale must be allowed for equal numerical units.

The bar graph is the simplest type, with bars of uniform width usually arranged according to magnitude (Fig. 10-3). It is useful in comparing quantitative data or qualitative data of discrete type.

The histogram is a bar chart showing frequency distributions of quantitative and continuous data. It is a series of adjacent rectangles, and the frequency of observations in the various bars, when added up, equal the total distribution of the variable being displayed. When the class intervals are of an unequal size, the relative frequency distribution may be used. The relative frequency is expressed in percent. It is calculated by taking the number of times a weight class occurred, dividing by the total

Table 10-3 Relative frequency distribution of weight in pounds of 65 senior nursing students at school X

Weight, pound	Frequency	Relative frequency, %
100–104.99	1	1.54
105–109.99	1	1.54
110–114.99	5	7.69
115–119.99	11	16.92
120–124.99	12	18.46
125–129.99	19	29.23
130–134.99	10	15.39
135–139.99	4	6.15
140–144.99	1	1.54
145–149.99	1	1.54
Total	65	100.00

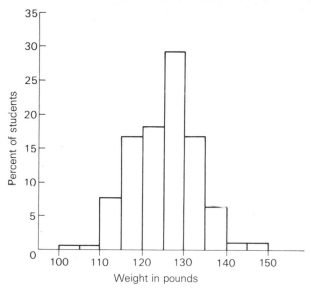

Figure 10-4   Histogram of weight in pounds of sixty-five students.

observations in the entire group, and multiplying by 100. The relative frequency of the weight in pounds of the example in Table 10-1, is shown in Table 10-3 and in the histogram in Fig. 10-4.

The frequency polygon is essentially the same as the histogram; the data are computed in the same way. In the frequency polygon, the frequency is plotted at the midpoint of the class interval and each point is connected by a line. The rectangles of the histogram are replaced by the connecting lines at midpoint of the interval, resulting in a continuous line. Using the same data as in Fig. 10-4, a frequency polygon is plotted in Fig. 10-5. When the frequency polygon is superimposed on the histogram, it is evident that the frequency polygon is an approximation of the area of the histogram (see Fig. 10-6).

ANALYZING THE DATA

Analysis of data is a process for the purpose of drawing pertinent conclusions from them. The analysis of data is one of the most important parts of any study. The techniques used for drawing conclusions vary according to the hypothesis and the type and amount of data collected. This is why the problem must be clearly defined and the data carefully obtained and well organized.

Vital statistics furnish data on quantity, quality, and composition with respect to a population. The data give a picture of the population and

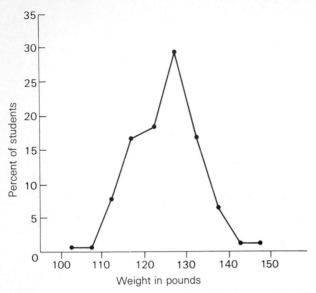

Figure 10-5 Frequency polygon of weights in pounds of sixty-five students.

allow for comparison, e.g., comparing the mortality of one group treated with a certain drug with that of another group not treated with the drug, or comparing the incidence or prevalence of disease in a given area with the incidence and prevalence in another area.

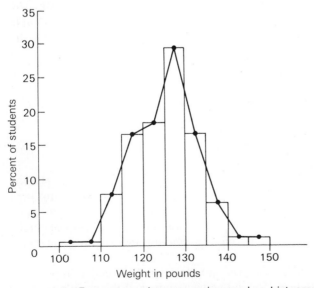

Figure 10-6 Frequency polygon superimposed on histogram.

Data with qualitative characteristics usually are summarized in rates or ratios. A rate is really a proportion, and refers to the rapidity with which a specific event is occurring. The mortality rate tells at what speed people are dying. A ratio describes the relationship between two distinct, separate numerical quantities; neither is included in the other, e.g., the ratio of women to men. It is often used as an index or comparative summary.

Many different kinds of rates are used in studying the various factors involved in the causation and control of disease. Each rate serves a different purpose and is subject to different interpretation. In calculating a rate, the numerator and denominator must be from the same population, and the numerator is included in the denominator. The numerator is usually the number of events that have occurred over a specified period of time, and the denominator is the population at the middle of that time period. This is considered to be the population at risk. When the rate is an annual rate, the population as of July 1 of the specific year is used. The population is usually divided into units of 1,000, and the rate expresses how rapidly a particular event is occurring in every 1,000 people at risk. The denominator base unit is selected in order to give reasonable rates, neither too large nor in small figures of less than one. The unit selected for all deaths, the crude mortality rate, is 1,000. The crude mortality rate can be expressed as 11.6 deaths per 1,000 people in 1970, or 1,160 per 100,000 or 1.16 per 100; they all show the same speed, but the 11.6 rate is more convenient to use. Morbidity, or disease incidence, rates are usually calculated for population units of 100,000. A case fatality rate is expressed as the number of deaths due to the specific disease per 100 cases of that disease, a percent. The crude death rate illustrates the principles involved. The rate is calculated according to the following formulation:

Crude death rate:

$$\frac{\text{Number of deaths reported in a given year}}{\text{Estimated population July 1, same year}} \times 1000$$

The rate is easy to calculate. The numerator is found by adding up the number of deaths from all causes that occurred during a given period, usually one year. The denominator is the estimated population as of July 1 of same year, and the base usually is 1,000. The following example gives the calculation of the crude death rate for Seattle, Washington, in 1970:

$$\frac{\text{Total deaths in 1970}}{\text{Estimated population, 1970}} \times 1,000 = \frac{6,092}{524,263} \times 1,000 = 11.6$$

The findings are interpreted as indicating that, on the average, for every 1,000 persons in the population of Seattle in 1970 there were 11.6 deaths from all causes.

Specific rates for deaths, diseases, age, sex, race, or any combination of these factors may be found as long as the numerator can be related to the same population. The following example gives the formula for the specific death rate from neoplasms in the state of Washington, 1969:

$$\frac{\text{Number of deaths caused by a particular disease}}{\text{Estimated population, 1969}} \times 100,000$$

$$\frac{4,953 \text{ deaths from neoplasms}}{3,203,218 \text{ estimated population}} \times 100,000 = 154.6$$

The specific rate is interpreted as indicating that, on the average, 154.6 persons died from neoplasms per 100,000 population in the state of Washington in 1969.

Incidence and prevalence rates often are used to express the frequency with which a disease is occurring in a population. They have distinct meanings. The incidence rate refers to new cases of a disease which arise during a given time period, usually a year. The prevalence rate refers to the total number of cases of a disease in a population at a given point in time. For chronic diseases, such as tuberculosis, the prevalence rate is higher than the incidence; for acute diseases, such as the common cold, the incidence is greater than the prevalence. The formulas for the two rates are as follows:

Incidence rate:

$$\frac{\begin{array}{c}\text{Number of new cases of disease X}\\ \text{occurring during a given time period}\end{array}}{\text{Estimated population at risk at midpoint same time period}} \times 1000$$

Prevalence rate:

$$\frac{\text{Number of cases of disease X at a point in time}}{\text{Estimated population at risk at that point in time}} \times 1000$$

It is important to distinguish between these two rates, and their names indicate their function.

Adjusted rates are often necessary when you want to compare rates of two or more geographic areas. Both the incidence and fatality of many

Table 10-4   Morbidity from disease K in communities A and B

| | Community A | | | Community B | | |
Sex	Cases	Population	Morbidity rate per 10,000	Cases	Population	Morbidity rate per 10,000
Males	50	10,000	50	50	15,000	33.3
Females	10	10,000	10	10	5,000	20.0
Total	60	20,000	30	60	20,000	30

diseases are influenced by certain characteristics, such as age, sex, and race. Rates are adjusted in order to eliminate the influence of one or more of these factors, as the unequal sex distribution of the hypothetical populations illustrated in Table 10-4. The morbidity rate of thirty cases of disease K is the same for both communities, which would indicate that the experience with this disease was equal in them. Further examination shows the incidence of disease K is greater in males than in females, and the female/male ratio is not similar for Community A and Community B. To compare the true impact of disease K in the two communities, the rates must be adjusted for sex.

A simple method of adjustment of rates is to select a standard population and to apply the sex-specific rates of Communities A and B to this population. The last census can be used for the standard population, or the population of the two areas can be combined. The method for calculating these rates and the sex-adjusted rates for Table 10-4 is as follows:

1 Morbidity rate:

$$\frac{\text{cases of disease}}{\text{population}} \times \text{base}$$

Community A:

$$\frac{60}{20,000} \times 10,000 = 30 \text{ cases per } 10,000 \text{ population}$$

Community B:

$$\frac{60}{20,000} \times 10,000 = 30 \text{ cases per } 10,000 \text{ population}$$

2. Sex-specific case rate $= \dfrac{\text{no. of cases per sex group}}{\text{population of sex group}} \times \text{base}$

Community A (males):

$$\frac{50}{10,000} \times 10,000 = 50 \text{ males}$$

Community A (females):

$$\frac{10}{10,000} \times 10,000 = 10 \text{ females}$$

Community B (males):

$$\frac{50}{15,000} \times 10,000 = 33 \text{ males}$$

Community B (females):

$$\frac{10}{5,000} \times 10,000 = 20 \text{ females}$$

3. Specific sex population = Community A males
                                        + Community B males

Specific sex population = Community A females
                                        + Community B females

Community A + B males = 10,000 + 15,000 = 25,000 males

Community A + B females = 10,000 + 5,000 = 15,000 females

4. Expected cases $= \dfrac{\text{sex-specific rate}}{\text{base}} \times \text{specific sex population}$

Community A (males):

$$\frac{50}{10,000} \times 25,000 = 125$$

Community A (females):

$$\frac{10}{10,000} \times 15,000 = 15$$

Community B (males):

$$\frac{33}{10,000} \times 25,000 = 82$$

Community B (females):

$$\frac{20}{10,000} \times 15,000 = 30$$

5. Sex-adjusted rate $= \dfrac{\text{total expected cases of each group}}{\text{total specific sex population}} \times$ base

Community A:

$$\frac{140}{40,000} \times 10,000 = 35$$

Community B:

$$\frac{112}{40,000} \times 10,000 = 28$$

These sex-adjusted rates of thirty-five and twenty-eight are now comparable. They reflect a higher rate for Community A than for Community B. For the sake of simplicity, race was considered to be similar in both communiites. The age distribution for a disease or condition is often important, and it becomes necessary to adjust the rates according to age groups.

Age Groups

The age groups frequently used for all causes of morbidity and mortality are:

Under 1 year: infant   25–44 years: young adult
1–4 years: preschool   45–65 years: middle age
5–15 years: school   66 plus: old age
15–24 years: adolescent

However, computing the age-specific rates of two populations from the above groupings is difficult; therefore ages may be regrouped into a greater span of years. The important principle is that the groupings must be the same for the two populations.

Some of the formulas for computing rates and ratios commonly used in public health have been given. Others include:

Infant mortality rate:

$$\frac{\text{Number of deaths under 1 year reported during given year}}{\text{Number of live births reported during the same year}} \times 1,000$$

Neonatal mortality rate:

$$\frac{\text{Number of deaths under 28 days reported during given year}}{\text{Number of live births reported during the same year}} \times 1,000$$

Maternal mortality rate:

$$\frac{\text{Number of deaths from causes of pregnancy during a given year}}{\text{Number of live births reported during the same year}} \times 1,000$$

Fetal death ratio:

$$\frac{\text{Number of fetal deaths during a given year}}{\text{Number of live births reported during same year}} \times 1,000$$

Case fatality rate:

$$\frac{\text{Number of deaths from spec. disease during a given time period}}{\text{Number of cases of the disease during the same period of time}} \times 100$$

Proportional mortality rate:

$$\frac{\text{Number of deaths from a specific cause during a given year}}{\text{Number of deaths reported from all causes during the same year}} \times 100$$

MEASUREMENT DATA

Data of all types, especially quantitative variables such as age or height, are summarized in terms of their distribution. Measures of central tendency describe this distribution, as measurements of variables tend to cluster around the highest point and will form a specific shape. The measures of central tendency are the mean, median, and mode.

The *mean* is the arithmetic average of a set of observations. It is calculated by adding up the value of each of the observations in a series and dividing by the total number of observations. Suppose that there is an outbreak of a waterborne disease in your district, and you want to determine the mean age at onset. To find the average of the sum of the ages in years, add the ages as follows: 12 + 15 + 16 + 16 + 17 + 18 + 18 + 19 + 20 + 20 + 20 + 22 + 24 + 25 + 28 + 30 = 320; then divide the sum by the total number of observations (16), i.e., 320 divided by 16, which equals 20 years. Each of these numbers has had equal weight in determination of the mean. If the mean of all the observations is subtracted from each of the observations, the sum of the differences or deviations is equal to zero, which is the center of the distribution. An example of the deviation from the mean of 20 years is shown in Fig. 10-7. The distribution in this situation is fairly symmetric, as the frequencies on each side of the mean are similar.

The *median* is the middle observation of a series of observations when the observations are arranged in order of magnitude. If there is an even number of observations, the average of the two middle numbers is the median. For example the median number for the age at onset of the waterborne disease is 19.5 years.

The *mode* is the observation occurring with the greatest frequency in a set of observations. Thus in the example of age at onset of this

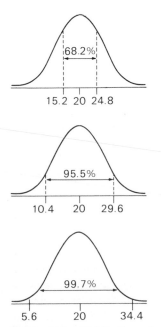

Figure 10-7 Distribution of normal curve with standard deviation of 4.8 years.

Table 10-5   Cases of waterborne disease

Age at onset, years		
	12	
	15	
	16	
	16	
	17	
	18	
Range = 18 years	18	
	19	Median = 19.5 years
	20	
	20	
	20	Mode = 20 years
	22	
	24	
	25	
	28	
	30	
	320 ÷ 16 = 20.0 years, arithmetic mean	

Arithmetic mean: The sum of the observations in a series divided by the total number of observations.

Median: The middle observation when observations are arranged in order of magnitude. In an even number of observations, the average of the two middle observations is taken.

Mode: The observation occurring with the greatest frequency.

Range: The difference between the largest and smallest observations.

waterborne disease, the mode is equal to 20 years. A summary of these three measurements is shown in Table 10-5.

The mean is the central measure of choice except when the distribution is asymmetric or skewed. The median is used when the distribution is asymmetric or when observations include occasional extreme values. For a more detailed discussion of the use and of the calculation of the measures of central tendency, the reader is referred to the work of Hill, listed at the end of this chapter.

It is beyond the scope of this chapter to present the numerous statistical methods appropriate for analysis of different types of samples. It is suggested that the reader consult a statistician within the agency or a statistical consultant from the state health department for planning and analyzing data.

Mention will be made of one measure of variation, the standard deviation, which is commonly used. The standard deviation is most useful with reference to the normal frequency distribution. The measures of central tendency will vary from sample to sample, giving a distribution of the sample mean. These will vary around the true mean of the population from which the samples were drawn. The standard deviation of the distribution of means gives the measure of the degree of chance variation or sampling within the population. The standard deviation is found by taking the square root of the sum of the squared deviations about the mean and dividing by the number in the sample or by the number of measurements. The formula, then, is:

$$\text{S.D.} = \sqrt{\frac{\text{sum of squared deviations}}{\text{no. of measurements}}}$$

or

$$Sx = \sqrt{\frac{\Sigma(x - \bar{x})^2}{n}}$$

When the standard deviation is calculated for a sample rather than for a population, the standard deviation is computed in the same way except that 1 is subtracted from the number of measurements, as a better estimate of the population is provided if the numbers are small. This would be the situation in the sample of age at onset of the waterborne disease. The formula would be:

$$\text{S.D.} = \sqrt{\frac{\text{sum of squared deviations}}{(\text{no. of measurements} -1)}}$$

Even though the measures in the sample are discrete, the pattern is characteristic of the normal frequency distribution and is approximated by it. Substituting numbers from the same example, the formula is:

$$\text{S.D.} = \sqrt{\frac{\text{sum of squared deviations}}{(\text{no. of measurements} -1)}} = \sqrt{\frac{348}{16 - 1}} = \sqrt{\frac{348}{15}} = 4.82$$

$$\text{or 4.8 years}$$

A summary of the distribution from the example is presented in Table 10-6. Since the sample is small and only approximates the frequency distribution, one is unable to generalize from the findings to large populations. The larger the sample, the closer is the approximation to normal frequency distribution.

Table 10-6   Distribution of 16 cases of waterborne disease according to age in years

Age at onset, years	Deviation from mean of 20 years	Squared deviation
12	−8	64
15	−5	25
16	−4	16
16	−4	16
17	−3	9
18	−2	4
18	−2	4
19	−1	1
20	0	0
20	0	0
20	0	0
22	+2	4
24	+4	16
25	+5	25
28	+8	64
30	+10	100
	0	348

Range: The difference between the largest and smallest measurements, e.g., $30 - 12 = 18$ years.

Standard deviation: The square root of the average of the squared deviations of the measurements from the mean.

$$\sqrt{\frac{348}{16}} = \sqrt{21.75} = 4.66 = 4.7 \text{ years}$$

When the standard deviation is being computed for a sample, rather than for a population, it is computed as follows:

$$\sqrt{\frac{348}{16-1}} = \sqrt{\frac{348}{15}} = \sqrt{23.2} = 4.82 = 4.8 \text{ years}$$

If measurements are normally distributed, 68.26 percent of them will fall within 1 S. D. on either side of the mean, or approximately two-thirds of the measurements will not deviate from the mean by more than 1 S. D. In other words, in the same example, within 1 S. D., two-thirds of the observations will occur 4.8 years on either side of the mean of 20 years (Fig. 10-7).

Also, 95.5 percent of the measurements will fall within 2 S. D. on either side of the mean, or approximately 95 percent of the measurements will not deviate from the mean by more than 2 S. D. Therefore, continuing with the same example, 9.6 years on either side of the mean equals 2 S. D.

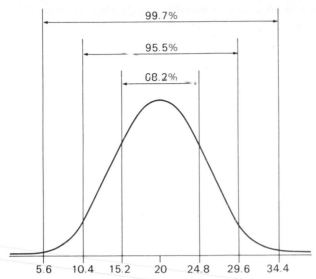

Figure 10-8   Distribution of normal curve with standard deviation of 4.8 years.

Last, 99.7 percent of the measurements will fall within 3 S.D. on either side of the mean. Applying this principle to the example, almost all the measurements will be within 14.4 years of the mean. Figure 10-8 summarizes the measurements of normal distribution.

SUMMARY

A brief discussion with illustrations of some epidemiologic principles and statistical concepts useful to the nurse in conducting studies is presented. Variation in people, behavior and environment influences health and disease and make it necessary to study the influence of special characteristics within the population. The purpose of the study, or the hypothesis, determines the study design, observational or experimental, and the type of data, quantitative or qualitative, to be collected. When planning the study, attention is given to the population and sample. After collecting the data, the findings must be systematically organized to show the interrelationships among the variables studied. Analysis of the data is the process of drawing conclusions so that intelligent judgments may be made. Rates and ratios allow for comparison of data with qualitative characteristics. Measurement data of all types, especially quantitative data, are summarized in terms of their distribution, e.g., measures of central tendency. Use of the data collected on a sample, as a basis for generalization to the entire population, requires statistical methods appropriate to different data. The standard deviation is the most useful in normal frequency distribution.

It is suggested that the nurse interested in conducting a study of her own consult with an epidemiologist and a statistician. This chapter provides an elementary discussion of both disciplines.

SUGGESTED READING

Bahn, Anita K.: *Basic Medical Statistics,* G. P. Putnam's Sons, New York, 1968.

Fisher, Ronald A., and Frank Yates: *Statistical Tables for Biological, Agricultural and Medical Research,* 6th ed., Hafner Publishing Company, Inc., New York, 1963.

Fox, John P., Carrie E. Hall, and Lila R. Elveback: *Epidemiology: Man and Disease,* The Macmillan Company, New York, 1970.

Friedman, Gary D.: *Primer of Epidemiology,* McGraw-Hill Book Company, New York, 1974.

Hill, Sir Austin Bradley: *Principles of Medical Statistics,* 9th ed., Oxford University Press, New York, 1971.

Ipsen, Johannes, and Polly Fiegl: *Bancroft's Introduction to Biostatistics,* 2d ed., Harper and Row Publishers, Incorporated, New York, 1970.

Kilbourne, Edwin D., and Wilson G. Smillie (eds.): *Human Ecology and Public Health,* Collier-Macmillan Limited, London, 1969.

Lester, Mary R.: "Every Nurse an Epidemiologist," *American Journal of Nursing,* **57:**1434–1435, November 1957.

Mausner, Judith S., and Anita K. Bahn: *Epidemiology: An Introductory Text,* W. B. Saunders Company, Philadelphia, 1974.

Maxcy, Kenneth F., and Milton J. Rosenau: *Preventive Medicine and Public Health,* 19th ed., Philip E. Sartwell, (ed.) Appleton-Century-Crofts, New York, 1973.

McCall, Robert B.: *Fundamental Statistics for Psychology,* 2d ed., Harcourt Brace Jovanich Inc., New York, 1975.

Remington, Richard R., and M. Anthony Schork: *Statistics with Applications to the Biological and Health Sciences,* Prentice-Hall Inc., Englewood Cliffs, N. J., 1970.

Roberts, Doris E., and Helen H. Hudson: "How to Study Patient Progress," Public Health Service Publication 1169, U. S. Department of Health, Education, and Welfare, Washington, D. C., 1964.

Seattle-King County Health Department, Annual Report, 1970, Seattle, Washington, 1971.

Terris, Milton: "Approaches to an Epidemiology of Health," *American Journal of Public Health,* **65:**1037–1045, October 1975.

Washington State Department of Health, Vital Statistics Summary 1969, Olympia, Washington, 1969.

Chapter 11

Looking Back and into the Future

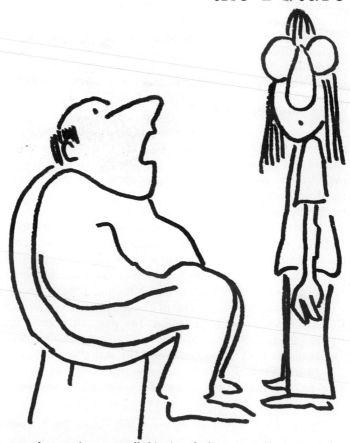

"Alright son . . . now that you've spent all this time finding yourself—let me in on it . . . who are you anyway?"

HISTORY OF COMMUNITY HEALTH NURSING

Early History

"Concern with matters of personal and community health appears to have been widely reflected in the records of every major civilization and the majority of cultures known to man."[1]

Similar references are to be found in the general literature and in the Bible. The Old Testament cites the efforts of Moses to prevent the spread of disease among his people by curbing their use of shellfish and pork as food. He did not know specifically why the ingestion of certain shellfish caused dysentery (probably typhoid) and death, or why the ingestion of pork caused illness and disability (probably trichinosis), but he did observe that when he prohibited the use of these foods, the incidence of these diseases declined among his people.

Community health nursing is also an outgrowth and a development of an ancient practice, that of visiting the sick. About 60 A.D. St. Paul mentions in his writings Phebe, a deaconess in the early Christian church, whose duties included a combination of parish work, friendly visiting, and district nursing. She has often been called the first visiting nurse; "from her day the work of visiting nursing has never been unknown."[2]

Nursing in Europe

For more than a thousand years after the time of Phebe, most of the nursing was done by men and women motivated by their religious faith. During the Crusades, illness and death were the fate of many pilgrims on their way to the Holy Land. Monasteries were established on some routes to provide care for these sick and travel-worn pilgrims. Here was the beginning of hospitals and nursing.

Following the Crusades, a spirit of great unrest dominated Western Europe. Many who had visited eastern Mediterranean countries, while on their pilgrimages, returned with a knowledge of new and easier modes of living, with stories of the luxuries of the East, its spices, jewels, and unfamiliar ideas about art and architecture. Important aftermaths of the Crusades were the improvement of economic conditions in many Western European countries; for example, the rise of the great maritime powers, Britain, France, Spain, and Italy, with their wealthy merchant class, and an eagerness for knowledge, especially in the sciences, in the universities.

Marked social reforms came with the end of the sixteenth century and the beginning of the seventeenth. This was also a period of creativity,

---

[1] Edward S. Rogers, *Human Ecology and Health*, The Macmillan Company, New York, 1960, p. 155.

[2] M. Adelaide Nutting and Lavinia L. Dock, *History of Nursing*, G. P. Putnam's Sons, New York, 1907, vol. 1, p. 102.

resulting in an increased production in literature and the other arts, a broadening of the horizons of science, and, even more important to community health, a notable increase in social understanding, with a growing recognition of social responsibilities by those on different levels of power. The concept of the brotherhood of humanity and other such revolutionary ideas, for those times, as that people are born free and equal and entitled to equal chances, were gaining acceptance. Improvement in living conditions continued, resulting in better housing, improved sanitation, and more nutritious food. In some instances these gains were the results of the English Poor laws of 1601 during the reign of Elizabeth I.

The sense of social responsibility for the welfare of others was demonstrated also by the sporadic attempts to provide nursing care for the sick, both in their homes and in hospitals. In 1610, in the little town of Annecy in eastern France, St. Francis de Sales (1567–1622) with the aid of Madame de Chantal, organized a nursing service for the care of the sick in their homes, the care to be given by a recently founded order of nuns drawn from women of the upper classes in the surrounding countryside. Unfortunately after five years, this order of nuns became cloistered and their home care of the sick was discontinued. Even though their project failed in such a short time, the work of St. Francis de Sales and Madame de Chantal created an interest in the venture, for in 1617 St. Vincent de Paul (1567–1660) founded a religious order of French women near Chatillon, France, to care for the sick on a home visiting nurse basis. St. Vincent de Paul had given much thought and study to the founding of this new organization while a university student in Paris. He introduced modern principles of social work and placed visiting nursing on a plane not reached in previous experiments of this nature. His order of nuns served local communities for many years, but after his death, it, too, became cloistered and could carry out its original purpose no longer.

Much of St. Vincent de Paul's philosophy of service to others is to be found in his writings, among which is the following, quoted from Nutting and Dock, which has significance and meaning for community health nurses today. "Lay off your jewels and fine clothing to visit the poor," said Vincent, "and treat them openly, respectfully and as persons of quality, avoiding all familiarity or stiffness. To send money is good, but we have not really begun to serve the poor until we visit them."[3]

In the centuries that followed, three movements or forces that stimulated interest in community health nursing were developing, slowly and unevenly, throughout Western Europe and were being carried to the New World.

These were (1) a sense of humanity, a deepening consciousness of

[3]Ibid., p. 414.

the social problems affecting the lives of many people, such as poverty, inadequate housing, evils of the industrial revolution, child labor, deplorable prison conditions, and lack of opportunities for education; (2) the growth of medical science, which was developing from the curing of disease to the prevention of disease and the promotion of health; and (3) the development of nursing as a profession and a discipline.

Social conditions in England showed definite improvement in the late eighteenth and early nineteenth centuries because of the work of both John Howard and Octavia Hill. John Howard (1726–1790), a sheriff of Bedfordshire, brought about, through his observations and writings, outstanding prison reforms, not only in his native England but in many countries in Europe as well. He has been called an "inspiration to the whole Humanitarian Movement." Octavia Hill (1838–1912), a social worker and contemporary of Florence Nightingale, instigated practical housing reforms in the Liverpool and London slums, bringing comfort, safety, and health to thousands of poor families.

Another evidence of a growing sense of social justice was the founding of the International Red Cross in Switzerland in 1863, through the efforts of Henri Dunant, a young man interested in promoting the welfare of others. As the Red Cross societies developed in each country, their emphasis on humanity and their efforts to prevent and to alleviate human suffering wherever it existed widened opportunities for providing nursing care in hospitals and in the community, particularly in many European countries.

The concept of present-day nonreligious community health nursing service was introduced in 1859 under the aegis of William Rathbone of Liverpool, England, who saw visiting nursing as a service that encompassed the new perception of humanity, the knowledge of modern medical science, and the "renewed art of nursing." He was actively supported in his work by Miss Nightingale.

Brainard has summarized the development of the three movements as follows:

> . . . the "new humanity" had taught that universal brotherhood is but a name, unless it seeks to remove the causes of one's brother's degradation; and the new science had taught that disease and suffering are not a visitation from an angered God, but are the direct results of our own carelessness in not following the right principles of hygiene, sanitation and healthful living; and finally, the care of the sick had been raised from the despised occupation of unskilled, untrustworthy women, and placed in the hands of women of refinement and character, who looked upon it as a vocation, and were trained, not only to the gentle ways of the early nuns and deaconesses, but to the scientific care and treatment of the patient as well.[4]

[4]Annie M. Brainard, *The Evolution of Public Health Nursing,* W. B. Saunders Company, Philadelphia, 1922, pp. 102–103.

Community Health Nursing in the United States

Nursing care of the sick in their own homes by a graduate nurse was commenced in New York City in 1877, sponsored by the Women's Board of the New York City Mission. The nurse was Frances Root, a graduate of the newly established Bellvue Training School for Nurses. The visiting nurse program, though modest, was a success, and similar ones were initiated on a sporadic basis in a few other American cities. Even in those early years, while providing bedside nursing care in city slums, these pioneer nurses recognized that many illnesses were caused by faulty economic and social conditions under which their patients and families lived, such as inadequate housing, lack of sanitation, insufficient food, and unfair, often vicious, labor conditions, and that measures for the prevention of these abuses were a necessity.

Nine years later the first district nursing associations were started, one in Boston and one in Philadelphia. They reflected a knowledge and understanding of the experience of the visiting nurse programs commenced previously in England. This was the period of prosperity in the reconstruction era following the Civil War. Standards of living were rising, and opportunities for education and travel, both in the United States and abroad, were becoming available to many people. Communication of ideas by post, telegraph, newspapers, and magazines were becoming a part of daily living. The idea of an organized district or visiting nurse service for the city poor spread rapidly west and south, and by 1900, twenty such agencies had been established in major cities.

Robert Koch, director of the Imperial Health Bureau in Berlin, in 1882 reported on his studies and those of his confreres, which demonstrated that tuberculosis was a transmissible disease, caused by a specific organism. This new concept of the cause of tuberculosis, with its bearing on the care and control of the disease, was quickly accepted by a large part of the medical profession, both in Europe and in the United States. Koch's discovery brought a new approach to the control of tuberculosis, that of public health measures, e.g., epidemiology and health education. The contribution that community health nurses could make to the control of this disease was recognized soon by the medical profession and the community. Community health nurses became responsible for much of the case finding and case holding, for teaching patients and their families, and for providing both pre- and postsanatorium home nursing care. Nurses soon discovered that the families of their tuberculous patients, many of them in the upper socioeconomic brackets in the community, had other health problems, too. This widened the scope of the community health nursing program at the beginning of the twentieth century. This new aspect in the care and control of a specific disease by community health measures was important in the early development of community health nursing.

The leadership of Lillian Wald (1867–1940), both a nurse and social worker, at the beginning of this century was responsible for many developments in community health nursing. Miss Wald brought to her work a basic love of and faith in mankind, a brilliant mind trained in the sciences, a sense of the practical, and a vision of what community health nursing and social work could do for communities and their people. In 1893, she and Mary Brewster established a visiting nurse service as a part of their Henry Street Settlement in New York City. This became a model for similar organizations and a training center to which community health nurses were sent for many years, both on an apprenticeship basis and for advanced work in supervision and administration.

Miss Wald, in 1909, persuaded the Metropolitan Life Insurance Company to begin, at first on an experimental basis, a home nursing service for its policy holders through a working arrangement with the Henry Street Settlement. Twelve years later, a study and review of the project showed that the program had been highly successful and had been adopted by community health nursing agencies in many communities. When the number of policy holders warranted it and no community health nursing agency existed in the area, the company set up its own visiting nurse service to care for its policy holders. This program, with some variations, was adopted by other insurance companies in succeeding years.

With the assured income from the provision of nursing services to policy holders for which the insurance companies paid full cost, community health nursing agencies had a firm basis on which to build their overall budget. The remainder of the budget could then be raised in the community by charging full or part fees for visits to nonpolicy holders who could afford to pay, by gifts, and by allotments from community funds. This contributed to a healthy and steady growth of privately supported visiting nurse agencies throughout the country. With a group of persons (the insurance company policy holders) who were fairly secure economically and who were receiving home nursing service in times of illness from the visiting nurse, the feeling that nursing services were only for the sick poor began to change in many communities. Community health nursing organizations began to note an increase in requests for nursing services from families able and willing to pay for them.

The programs of caring for insurance companies' policy holders continued on a nationwide basis until several years after World War II, when changing social, economic, and health conditions made them no longer feasible. Many communities, however, had learned the value of community nursing services and had come to realize responsibilities for supporting, by both public and private means, this health service to the community.

Lillian Wald, while on a visit to London, had an opportunity to observe a school nursing program that had been functioning in the London schools for nearly ten years. She was impressed to see that the nurses' work showed an improvement in school attendance and a reduction in the spread of communicable diseases among the children, especially skin diseases such as scabies and impetigo.

Through the efforts of Miss Wald, school nursing as a full-time program for a community health nurse was demonstrated and adopted in the New York City schools in 1902. This had followed by a few years the beginning of an industrial or occupational health nursing program in 1895 and was succeeded later by the development, on a specialty basis, of tuberculosis nursing in 1904, following the founding of the National Tuberculosis Association, and of venereal disease nursing as a specialty in 1909, when improved laboratory methods of diagnosis and treatment for syphilis and gonorrhea were developed through the work of Ehrlich.

Maternal and child health had its beginning as a specialty following the first White House Conference on Children called in 1909 through the interest and support of President Theodore Roosevelt. The program received an impetus in its development with the founding of the Children's Bureau by the federal government in 1912 and 1913. Outstanding landmarks in the development of maternal and child health followed rapidly. The New York City Health Department had established a Division of Child Hygiene in 1908, and the New York State Health Department followed in 1914. In 1922, Congress passed the Sheppard-Towner Act for federal aid for local infant welfare work. This money was distributed nationwide, generally through the state departments of health. The Social Security Act of 1935 and its amendments in succeeding years included, among other measures, provisions for public assistance, social services, and means of strengthening family life. These all had an important bearing on maternal and child health work in all parts of the country, rural and urban.

During the 1960s, additional health and welfare programs were initiated by Congress and state legislatures, such as the provisions for medicare, medicaid, and similar programs sponsored by individual states. All this social legislation has increased the opportunities for the community health nurse to provide nursing care and health teaching to patients and families in all age groups.

In the years immediately preceding World War I, certain social, economic, and humanitarian forces, implemented by such leaders as Annie W. Goodrich, Lillian Wald, and Edith Abbott of the Children's Bureau, brought about several events that were important in the development of community health nursing. In 1910, Mrs. Helen Hartley Jenkins, a friend of Miss Wald's, gave funds to Teachers' College, Columbia

University, to establish an academic program of study in community health nursing. Thus a little more than thirty years after Frances Root began her work in district nursing, college preparation in that field became available to nurses. Prior to this, whatever preparation nurses had been able to secure had been provided on an apprenticeship basis by some of the big city nursing agencies, such as the Henry Street Settlement and the Instructive District Nursing Association of Boston.

Following World War I, many colleges and universities initiated study programs in community health nursing for graduate nurses. These were discontinued as community health nursing preparation became recognized as an integral part of the preparation for *all* nurses in the collegiate programs for nursing.

The National Organization for Public Health Nursing was founded in Chicago in 1912. Miss Wald was its first president. The new organization had three types of membership: nurse members, lay members, and corporate members. The key word in the name of the organization was "for." Lay members were active participants and were considered important to the new organization. They worked closely with community health nurses for forty years to improve the standards of nursing service and education. In 1952, the organization became a part of the National League for Nursing at the reorganization of the nursing organizations.

At the time of its founding, the National Organization for Public Nursing received a small but successful quarterly publication from the Cleveland, Ohio, Visiting Nurse Association. This became the official national magazine of the young organization, and was best known as *Public Health Nursing.* It devoted its contents to the interests of those in the public health field. In 1953 it was absorbed by a new publication, *Nursing Outlook,* founded to meet, on a broader basis, the needs of an expanding profession.

The American Red Cross pioneered in rural community health nursing when, in 1912, it provided demonstrations of community health nursing care to people in the villages and on the farms. Much of the work was done by "itinerant nurses," who were sent to an area for a period of several months to demonstrate home care of the sick, school nursing, and well-baby conferences. These nurses also conducted mothers' classes and home nursing classes. It was hoped that the communities would recognize the need to employ full-time community health nurses to carry on the program.

Following the introduction of the Red Cross program, rural nursing developed rapidly. County health departments, particularly in the Southern and Western states, were established. Nearly every county health department had a full-time nurse on its staff, though often she was the only full-time professional member of the department. Rural nursing was facilitated further by the production and marketing of the first inexpensive automobile, which made it possible for many nurses to reach patients and families on distant farms and ranches. Putting nurses "on wheels" opened up many new opportunities for nursing services in both rural and urban areas.

The organization of the Children's Bureau by the federal government was completed in 1913. The Bureau stimulated programs of mother and child care by preparing and distributing health literature, e.g., *Prenatal Care,* by investigating unsatisfactory conditions relating to mothers and children, and by assisting with community health studies. The Children's Bureau programs expanded rapidly following the Social Security Act of 1935. The Bureau is now a division of the Department of Health, Education, and Welfare.

Following World War I, a trend from specialization toward generalization occurred, with the staff nurse being responsible for all types of community health nursing services in her district, and the agency providing her with consultant service. This shift from specialization to generalization, and an increasing demand for community health nursing services, contributed to the rapid expansion of community health nursing programs of study for graduate nurses, as previously mentioned, in colleges and universities. The National Organization for Public Health Nursing offered consultant service in the development of such programs and helped to promote standards by an accreditation service and by studies and surveys.

For many years Annie W. Goodrich had pointed out that although nursing had a place in the institutions of the sick, it could not render its full service to the community until it had found a place also in colleges and universities. In 1923 Miss Goodrich founded the Yale School of Nursing as a collegiate school, and for the first time adequate preparation for community health nursing was included in the basic curriculum. This was an innovation closely watched by other collegiate schools of nursing. Slowly they adopted the program, but it was not until after World War II that community health nursing preparation became an integral part of the basic collegiate curriculum and a requirement for national accreditation for a collegiate school of nursing.

During and after World War II, the increased demand for nursing services by the military and by the civilian population made mandatory many improvements in the utilization of nursing services, both in hospitals and in community health agencies, including a discriminating use of the professional nurse's knowledge, abilities, and time. Wider use of the team concept and more carefully planned services by auxiliary personnel were instituted in many hospitals and community health agencies.

Across the country, there was a growing effort to prevent duplication of services offered by the official and nonofficial agencies, wherever possible, thereby conserving the nurses' time and efforts and reducing such overhead costs as those of rent, administration, and travel. Knowledge regarding health practices acquired by the laity during and since World War II and the new public health and community health nursing practices that developed from the nation's war experiences facilitated the movement for the combining of community health nursing agencies.

Some nursing studies had been made in the period between World War I and World War II, such as *Nursing and Nursing Education in the United States, Nurses, Patients and Pocketbooks,* and the *Survey of Public Health Nursing.* In order to determine how to meet adequately the country's needs for nursing in the period following World War II and how to provide the kind of professional education and preparation required by nurses, it was recognized that more studies and research regarding nursing and nursing education were needed. Such additional studies, e.g., *Nursing for the Future, Collegiate Education for Nurses, Twenty Thousand Nurses Tell Their Story,* and *Toward Quality in Nursing,* have been published. Many other studies relating to curriculum needs and development have been made; these have pointed out the need for deepening the content of the preparation for nursing, for supporting nursing knowledge with contributions from other disciplines in the natural and social sciences and the humanities, for developing skills and abilities in the problem-solving approach, and for preparing students in collegiate programs in basic nursing for beginning positions in both hospitals and community health agencies. Current developments in nursing education attempt to meet these needs on both basic and graduate levels of study.

The nursing profession recognized the need also for continued research in other aspects of nursing, nursing practice, and research methodology as well as education, thus the founding in 1952 of the periodical *Nursing Research Report,* sponsored by the National League for Nursing and later by the American Nurses' Association also. Through its pages, *Nursing Research* has made the results of many studies in the various fields of nursing available to the profession as a whole and to allied disciplines. In 1955, the American Nurses' Association created the American Nurses' Foundation to meet the needs for a permanent nonprofit organization devoted to research in nursing.[5] Research programs to determine community needs for nursing in all its aspects and ways for meeting these needs will continue for years to come.

[5]Susan D. Taylor, "American Nurses' Foundation, 1955–1970," *Nursing Research Report,* 5(4):1–6, December 1970.

TRENDS IN COMMUNITY HEALTH NURSING

"The most frustrating fact of life is this: the more progress we make, the more we must make. The more needs we satisfy, the more needs we develop."[6]

Trends in community health nursing are part of the overall trends in general nursing and reflect those evidenced in current medicine. Furthermore they are closely allied to the social, economic, and political trends of the times. A distinction should be made between a tendency and a trend. A trend is a turn toward a specific direction; a tendency is an aptness to move or act in a particular way. A tendency should be watched, as it could be the beginning of a trend. An alert nurse might note a tendency in a family or a neighborhood which could become a trend, e.g., if two or three families with school-aged children move from the neighborhood, the nurse might wonder if this tendency could become a trend, producing a change in the average age of those living in the neighborhood and requiring a different type of nursing service, with more emphasis on geriatrics and less on preschool and school-age child health programs.

Comprehensive Health Care for All Citizens

Community health nursing practice is a changing and evolutionary concept of our time, and nurses must prepare and adapt to the needs of a dynamic society, which itself is in a continuous state of change and new order. Community health nurses are expected to assume many new duties and functions in America's move toward comprehensive health care, not only for the poor, but for the entire community.

The outstanding trend in community health programs is that of establishing the delivery of a comprehensive, effective system of health care for every citizen. This trend is in response to demands that have been made in the past few decades by leaders in community health and other groups of society. For all citizens to receive health care as needed, they must have access without financial or other barriers, to the whole spectrum of health services, and have access to a meaningful personal relationship with at least one health professional who will provide continuity.[7] Identification with a health professional might be with a physician, a nurse practitioner, a paraprofessional, or a member of an interdisciplinary team through whom coordination and referral to appropriate resources would be instituted. For clientele representing under-

[6]Richard E. Farson, "Bill of Rights for 1984," *Worlds in the Making,* Maryjane Dunstan and Patricia W. Garlan (eds.), Prentice-Hall Inc., Englewood Cliffs, N.J., 1970, p. 367.

[7]Anne R. Somers, *Health Care in Transition: Directions for the Future,* Hospital Research and Educational Trust, Chicago, 1971, p. 100.

served populations in the United States, the need for health personnel to give primary care services as needed is worthy of emphasis.

In preparation for and preceding the forthcoming decision regarding the adoption of a National Health Insurance plan in the United States, the National Health Planning and Resources Development Act (PL 93-641) was signed into law January 1975. Nurses should be well acquainted with the provisions of the act and functioning in capacities where they are determining the nursing roles to be enacted in relation to this and future national health legislation.

PL 93-641 created a system of regional health planning agencies throughout the nation. They were to determine the population's health service needs and the necessary manpower and facilities needed. Every state was required to enact a certificate-of-need law in an effort to decrease the number of excess hospital beds and eliminate construction and/or modernization of unneeded health facilities.

In addition, health-systems agencies were delineated by the governors of the states. Under the Secretary of HEW's guidelines, comprehensive health planning was developed within health service areas (HSAs). Working in conjunction with HSAs, state health planning and development agencies assisted state governments in developing and funding state health planning and development.

Objectives of the law were to:

1   Develop a comprehensive, rational, and coordinated approach to health planning and resources development
2   Provide meaningful consumer and provider participation in the planning process
3   Lay the groundwork for national health insurance

Under the health planning and resource development system, establishment of national health priorities was designated as follows:

1   The provision of primary care services for medically underserved populations, especially those located in rural or economically depressed areas
2   The development of multi-institutional systems for coordination or consolidation of institutional health services (including obstetric, pediatric, emergency medical, intensive and coronary care, and radiation therapy services)
3   The development of medical group practices (especially those whose services are appropriately coordinated or integrated with institutional health services), health maintenance organizations, and other organized systems for the provision of health care
4   The training and increased utilization of physician assistants, especially nurse clinicians

    5 The development of multi-institutional arrangements for the sharing of support services necessary to all health service institutions

    6 The promotion of activities to achieve needed improvements in the quality of health services

    7 The development by health-service institutions of the capacity to provide various levels of care (including intensive care, acute general care, and extended care) on a geographically integrated basis

    8 The promotion of activities for the prevention of disease, including studies of nutritional and environmental factors affecting health and the provision of preventive health-care services

    9 The adoption of a uniform cost accounting, simplified reimbursement, and utilization reporting systems and improved management procedures for health-service institutions

    10 The development of effective methods of educating the general public concerning proper personal (including preventive) health care and methods for effective use of available health services[8]

The priority list spells out the need for assessing, planning, implementing, and evaluating services on a continuous basis to insure that the health system gives quality care and is accessible to the population it serves. Nurses play a significant role in providing quality health care for citizens and must be participants in decision-making bodies whose purpose is to fulfill the functions designated by the act.

Implications for Nurses

When viewed from a nursing perspective, the national health priorities point out the essentiality of preparing nurse practitioners of sufficient numbers to fulfill the need for primary care services for underserved populations, coordinating health-care practices with other health professionals and team members and/or interdisciplinary teams so that support services are shared and utilized, providing for quality assurance of health-care services, producing creditable research based on factors affecting health and leading to preventive health-care services, assuring that consumer's or patient's rights are advocated and maintained, providing health education designed to educate and motivate clients to voluntarily participate in changing health behavior or health concerns, and upgrading nursing competence and skills through ongoing continuing education.

    Nurse practitioners Nurses on a whole are committed to providing primary care services for citizens for whom health care is not easily accessible. They are also well educated and skilled in providing health-

---

[8]Maxine I. Haynes, "What Is an HSA?" *Washington State Journal of Nursing*, **47**(4):3–8, Fall 1975.

care services designed to maintain or regain health and wellness. However, Hinsvark pointed out a deficiency area that nursing students complain about—that of being taught to be "non-decision-makers." She recommended that nurses must look at themselves and at their nurse peers and must consciously imbue themselves and others with a sense of worthiness as independent practitioners who can work *with* other health professionals, not for them. "We must also respect the differences among nurses and be supportive of each other."[9]

To meet the health-care needs of the American population in a wide variety of community settings requires specialized knowledge and skills which increasing numbers of nurse practitioners can fulfill. The management of chronic illness, patient and family teaching, community education programs, case findings, health counselling, well-care supervision, prenatal and postnatal care are just a few of the areas which can be managed effectively and efficiently by qualified nurse practitioners.

With the development of a health-care delivery system designed to reach consumers who are receiving inadequate or incomplete health care, nurse practitioners will provide the essential manpower, skill, and expertise as required in concentrated and rural population areas. They will become increasingly visible in leadership and will be accepted as competent health-care providers by clients. In this expanded role, their practices in many instances, will require independent and responsible decisions and risks for which they will be accountable.

Through the professional organization (ANA), certification programs for various classifications of nurses assure quality of care for clients. Certification is the process by which the association grants recognition to nurses who have met certain predetermined qualifications attesting to their proficiency and excellence in an area of practice as specified by the association. The ANA certification program has recognized many nurses for their excellence, individual achievement, and superior performance in clinical practice. The certification program is national in scope, is based on authoritative standards of practice, is cohesive and comprehensive with reasonable uniformity in the criteria in the various sets of the areas, and is based on the philosophy that every professional has the obligation to be accountable for establishing and implementing standards of practice.[10] As certification proceeds, directories of well-qualified proficient nurse practitioners will be published and kept current for purposes of assuring quality of care for clients. In the meantime, ongoing research on

[9]Inez G. Hinsvark, "Implications of Action in the Expanded Role of the Nurse," *The Nursing Clinics of North America*, "Current Legal and Professional Issues," Helen Creighton (ed.), **9**(3):418, September 1974, W. B. Saunders Company, Philadelphia, 1974.

[10]Pearl Dunkley, "Around the Country in Sixty Minutes," *Washington State Journal of Nursing*, **47**(2):3–9, Spring 1975.

quality of nurse practitioner care will focus on legitimating the nurse practitioner as an acceptable new professional in the health-care delivery system.

Coordination of health-care practices With the declaration that health is a right of all individuals, many concerns that are directly or indirectly related to health are being accepted as part of the domain of activities associated with health care. At the same time there is a proliferation of manpower in the health professions and allied disciplines. Many of the health professionals who are prepared in specialty areas have their own territory and expertise which must be coordinated with other skilled practitioners if the client is to receive comprehensive health services. Teamwork or team approaches are based on the assumption that clients' problems are complex and involve facets that can be better understood and ameliorated through specialized knowledge and skills possessed by the various professsions.[11] Health care which is coordinated on an interdisciplinary basis is recognized as having dimensions potentially enhancing and productive of quality of care for clients. Again, research as to the efficacy of interdisciplinary teamwork and coordination efforts of health professionals will be ongoing. If data support the claims of improved or quality health-care services for clients, then new curricula and educational experiences of a cooperating, coordinating nature will be made available to the various students who must learn about the many domains of health professions.

Quality assurance The trend toward quality assurance has been accepted and encouraged by the American Nurses' Association which published standards of nursing practice in 1973. Many institutions and agencies use the nursing audit to evaluate patient care compared to the standards for practice. Peer review is another method which is receiving wide endorsement throughout the profession. Peer review is a refined form of planned observation for review of nursing process, nurse performance, patient outcomes, or other activities which may directly or indirectly relate to patient care. Individual involvement in the peer review process is an essential characteristic for nurses since personal growth is one of the ultimate goals.[12] As stated by Zimmer, peer review is nurse peers' review of the health/wellness outcomes of a population of patients—of nursing activities that assisted patients to attain these

[11]Saad Z. Nagi, "Teamwork in Health Care in the United States: A Sociological Perspective," *The Milbank Memorial Fund Quarterly,* "Health and Society," **53**(1):75–91, Winter 1975.
[12]"Guidelines for Peer Review," *Washington State Journal of Nursing,* **48**(1):10–12, Winter 1976.

benefits, and observable evidence of patients' progress toward these results. Quality assurance guarantees excellence in patient health/wellness outcomes which involves *both* evaluating the degree of excellence of the results of delivered care and taking action to make improvements that in the future will result in a higher degree of quality. A patient health/wellness outcome is an alteration in the health status of the patient that is the end result of care given.[13] Assessment of outcomes of care is a powerful means for quality assurance. When outcomes are below criteria level, research must be done to search out new knowledge and provide direction for measuring productivity in ways that assure predictable satisfactory outcomes.[14]

Research   The professional practice of nursing requires the active and creative use of a knowledge base pertinent to the care of the ill and to the maintenance and promotion of health. Research, through its conduct, dissemination, and utilization is one means through which renewal or refurbishing of knowledge can occur. The goal to be achieved is professional practice which addresses consumer needs and concerns in health services and provides quality care with quality outcomes.

For research to be viable and respected as an indispensable reference source, it must be studied and utilized by all nurses practicing in educational and clinical settings. In many instances, research findings will provide support for current practices or will imply a change of established practices or ways of thinking about practice. For change to occur, legitimization of a proposed innovation must be provided by those persons in leadership positions, who can manage organizational conditions as feasible to ensure that implementation is carried out as suggested by the research finding, and rewards given for reinforcing the desired new behavior.

When a research finding is utilized, it must be evaluated in terms of its quality of process and quality of outcome. The purpose of quality of process evaluation is to identify points to maximize the quality of professional practice. Criteria must be used or developed as a basis for making judgments about quality. The quality of outcome evaluation asks the difference which the use of the innovation makes on the outcome of practice. Evaluation on an ongoing basis is imperative when improvement of quality of care is the goal. Concurrent with ongoing evaluation of research, nurses must be alert to and protective of the consumer's human

[13]Marie J. Zimmer, "Quality Assurance for Outcomes of Patient Care," *The Nursing Clinics of North America*, "Quality Assurance," Marie J. Zimmer, (guest ed.), W. B. Saunders Company, Philadelphia, 9(2):305–315, June 1974.
[14]Marie J. Zimmer, "Guidelines for Development of Outcome Criteria," *Ibid.*, 9(2):317–321, June 1974.

rights. Securing the consumer's understanding, consent, and assuring confidentiality regarding his or her participation in a study must never be forgotten or overlooked.

For research to have an impact on health-care delivery processes, reports and findings must be studied and utilized by all nurses. There must be active sharing of ideas, viewpoints, knowledge, findings between nurses in education and clinical practice on a mutually cooperative basis.[15]

Rights of consumers The role of the health-care consumer is expanding from that of patient to include the roles of planner, implementer, and assessor of the evolving health-care system. As national health legislation is developed, clients will have a voice and vote in the deliberations of planning, developing, implementing, and evaluating programs and services.[16] They are concerned about coordination of services, elimination of gaps and priorities in services, and definition of ethical and moral issues that pervade advances in medical technology.[17] By making patients, potential patients, or their advocates an integral part of the health-care decision-making process, the patient's viewpoint is reflected in health-care policy decisions aimed at improving the quality of care and increasing patient satisfaction.

The popularity of health information and do-it-yourself medical care books, newspaper articles, television, and radio broadcasts grows day-by-day. With increasing consumer knowledge and sophistication as to health problems and medical care, their participation with the health-care delivery system will be influential in affecting the following results: (1) The health status of the American people will improve significantly; (2) Pressures on, and criticism of, the health professions will decline substantially; and (3) There will be opportunity for nurses and paraprofessionals to practice to their fullest potential and gain understanding, acceptance, and respect in so doing.[18]

Consumers play an active advisory role within health maintenance organizations (HMO's). They are a part of the ongoing intercommunication system which is vital to the development of these programs. The success that these organizations are demonstrating is due partly to the fact that comprehensive health-care services, including prevention, are

[15]Marjorie V. Batey, "Research: Its Dissemination and Utilization in Nursing Practice," *Washington State Journal of Nursing,* **47**(1):6–9, Winter 1975.

[16]Report of the NLN Committee on Perspectives, *Perspectives for Nursing,* National League for Nursing, New York, July 1975, pp. 9–10.

[17]Eleanor C. Lambertsen, "The Changing Role of Nursing and Its Regulation," *The Nursing Clinics of North America,* Creighton, op. cit., p. 395.

[18]Nancy Quinn and Anne R. Somers, "The Patient's Bill of Rights," *Nursing Outlook,* **22**(4):240–244, April 1974.

given at a central location, costs are reasonable, and consumers play a participatory role. HMO's are a kind of health-care delivery system which provides the most appropriate level of quality medical care at a reasonable cost and is run by ethical, skilled professionals. Specifically, the HMO consists of the following:

1   An organized health-care delivery system that includes health manpower and facilities capable of providing or at least arranging for all the health service a patient population may require
2   An enrolled population consisting of individuals and groups of individuals who contract with the delivery system for the provision of a range of health services, for which the system assumes the responsibility
3   A financial plan that incorporates underwriting the costs of the agreed upon set of services on a prenegotiated and prepaid per-person or per-family basis
4   A management organization that assures legal, fiscal, public, and professional accountability[19]

The HMO concept is one answer which consumers have accepted for securing health-care services as needed. When a national health insurance plan is ultimately adopted, the implications it will contain for HMOs are yet to be seen.

Health education   Changing the delivery of health-care services so that requirements, desires, and wants of United States citizens are met means the involvement and intelligent participation of consumers. The issues of health legislation which are in the process of being debated nationally must be shifted to the local level where consumers can talk about and determine the options they desire. Becoming aware of available alternatives inherent in specific national health insurance plans must be discussed and internalized through community groups, local television, or other media. Consumers must become knowledgeable of the issues so that they can make their desires known to their legislators through letters, telegrams, or group action. Nurses can and must educate and/or collaborate with consumers in contributing toward a changed health-care system that is viable and equitable for all citizens. The challenge in this type of health education is in arousing an indifferent or apathetic consumer population to awaken and act. A small vocal minority can be heard and can influence.

Continuing education   Since nursing is concerned with the welfare of human beings, individual practice should be based on a continuously

[19]From Robert Gumbiner: *HMO: Putting It All Together*, 1975, The C. V. Mosby Company, St. Louis, pp. 1–3.

expanding and updated body of knowledge. It should incorporate ever-changing personal and societal values and needs. This requires a commitment to lifelong learning.

Continuing education is formalized learning experiences or sequences designed to enlarge the knowledge or skills of nurses. Its purpose is to ensure to the public that there will be a basic standard for the quality of nursing practice.[20]

Through the American Nurses' Association, a continuing education recognition program (CERP) was established to design and implement a system whereby nurses' accountability and quality continuing education activities would be recorded, recognized, and documented in the event that mandatory continuing education becomes a reality. Guidelines were developed for continuing education recognition programs in each state so that uniformity and reciprocity of recognition would be consistent throughout the nation. CERP committees review proposed educational offerings in terms of specific criteria and factors assessed to be essential and determine a particular number of points to be granted by CERP for each continuing education offering. For individual nurses seeking recognition points and proof of maintenance of professional competency, enrolling in a CERP program is advantageous. Records of continuing education activities for which recognition points have been awarded can be maintained and retrieved through a computerized databank. Recognition points can be earned by attending CERP approved offerings or pursuing an approved plan of independent study. In determining criteria for quality continuing education, nurses are demonstrating their commitment for seeking new knowledge and providing quality health care to consumers.[21]

Community health nursing and international health International health is a new responsibility on the world scene and one of today's major health problems. Community health nurses in all parts of the world share the concerns of their governments for improving the health of their own people. It is well known in public health that health or the lack of it in *one* country can affect directly the health of people in *other* countries. One country's communicable disease incidence can quickly become a serious matter to other nations, because of modern transportation, international commerce, and increased global travel.

It is necessary for all nations and their health professions to work together to protect the health of the world. Many governments and their leading health personnel do this through participation in the specialized

---

[20]Judith G. Whitaker, "The Issue of Mandatory Continuing Education," *The Nursing Clinics of North America*, Creighton, op. cit., pp. 475–478.

[21]Cecilia Smith, "CERP: Where We Have Been, Where We Are, and Where We Are Going," *Washington State Journal of Nursing*, 47(1):17–18, Winter 1975.

agencies of the United Nations, e.g., the World Health Organization and the Food and Agricultural Organization.

The International Council of Nurses provides channels for nurses of many countries to work together and to share their knowledge and skills. The basic desire to help others, which is a part of nursing, provides a common bond between nurses of every country. Since the days of Miss Goodrich, Miss Wald, and Miss Nutting, American nurses have taken a deep interest in the responsibilities they share with nurses of other countries, such as care and teaching of the patient, nursing service administration, nursing education, and community health nursing. They participate in the study and development of these subjects on an international basis through the International Council of Nurses, the World Health Organization, and other agencies of the United Nations.

Helen Nussbaum, the former general secretary of the international Council of Nurses, pointed out the barrier of language in achieving understanding of problems in nursing education and nursing service in various countries, citing the word "welfare" as being difficult to translate into certain languages. She believed that understanding between nurses of different countries could be reached by developing insight into the cultural background of others, by being tolerant, by having patience in trying to understand the philosophy and beliefs of others, particularly as they pertain to health matters, illness, and death, and finally, by gaining *wisdom.* The latter she considered to be the supreme quality in the definition of understanding.

Nurse power   Nurse power is an idea whose time has come. Changes in nursing education and health-delivery systems have contributed to the fact that large numbers of nurses have specialized expertise in practice. Through their commitment to improved practice, these nurses are realizing their own potential influence on the machinery of health-care delivery and are asserting themselves in the formulation and implementation of policy in primary health-care centers, critical-care facilities, and independent and joint practice settings. Individually and in groups, they are exercising their power as practitioners.

Nurses have not yet achieved a unified spirit, but their growing awareness of common concerns about patient advocacy, standards of practice, continuing education, certification, accountability, and other issues constitute what can be called superordinate goals for the profession. The fulfillment of these goals demands the cooperative efforts of all concerned.[22]

[22]Rosemary Amason Bowman and Rebecca Clark Culpepper, "Power: Treatment for Change," *American Journal of Nursing,* **74**(6):1053–1056, June 1974.

Tomorrow As stated by Glasser, everyone tries to use work, service, or play to gain a successful identity through involvement with others and through goals that help them to be successfully involved. Three factors have contributed to the emergence of our identity society—affluence (either a realization of or an illusion of abundance), political enlightenment for human rights, and the media (particularly television). If we are to succeed in our identity society, we must cooperate intelligently and become involved with one another for our common good. When people experience satisfaction of their need for involvement, an independent or a mostly independent role becomes possible. This independent role is potentially about the same for everyone; we gain a successful identity as a human being separate from what we do. Enjoying ourselves as people, we help others do the same. We can give free vent to what we feel and what we wish to do as long as we do not deprive others of the same choice. We feel successful, wanted, and valuable as people.[23] We also become successful as nurses, wanted by consumers, and valuable as professional colleagues in the delivery of quality health-care services to clientele.

SUGGESTED READINGS

Bailit, Howard, Judy Lewis, Louis Hochheiser, and Nancy Bush: "Assessing the Quality of Care," *Nursing Outlook,* 23(3):153–159, March 1975.

Bennis, Warren G., and Philip E. Slater: *The Temporary Society,* Harper & Row, Publishers, New York, 1968.

Bierman, Jessie M.: "Some Things Learned," *American Journal of Public Health,* 59:930–935, June 1969.

Brandner, Patty: "A Matter of Identity—New Horizons," *Nursing Outlook,* 22(3):188–191, March 1974.

Christy, Theresa E.: "Portrait of a Leader: M. Adelaide Nutting," *Nursing Outlook,* 17:20–22, June 1969.

Christy, Teresa E.: "Portrait of a Leader: Annie Warburton Goodrich," *Nursing Outlook,* 18:46–50, August, 1970.

Christy, Teresa E.: "Portrait of a Leader: Lillian D. Wald," *Nursing Outlook,* 18:50–54, March 1970.

Cooper, Signe S.: "This I Believe—About Continuing Education in Nursing," *Nursing Outlook,* 20(9):579–583, September 1972.

Craig, James H., and Marge Craig: *Synergic Power beyond Domination and Permissiveness,* Proactive Press, Berkeley, California, 1974.

Dunstan, Maryjane, and Patricia W. Garlan: *Worlds in the Making,* Prentice-Hall, Inc., Englewood Cliffs, N. J., 1970.

---

[23]William Glasser, *The Identity Society,* Harper & Row, Publishers, New York, 1972, 1975, pp. 6–247.

George, Madelon, Ide Kazuvoshi, and Clara Vamber: "The Comprehensive Health Team: A Conceptual Model," *Journal of Nursing Administration,* **1:**19–13, March–April 1971.

Glasser, William: *The Identity Society,* Harper & Row, Publishers Incorporated, New York, 1972, 1975.

Lowen, Alexander: *Pleasure,* Penguin Books Inc., Baltimore, 1970.

Miller, C. Arden: "Societal Change and Public Health: A Rediscovery," *American Journal of Public Health,* **66**(1):54–60, January 1976.

"On the Health Care Horizon: Nursing Issues," *American Journal of Nursing,* **75**(10):1834–1859, October 1975.

Roberts, Mary M.: *American Nursing: History and Interpretation,* The Macmillan Company, New York, 1954.

Rubin, Irwin, and Richard Beckhard: "Factors Influencing the Effectiveness of Health Teams," *Milbank Memorial Fund Quarterly,* **3:**317–335, July 1972.

Smith, Richard A., and James E. Banta: "Global Community Health—A New Health Direction," *American Journal of Public Health,* **59:**1713–1719, September 1969.

"The Ten-Year Health Plan for the Americas," *American Journal of Public Health,* **65**(10):1046–1059, October 1975.

Part Two

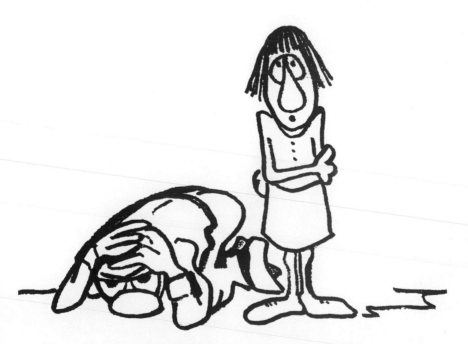

"I think he is trying to tell me something . . ."

INTRODUCTION

Case situations, experiential exercises, and case studies are provided in the following section to be used as examples for discussion and learning. It is hoped that these descriptions of community health situations will provide insight about aspects of community health nursing, will arouse thought regarding the effective use of self as a nurse with families in communities, and will demonstrate the utilization of selected theories with consumers.

The case studies are based on papers written by nursing students and are descriptive of actual situations encountered with families in the local community. Grateful acknowledgment is expressed for the direct and indirect contributions of the following students: Janet Arusell, Diana Ciganik, Lynda Gentz, Nancy Hoover, Sandra Kennedy, Michelle Kroll, Sonia Mounsey, and Sandra Withers.

Community Study

USING ROSS'S COMMUNITY ORGANIZATION PROCESS

In searching for an idea which would be acceptable in fulfilling the requirements of a community project, a small group of senior nursing students enthusiastically decided to start working toward the establishment of a drop-in center for teen-agers in the local community. They felt a deep concern and empathy for the youth in the community because recreational and social facilities were limited. They thought that if a drop-in center for teen-agers were available where they could "come and rap," perhaps some would be prevented from choosing self-destructive alternative life-styles (drugs and alcohol).

Their first steps in proceeding to identify the needs of the community in regard to youth were to investigate the existence of resources currently in operation. They found that the youth in the community had no "constructive" recreational or social facilities. There were no resources

373

dealing with drug and alcohol problems. There were facilities for youth in nearby communities; however, because of the rivalry of community competition, the youth did not feel welcome in nearby community facilities. The next activities of the nursing students were to interview a cross section of local community citizens. They interviewed school teachers and administrators, psychologists, police, clergy, representatives of the local coordinating and planning agencies, and a member of the YWCA. The nursing students returned from these interviews either depressed or enthusiastic, depending upon to whom they talked. As they discussed their goal and experiences among themselves, regardless of the up-and-down swings of emotion, they became increasingly convinced that a drop-in center was desperately needed in that community. An empathy for the plight of the local teen-agers was particularly poignant at that stage of the community organization process. An opportunity arose to attend an evening community meeting sponsored by the local YWCA in relation to the need for a drop-in center in the community. The director and two high school students from a nearby community facility were on the agenda to explain their organization, purpose, and functions. During the meeting the local citizens were informed that all that was necessary to start a drop-in center was a group of interested young people and a house, and other details could be worked out thereafter. The discussion during the meeting accepted the assumption that a drop-in center was needed; however, the securing of a house and the financial and legal implications involved a risk with which no one wanted to deal. As the meeting terminated on an indecisive note, a young woman counselor of the local community recreational center volunteered her services to work toward the goal of a drop-in center. At a subsequent meeting with the counselor, the nursing students were advised to contact a clergyman who had expressed an interest in the project. It was at this point that the nursing students were searching for potentially productive local resources to deal with their objectives. They were also vacillating in emotions about the behavior of local citizens at meetings. With uncertainty, but with hope, they met with the local clergyman who had with him a public school counselor and physical educational coordinator. In their report of this meeting they described the discussion as follows:

> We discussed the drop-in center in abstract terms. Father —— and Mr. ——
> mentioned influential people in the community who might be of some aid to
> our project. Father —— stated that if he was going to help us financially, he
> wanted to know more about how we were going to be organized. He
> mentioned lawyers, incorporating the center, and made what we thought to
> be a relatively simple organization a very complex endeavor. However, his
> assistance was vital in making us aware of the problems that would arise.

A series of meetings were held with the clergyman and school counselor at regular intervals thereafter, and an increasing number of local citizens were drawn into the project, including a lawyer, a judge, a policeman, a Catholic clergyman, a local businessman, a physician, representatives from the local school district, local service clubs, and the local coordinating agency, as well as local high school students. All aspects of planning and implementing the project were discussed thoroughly. The nursing students learned many things, including the following: (1) The importance of planning which envisions all obstacles, possibilities, and events that may aid or infringe upon the project, (2) How citizens behave and talk when dealing with a controversial project during community meetings—the desire of some citizens to become involved in changes when they are asked to assume some responsibility. (3) Action seems slow when a large number of citizens are involved. (4) When asking for support, words must be carefully chosen; for instance, if comparison is made with facilities of nearby communities, citizen response is inclined to be negative. (5) Influential persons are essential because of their emotional support, financial backing, and knowledge about existing local politics. (6) Risk taking is involved in any project and some citizens assume more responsibility and risk than others. (7) Organization is a must; all procedures are best anticipated in advance and planned for before implementation of action takes place. (8) There is an orderly procedure involved in establishing a center, which takes into consideration the need for rules and regulations, criteria for eligibility of staff workers, an advisory board, a board of directors, and other considerations. (9) With a firm foundation, a newly established center is less vulnerable to negative legal procedures or negative public opinion.

A center was opened in the local community eight months after the first nursing students became actively involved in initiating the establishment of such a facility. The nursing students participated actively in the community organization process. In their evaluation of their activities they stated:

> The students' efforts in organizing this project have had a tremendous influence on our ideas about how to organize a community, how to contact key people in the establishment, and how to become involved. As nurses, we find that our training and our individual personalities can lead us far from the emergency room or the operating room of a large hospital, and very much into the community to work with the people with whom we live. We can work at any level of community organization, in that we have the ability to recognize problems, to make people aware of them, and then to do something about them.

DISCUSSION

1 Identify the steps of the community organization process as outlined by Ross in this community study.
2 In reading this community study, what factor or factors were most important in accomplishing the desired end-result?
3 If you were to critique this community study, what points or steps would you emphasize as needing further investigation?

Using Social Learning Theory and Festinger's Theory of Cognitive Dissonance

Mrs. F., a sixty-nine-year-old widow who had been living alone for twelve years, was referred for a visit by the community health nurse to assess her ability to continue living independently. Mrs. F. was in desperate need of help financially and physically. She was having blackout spells almost daily. She had a 2-inch pile of medical bills from recent hospitalizations for a CVA and later hospitalizations for smoke inhalation, from a fire she caused by dropping a lighted cigarette on her mattress.

When I first went into her home, Mrs. F. and I were aware that I was evaluating her ability to be independent. On a series of visits, from interviews and personal observations, I found that Mrs. F. was existing on a diet of Chinese noodles and canned milk. She was not taking medication for her hypertension, ulcers, anxiety, or osteoporosis in the proper dosages or time intervals.

She was highly motivated to change her behavior because of the high value she placed on independent living. She stated, "I'd rather die right here in this house, than have to leave right now." I believe one reason she

wanted to stay so badly was because of her dog, whom she had raised for
nine years in this same home. She loved him as a mother loves a child, and
would rather feed him than herself. She therefore was receptive to the
idea of setting mutual goals for demonstration of capability of independent living, and together, we established a contract.

I decided to use the social learning theory because social reinforcement is an important source of motivation for human behavior. Social
learning also considers environmental factors and their effect on behavior. Verbal and nonverbal attention and recognition can serve as social
reinforcers.

Application of Theory

Mrs. F. and I decided to attempt to change two basic behaviors—eating
habits and taking medications—both being essential to her health maintenance and ability to care for herself competently and safely. I suggested
that we employ the use of flow charts, in the hope that this would enable
Mrs. F. to actively participate and assume maximum responsibility for her
own daily activities. In addition, the charts would serve as a reminder to
take her medications at the proper times. Modification of dietary patterns
is difficult. Therefore, we felt it was most realistic to include one new food
each week, and gradually build until a varied, well-balanced diet including
all food groups was achieved.

I had two basic hypotheses. The first was that my verbal recognition
of her efforts to achieve independence and the attention she received
weekly from me during my visits were social reinforcers which could
motivate Mrs. F. to change her behavior. I held this to be true because
Mrs. F. was a lonely woman, unable to get out of the house and actively
seek companionship, and was blessed "with the gift of gab" and loved to
converse. I fulfilled her desire and need for companionship so she would
act in a manner pleasing to me in order to achieve the reward of my
continued visits and pleasure in her successes.

My second hypothesis was based on Festinger's theory of cognitive
dissonance which states that a person's related beliefs are mostly
consistent with each other, and if they are not, the person feels discomfort
which often motivates him or her to change. Festinger sees the inconsistency as a motivating drive. When the nurse introduces dissonance as a
motivating factor, she states her view of the situation, as opposed to the
view of the client, and examines the differences in viewpoints. If rapport
has been established, these differences are likely to cause unpleasant
psychological tension (cognitive dissonance). The inconsistencies felt
should prompt action in such a way that the unpleasant tension will be
reduced.

In Mrs. F.'s case, her lack of responsibility in self-care, specifically in preparing nutritious meals and taking her medications as prescribed, is inconsistent with the concept of independence. It was my hypothesis that this inconsistency would produce cognitive dissonance, and serve as a further motive for Mrs. F. to change her behavior, in order to decrease psychological tension and behave within the context of independence.

Social reinforcement was very effective in Mrs. F.'s case. We initially discussed the basic elements of good nutrition, inexpensive yet high-protein dishes, likes and dislikes, planning for shopping, and her accessibility to stores. She asked many questions and showed a great deal of enjoyment in planning menus and shopping lists. I felt that she appreciated my acknowledgement that it was difficult to stretch a limited budget, but together we agreed on some economical, yet delicious, dishes.

We also spent time reviewing Mrs. F.'s medications, their purposes, proper dosages, and frequency. I was glad I took the time to explain these thoroughly and carefully because Mrs. F. had several misconceptions about both purposes and frequency of her prescriptions. At each visit, I would also take Mrs. F.'s blood pressure which on my initial visit was 180/110.

Twice a week I visited Mrs. F. to review her charts, take her blood pressure, and listen to her questions, concerns, and family problems. The biggest problem, I soon discovered, was her very limited vision, due to one glass eye and a severe cataract on the other. This posed a problem in reading medication labels, food cans, writing grocery lists, reading hospital bills that came in the mail, as well as reading the flow sheets. I had made the print very large on the sheets, so she was able to fill them in with little trouble, but this was not the case with bills or labels. I discussed this with Mrs. F., and she felt that a magnifying glass would be a great aid to reading. She had already discussed the visual problem with her physician, who said the cataract "was not ripe yet."

Only a week after my initial visit with Mrs. F., she blacked out and was taken to the hospital. The cause was probably a transient ischemic attack secondary to chronic hypertension, but it was an incentive for her physician to change her antihypertensive medication. Mrs. F. subsequently had no more blackout spells and her blood pressure remained at about 140/85 on all my later visits.

I found that as Mrs. F. kept the charts, she would recognize if she ate poorly, that she had indeed done so. "I was depressed after my son called because he was so drunk," she would state. I neither agreed with the excuses nor reprimanded her, but merely acknowledged the fact that she had eaten poorly, and allowed her to accept the responsibility. Mrs. F. also cut down tremendously on her ingestion of pain medications, stating that she only occasionally suffered severe pain. She could recall that no one ever explained what the pills were for but had said to take them four times a day. This is indeed what the label stated. They had made her groggy, so she decided to take them only at bedtime. Her other medications were now taken regularly in the proper dosage, and she could not explain the purpose of each.

I felt that Mrs. F. was making great progress in moving toward independence. An added benefit which evolved was that Mrs. F.'s granddaughter, who was pregnant, had assumed the job of cleaning Mrs. F.'s home twice weekly and was paid by the Department of Social and Health Services. She was there during my visits and became very interested in the nutritional guidelines I discussed with Mrs. F. at each visit—menu planning, budgeting, and buying a variety of economical, yet nutritious, foods. She asked questions, and when Mrs. F. and I reviewed the weekly flow sheet for food intake, she would reinforce my suggestions and augment my encouragement of Mrs. F., offer her own suggestions, and offer to shop for whatever Mrs. F. needed to follow through with her menu plans. She began to eat lunch with Mrs. F. two to three times a week.

This support by a family member was an essential step in Mrs. F.'s gain of independence. The focus of reward was gradually being turned away from social reinforcement by my presence and praise, to reinforcement by her granddaughter and an actual sharing by her in the learning experience.

DISCUSSION

1 Was social learning theory used appropriately with this client? Cognitive dissonance?
2 Specify other ways that the theories may have been used more effectively.
3 Were any principles of learning evident in this case study?
4 Identify the steps of the nursing process used in this case study.
5 If you were to critique this case study, what points would you emphasize as needing further investigation?

Using Rogers's Law of Interpersonal Relationships

Carl Rogers states that "It is the quality of the interpersonal encounter with the client which is the most significant element in determining effectiveness." He talks of several components which the counselor must have and utilize to facilitate such a relationship and to promote true growth of the client. The counselor must have genuineness or congruence, empathy, and positive regard. In addition, an important element in the interpersonal encounter is the client's perception of the counselor. How has the client perceived the attitudes that have been communicated to him or her?

Application of Theory

I used this theory with a client and her two sons with whom I had previously been ineffective. I initially began the relationship with this family by feeling that I was the "helper," and they were to be "helped." They would tell me what their problems were, and I would deal with those problems for them, and we would live happily ever after. Therefore, I entered the home with a preconceived idea of how I wanted them to talk and react, and I was actually fearful that they would not cooperate with my plans. I was surprised to find on our first two visits, the mother was very compliant to all my wishes, mechanically answered all my questions with all the "right" answers, and then promptly admitted herself in the local hospital, as she felt very depressed and suicidal. Although I realized that in such a short time, I as a counselor probably could never have prevented such feelings, it bothered me that I had not had an inkling during my visits of what was going on inside her.

I began thinking through step-by-step what our relationship had been and came to the conclusion that we had been sharing facades. I also sought help from people who had had dealings with my client. Her psychiatrist replied, "Talk to R."; her mother said, "Be her friend"; her psychiatric nurse answered, "Everyone makes plans for R. without consulting her." These answers reminded me of Carl Rogers's theory. They were saying, "R. is a person and she must be dealt with as a person."

In my next visit I tried putting Rogers's theory to practice. This required much inner thinking and searching as to my true feelings in regard to our relationship. This was the beginning of genuineness and congruence. I felt the best way to begin communicating this feeling of genuineness would be to tell R. these feelings, which include "I have been trying to be a helper to you without knowing your feelings. I have been acting as the Saviour to the sinner, and I have been wrong. I realize that you are very capable of seeking help for yourself, and I have stepped where I was not invited." It was somewhat uncomfortable at first but R. replied with genuineness. She replied that she felt most of the problem was that she could not be open because she did not want to be hurt; that she knew she could not help herself, but she hated people. With that, she burst into tears. It was at this moment that I truly saw R. as a person.

I found that this first act of true genuineness-congruence and openness led easily to the other elements. I did not have to consciously think about these next elements, but I could see them happening as our communication progressed. I found several ways of communicating empathy—through reiteration, such as "I feel that you are meaning this . . ." and clarification statements. For example, R. said, "I hate people." I replied, "Do you mean you hate all people?" She replied by saying that she did hate all people because they tell her what to do all the time without giving her a chance, but it was all right for me to tell her what to do because she needed help. I reiterated her statement, then said, "I feel that you mean you hate people who butt into your life and try to take command but as long as you are the one who first asks for help, you are still the one governing your life and therefore, have a feeling of worth." R. seemed to pick up the fact that I was really trying to understand her feelings and went on to describe some examples of real people she hated. It was difficult to be truly empathic at first as I could not know R.'s true feelings, but the fact that I let her know that I was trying to grasp an understanding told R. that I cared.

True positive regard was one of the most important elements of the "growing" relationship between R. and me. I looked at all the things which made R. a person—an individual—the fact that she cried, became nervous, smiled, had her own thoughts and feelings, loved her sons, had a special way of dealing with her sons, had her own unique facial features, walk, air of being. Something I said placed an absolute flow of pleasure on R.'s face—something I had not observed before. It was, "R., I am so glad that you do not want to live with your mother because you feel she dominates the children. I think that you are the most loving, caring, concerned mother. You know your children better than anyone else— they are a part of you—and you are the most able to care for them. I would hate to see that ability taken away from you." On paper, this sounds like a "buttering-up" routine. However, it was exactly how I felt about her as a person in the role of a mother. This kind of positive feedback truly seemed to bolster her morale and it seemed easier for R. to communicate her true feelings. Also, I felt she began to see herself as a worthwhile person with some positive strengths.

DISCUSSION

1 Was Rogers's interpersonal approach the appropriate one to use in this case study?
2 Are there other communication theories that may have been used more effectively?
3 Describe examples in the case study demonstrating the nurse's use of therapeutic interactions.
4 Identify the steps of the nursing process used in this case study.
5 If you were to critique this case study, what points would you emphasize as needing further investigation?

Using Maslow's Hierarchy of Human Needs

L. was referred to the community health nurse for the purpose of offering antepartum care and counseling. On the initial home visit it was obvious that there were explicit overwhelming needs which were not being met for the maintenance of a safe, comfortable, and healthy daily life. The observations and nursing history which I gained are itemized as follows:

1 Water was coming through the bedroom ceiling—the room was uninhabitable. The water was from an overflow of the toilet in the upstairs apartment.

2 Nothing could be stored in bottom cupboards of the kitchen because shelves were covered with "rat" droppings. The family had seen "rats" and had heard them at night.

3 Windows were broken and taped.

4 The porch and steps were collapsing—the porch had a 35° slant.
5 L. had fears about her fetus. She was eight months pregnant, had had x-rays during the first trimester, and was worried about her baby's normality.
6 One of the children had a skin rash.
7 L.'s husband had deserted the family three months previously.
8 The family was financially supported by welfare and owned no car.

I selected Maslow's theory because of its realistic approach and assistance in knowing how to proceed. I hypothesized that L. would not be able to experience and/or fulfill higher needs such as love and belonging, esteem, and self-actualization, until the lower, basic physiological and safety needs were met. By systematically going over each problem and determining the level of human need, I planned my activities with the family.

Application of the Theory

1 The environmental and living conditions. L. stated that her brother had been bitten by a rat as a baby and she did not want that to happen to her children. She had a choice of motivating the landlord to improve the environment or changing residences. This problem fell into the physiological and safety levels, and I gave it top priority by helping L. to find a new home.
2 L.'s pregnancy. When L. found out that she was pregnant, she had been advised to have an abortion, and all arrangements had been made. On the day it was scheduled, after completing some of the preliminary procedures, she could not go through with it because of moral and religious convictions. She subsequently had a fear that radiation had affected her baby. This problem represented a physiological need. I listened to L.'s feelings, gave explanations as appropriate, and encouraged her to visit the doctor for examination and reassurance.
3 L.'s feelings about her husband. "I still love him but can't live with him as we argue too much." This problem was of the higher level, that of love and belonging, so I deferred any action on this problem until a later time when the physical comfort and safety needs were met.

By using Maslow's theory I was impressed that some clients just accept and tolerate life on a day-by-day basis and are not motivated to act until they receive help, encouragement, and support from persons who can offer hope and direction. I was also amazed that clients do not realize that they themselves can change their predicament; they have the capabilities, but wait for stimulation or encouragement from an outside source.

DISCUSSION

1 Was the application of Maslow's theory appropriate in this case study?
2 At what phase of the nursing process was Maslow's theory most facilitative?
3 Are there other theories that may have been used effectively with this family?
4 Were any principles of learning evident in this case study?
5 If you were to critique this case study, what points would you emphasize as needing further investigations?

Using a Client-Centered Approach

In the clinical experiences I have had during the past year, I have become increasingly reluctant to use certain "techniques" in my approach to patients. I have felt particularly uncomfortable using those methods in which I formed a judgment about what was "good" or "acceptable" behavior in a patient and then proceeded to mechanically reinforce and reward that "desired" behavior, so that the patient would see it as desirable behavior also.

In my relationships with patients, with my son, and with mentally retarded persons, I have preferred to use a less manipulative, less mechanical approach—one that does not see the other as an object for control. I have frequently observed with my son that positive reinforcement is a very heavy burden for him to carry, and he frequently rejects my positive evaluation for one of his own that is less demanding and less threatening. He has taught me that the appropriate place for evaluation and judgment is within ourselves and that a truly helping, growth facilitating relationship must allow the individual space and freedom for this to occur.

In visiting a multiproblem family for the first time, I ran into problems with my own feelings at the very start. Mrs. O. is very obese, and I place a very high value on physical fitness. Mrs. O.'s house is in a state of total chaos—it appears that nothing is in place or even has a place. The entire house is very dirty and the smells are most unpleasant to me. I was repulsed by the conditions of the house and even by Mrs. O. herself. When I thought of trying to see the world through the client's eyes, I felt a little afraid and very reluctant. If I *really* saw her world through her eyes, how could I justify my own world: and if I felt this need for justification, how helpful could I be to her? If I saw her world through her eyes, would my feelings of compassion be touched, and would I not then perhaps be vulnerable to demands I could not meet?

As I made more visits to her home, I still had not come face to face with these feelings, and I could tell that my goal of forming a relationship with her that would increase her self-esteem was far from being met.

However, I found my regard for her was increasing as I observed her interacting with her children, and by their responses to her. She showed obvious pleasure in being with them, in playing with the baby, and in talking with each of them about their activities. The youngest, who is eighteen months, was born six weeks prematurely, and she was concerned about his developmental progress. I suggested a DDST and she agreed. It was during the administration of this test that our relationship became closer. Our mutual focusing on this child and the shared pleasure of seeing him perform each of the activities brought a dimension to our relationship that helped me to overcome some of my earlier negative feelings.

DISCUSSION

1 Was the client-centered approach an appropriate one in this case study?
2 Are there other theories or approaches that might have been used successfully?
3 Explain how the relationship with a client affects each step of the nursing process.
4 Were principles of learning evident in this case study?

A Family with a Newborn Baby

A description of a young family with a new baby who had been visited by a beginning student in community health nursing was written as follows:

Mrs. H. is an eighteen-year-old pale young girl with bangs hanging to her eyes, who was startled to have a nurse visit but accepted it compliantly. She stated that she had never had a nurse visit her before. She lives in a housing project and has two kittens. She states she feels OK. Her breasts have been engorged, but she has been wearing tight bras, and the discomfort is lessened. Her flow has been intermittent, varying from light to heavy. She admits to tensions, varying at times, because she wants to be a good mother. She says she gets enough rest. She does not want to be the same kind of mother as her own mother. She has done a lot of babysitting and likes having her own baby. Mrs. H. likes to read, but not books about mother-child care. She seems lonely. She was encouraged to give the baby a lot of love and not worry about spoiling the infant.

D. is a normal-appearing contented newborn who sleeps 3–4 hours and drinks 3–3½ ounces of formula every 3–4 hours. Birthweight: 6 pounds ¾ ounces. Mother is concerned about dry peeling skin and has been applying lotion. Skin appeared soft and nonpeeling to nurse. Baby was dressed warmly. Cord dropped off today. Mother plans to see physician this weekend. Would like to have cereal added to diet. Mrs. H. agreed to another visit next week.

DISCUSSION

1 How might this visit be converted to the problem-oriented style of recording?
2 What would be your plan for the next visit with this family?
3 Did the nurse give satisfactory service on this first visit to a "new" family?

Clarifying Nursing Visits

In meeting a family for the first time who had had nursing visits for the purpose of assisting with disciplinary measures with the children, I had this experience.

K. greeted me at the door and asked me into the dining area. She offered some tea, and while she was fixing it, she quite candidly asked me what the community health nurse is supposed to do. I was a little surprised by the question and in answering it, I simply told her that it was primarily up to the person or members of the family to decide or determine what kind of help was needed or what they wanted the community health nurse to help them with. She explained how the nurse happened to visit in the first place. When she had B. (one year old) at the pediatrician's for his immunizations, she mentioned to the doctor that some days she felt like she could discard the kids, especially S. (two and one-half years old). The pediatrician asked her if she would like a nurse to visit her and give some suggestions on how to manage the kids. She consented to have this done. Then she went on to explain what the nurse had done thus far. On her visits, the nurse had asked a few questions, commented about the sweet kids, given advice on how to handle S., marked things down on a clipboard, and left.

DISCUSSION

1 How would you clarify the purpose of nursing visits with clients?
2 Explain the bearing that perception has on relationships and interpretation of behavior.

A Family with Communication Problems

Mrs. A. is a nineteen-year-old mother of two children. She acts immature for her age and has had great difficulty just getting through the ninth grade (most of her school work was at a failure level). Mr. A. is presently unemployed. The family live with Mrs. A.'s parents and are on welfare for support. The oldest child is a little boy of three years and was born before the couple were married. He is not Mr. A.'s son. The second child is a little girl of eight months who is Mr. A.'s daughter. This child was diagnosed as having hydrocephalus. At the birth of the little girl, Mr. A.'s mother began blaming Mrs. A. for all the baby's problems.

On my first visit with Mrs. A., I sat on the front steps with her and devoted my attention to her. I listened to what she had to say and how she was feeling about her situation. She seemed depressed (did not smile much, kept her head down, and frowned whenever she spoke of her mother-in-law). In talking with her I could tell she had some very angry feelings toward her mother-in-law, as was indicated by gritting her teeth and by her glare. She said she could not talk to her mother-in-law about the baby's defect because her mother-in-law kept blaming her and making her feel guilty. I asked her if she did feel guilty. She replied, "No, not really." The reason she gave was because the doctors had told her it was a birth defect and that she was not to blame. I asked her if she was sure she felt this way, as she had been a little hesitant in her answer. She then said, "Yes," but that she felt bad because it was hard to take the blame which came from her mother-in-law. I agreed with her that it indeed would be hard to take. She said that the doctor had written Mr. A.'s mother a letter explaining about the baby's defect, and that she and her husband had tried talking with the mother-in-law; however, nothing seemed to change the mother-in-law's opinion that Mrs. A. was to blame. Mrs. A. said she was unable to communicate any longer because it always ended up with a lot of yelling and name-calling which emphasized the bad feelings between them.

In later visits, as I got better acquainted with Mr. and Mrs. A., I observed their supportive relationship with each other and Mrs. A's increasing acceptance of the baby, which was demonstrated by the spontaneity with which she played and talked with the baby. Imagine my surprise when, about this time, Mr. and Mrs. A. asked if I would please talk with the mother-in-law and see if somehow I could help her understand about the baby's condition. My first thought was, "You have got to be kidding, ME?—when already doctors have tried talking with her?" I told them I would see what I could do.

DISCUSSION

1 Describe examples of behavior description evident in this case situation.
2 Describe examples demonstrating the nurse's use of therapeutic interactions.
3 How would you plan a contact with the mother-in-law?

A Potentially "Abusing" Family

The L. family had initially been referred for a community health nursing visit by Dr. T., who wanted the nurse to assess the home situation for child-abuse potential. The baby boy in ten months' time had been cared for by Dr. T. in regard to a skull fracture, frequent bruising, allergy, and two episodes with pneumonia requiring hospitalization. The first community health nurse made a contract with Mrs. L. to visit the home to see how R. (baby boy) was recovering from his latest problem. Mrs. L. agreed to this, and the nurse made several visits to the home. At this point in time, the case was assigned to a student nurse.

After several home visits, my assessment of the family and observations of behavioral dynamics are described as follows:

N., the mother, has attractive hair and facial features. She has a flawless complexion but is obese, having a weight of 167 pounds and a height of 5'2". She is open to talking about herself and the family. N. was raised with a lot of responsibility and feels this is how children learn to cope with life. In the home many fragile and dangerous items are left out. N. will say "No, No!" to R. repeatedly as a warning not to touch something. If he touches it and the object breaks, she spanks him. If he hurts himself, she says to him, "I told you that you were going to hurt yourself." The baby is walking and bumping into things quite frequently. When he falls and hurts himself, he does not get picked up. If N. does anything at all, she will get him a bottle of juice and put it by him on the floor.

R. is a ten month old, pale, tense-looking baby. He is advanced for his age level developmentally. When he walks and falls, he really whacks his head frequently but rarely cries. If his mother screams at him, he just throws himself on the floor and bangs his head a few times. He has a phony kind of smile. He rarely smiles spontaneously. He will reach for his mother when he hurts himself. He is allowed to play with the coasters on the living room floor. The house is full of hazards. As an example, on my first visit, he fell off the rocker once, teetered and hit his head on the corner of the coffee table, hit his head on the stone corner of the fireplace ledge, and fell down, hitting his head again. After this episode, N. did nothing—as if the baby did not exist. R almost never verbalizes anything, unless it is with the cat.

C. (the five year old sister) is tan, attractive, slim, average height, and cannot pronounce some of her consonants because of a hearing loss due to colds. N. related C.'s daily tasks to me—feeding R. and getting him up, changing diapers, vacuuming his and her bedrooms, dusting the house, and feeding the animals. C. starts school this fall, and N. related she will really miss all the help around the house. C. picks out her clothes for each day and has always had matched clothing. C. seems devoted to her brother, giving him the physical affection he does not get from his mother. She will pick him up and carry him, although he is half her size. She looks out for him. When R. cracked his head on the corner of the coffee table again, C. put her hands on her hips, walked up to her mother pointing at the table, and told her mother that it was a "bad coffee table." N. relates there is only one thing with which she has trouble with C., and that is when C. just will not stop going up to R. and hugging him after she (N.) has disciplined him. C. minds well, seems to love her mother, and is happy.

B., the father, is 5'5", good-looking, medium build, and very quiet. He is very attentive to N., carrying in the groceries for her and performing similar activities. There is no physical greeting such as a kiss or hug when he returns from work. He is unassuming, affectionate with the children, plays with the children, and substitutes other toys for R. if R. is not to play with a particular toy.

DISCUSSION

1 Is this family a potentially abusing one?
2 What other information do you need to complete your assessment of the family?
3 What communication theory might be useful in working with this family?
4 What would be your approach as a helping person in working with this family?

Need—A Factor in Learning

The director of a home for single pregnant mothers asked a community health nurse to discuss venereal diseases with the young women in the home. The group ranged from thirteen to thirty years in age, with a median age of sixteen. The nurse, recognizing that this was a difficult assignment, prepared her outline with much care.

On the evening of the meeting, the group filed into the dayroom, looking bored and uninterested. They listened politely but with little change of expression. After about ten minutes, the nurse, seeing that they were not interested in what she was saying, brought the talk to a close and asked for questions. There was silence; then the thirteen-year-old girl raised her hand timidly and asked, "What kind of diapers do you think are best, the three-cornered ones or the long ones?" Realizing that the question indicated what the young women were interested in, the nurse hastened to answer the question. Before she had finished, other questions on baby care and growth and development came so fast that there was not time to answer them all, and she promised to return another evening.

DISCUSSION

1 What principles of learning were operating here?
2 What principles were not operating?
3 Since these young women had been exposed to venereal disease, would you have accepted the director's request for such a talk? Give reasons for your answer.
4 Outline the content of a talk to young people on venereal diseases.

Syphilis in an Itinerant Family

An itinerant construction worker, with his pregnant wife and two children, was en route from one job to another in a car and trailer. Late in the evening, while they were traveling on a lonely mountain road, the mother commenced her labor. The father ran to a nearby ranch house to inquire for the nearest hospital and was told that it was 30 miles down the valley but that there was a doctor in a small town 2 miles away. The rancher offered to call him.

The doctor arrived in time to deliver the patient by candlelight in the trailer. The delivery was quick and easy. He recommended that the family not move on for a few days and promised to ask the community health nurse to call in the morning.

The next morning the doctor called the local health department to request a nursing visit to the family, for the purpose of bathing mother and baby and checking their conditions. The nurse found them without difficulty. She bathed the baby. His physical condition aroused suspicions in the nurse. Then, while bathing the mother, the nurse noted some signs and symptoms which she thought might be caused by secondary syphilis. (Later, laboratory findings confirmed the nurse's suspicions.)

DISCUSSION

1 What steps should the nurse take at this point? List them in order of importance.
2 What precepts of community health nursing were important to observe in this case?
3 Name some possible signs and symptoms of secondary syphilis that the nurse might have observed while bathing this mother.
4 What symptoms might the nurse have observed in bathing the baby?

A Family with an Alcoholic Member

During a teacher-nurse conference one afternoon, the teacher mentioned Jean N.'s periodic absences from school for no apparent reason and said that she was falling behind in her schoolwork.

"I used to have her brother, Jimmie, in my class last year," the teacher commented, "and he was absent this way, too. Usually the mother telephones that the children will not be in school that day, but gives no reason. They come on the school bus, and I've asked the driver if he knows anything about them. He said the mother told him if the children were not at the bus stop in the morning not to wait for them. I'm sure it's not a matter of money, they are always nicely dressed. Do you think a home call would be in order?"

The nurse agreed that it would be; she, too, had wondered about the children lately, as neither of them looked well and both seemed unhappy. She planned for a home call that afternoon.

The nurse found the home, a large well-kept farmhouse, about 15 miles from the school. Mrs. N., a neat-looking somewhat tense woman, answered the nurse's knock. The two children were with her. The nurse introduced herself and was invited into a pleasant living room. The mother was courteous but unresponsive. She gave some vague excuses for the children's absences. After about ten minutes, the nurse, realizing that nothing was being accomplished, took her leave, baffled by the situation. She made another home call en route to her office. It was nearly five o'clock when she reached her desk, to find a note to call Mrs. N. as soon as she came in. Somewhat puzzled, the nurse returned the call. Mrs. N. was almost sobbing as she said, "I didn't know what to say to you this afternoon. My children and I are in great trouble. My husband is really a very good man, but often he drinks too much, and then I have to keep the children home on those days to help me with the chores. Could you come back in the morning to see me?"

The nurse promised to do so, and made an appointment for about ten-thirty the next day.

DISCUSSION

1 What should the nurse include in her preparation for the next day's visit?
2 How should the nurse approach the situation?
3 In reporting back to the teacher, what information should be shared with her regarding the family?
4 What can a nurse contribute to a family faced with problems due to alcoholism?
5 List the official and nonofficial resource agencies available in your community for helping a family with this sort of problem.

A Family's Reaction to Death

In May, Mrs. B. brought Mark to a preschool registration conference. While talking to the community health nurse, Mrs. B. said she expected a new baby early in October. When the nurse offered to call to help her plan for the baby, Mrs. B. eagerly accepted.

The nurse found the family living in an attractive duplex in a pleasant area, one block from the school. They had lived in this home about a year. Mr. B., age thirty, had been a federal government employee for the past nine years. He had been attending night school classes at a nearby college. The nurse did not meet him, but from his wife's comments, he appeared to be conscientious, stable, and intelligent. He helped at home when he could, took the children to the park to play, and seemed to understand the importance of physical and emotional health.

Mrs. B., twenty-eight, was a bright, energetic woman with a variety of interests, her main ones being her family and their welfare. The children, Eileen, seven, and Mark, five, appeared to be normal, healthy, and active.

Although Mrs. B. had seen her physician several times, she had questions relating to her pregnancy and was interested in having help. Her other pregnancies had been normal, and she had breast-fed her babies. With this pregnancy, she experienced great fatigue and was completely exhausted by evening. This concerned her. As she was talking, she suddenly interrupted herself and said, "I should tell you why we are having this baby, and why it is so important to us."

She explained that five months previously, their fourteen-month-old daughter had died of sudden infant death syndrome. She said that she and her husband did not talk about the tragedy, but that both of them got up at repeated intervals during the night to check and recheck that Eileen and Mark were all right. Since the accident, Eileen had refused to mention her baby sister, had frequent nightmares and unexplained severe crying spells, once at school. The doctor had ordered sedatives for her. The neighbors were supportive and included the family in their social activities.

The physician had advised the parents, shortly after the death, to consider having another baby as soon as possible.

DISCUSSION

1 How can Mr. and Mrs. B. be helped to accept the loss of their little daughter and to accept the new baby?
2 Is the frequent checking on the children during the night by the parents a normal reaction five months after the death?
3 What could be done to help Eileen overcome her sense of grief and loss?
4 Assume the role of the nurse. What is your reaction to this family's problems?

Cuban Refugee Family

Mr. F., age forty, laborer
Mrs. F., age thirty-five, mother
Manuel, age fifteen
Tito, age fourteen
Rosita, age twelve
Carlos, age seven, patient (cerebral palsy)
Maria, age five
Juan, age three
Panchita, new baby

The F. family, Cuban refugees, was referred by their social worker to the nursing service of the city-county health department. She reported that Mrs. F., about seven months pregnant, had been in the county hospital for a week because of high blood pressure, and was being discharged that day. The social worker said the parents spoke little English. They were living in a three-bedroom apartment in a large public housing complex. The family was Protestant.

Visit 1 The nurse made a home visit the next day. Talking in broken Spanish and English with Mr. and Mrs. F., the nurse learned that the family had been in the United States less than a year. In Cuba, Mr. F. had made a fairly comfortable living as a fisherman and had had additional employment in a factory. The family escaped from Cuba in Mr. F.'s small fishing boat, which was wrecked off the Florida coast. Two of their children were lost in the accident. After a short stay in Miami, the family moved to the West Coast. At the time of the nurse's visit, Mr. F. did not have steady employment and the family had been on welfare for three months. The three elder children attended a nearby grade school but were not doing well because of language difficulties.

During the visit, the nurse became aware of strange gutteral sounds and an unusual crying. Mrs F. finally left the room and returned with Carlos in her arms. The child was undersized, emaciated, unable to walk, and had uncontrolled head movements. The nurse thought he had a cerebral palsy condition. Throughout the visit, Maria and Juan clung, whimpering, to their mother and watched the nurse fearfully.

The nurse reviewed the doctor's orders for Mrs. F. regarding diet and rest with Mr. and Mrs. F. and felt there was little more she could do at the time because of language difficulties. She promised to return in a week. As she was leaving, the Protestant minister arrived. The nurse explained to him that her knowledge of Spanish was insufficient for her to help the family as she wished to do, and asked if there were someone who might act as interpreter. He suggested Mrs. L., a neighbor who spoke English and Spanish fluently and would be acceptable to the family.

Later The nurse called on Mrs. L., a friendly young woman of Spanish-American descent. She said she and her husband felt sorry for the F. family. Her husband had tried to help Mr. F. find work, but his lack of knowledge of English made it difficult. Mrs. L. worked part-time in a neighborhood grocery store. She said if the nurse could arrange her visits to the family when she was free, she would do all she could to help. She gave the nurse her telephone number.

Later The nurse reported to the social worker, who had not known of Carlos' condition. She offered to work with the nurse in getting him to the children's clinic for a diagnosis.

Later The nurse telephoned the school nurse, who reported the children were absent a great deal and were seriously handicapped in their school work by their lack of English. The teachers were concerned and wished the children could have extra help in learning English.

Visit 2 With Mrs. L.'s help, the nurse had arranged for another visit to the family a week later. With an interpreter, the nurse found it easier to build interpersonal relationships. She discovered Mrs. F. had been eating some foods not on her prescribed diet, but thought this resulted from a misunderstanding. With Mrs. L.'s help, she was able to explain the importance of following the doctor's orders. The nurse told the parents that the social worker had made a tentative appointment for Carlos at the children's clinic the latter part of the next week if they could take him at that time. The parents quickly agreed, and Mrs. L. said she would either take them herself or find someone who could provide transportation.

Later The nurse confirmed the appointment with the social worker and notified Mrs. L.

Because of unusual pressure of work in the agency, the nurse was unable to visit the family for two weeks. However, she telephoned Mrs. L., who said the family had taken Carlos to the clinic and that institutional care had been recommended for him. The family was given an application to River Falls, a state school for handicapped children about 20 miles away. A neighbor had taken them to visit the school and they were satisfied that Carlos would have good care there, and they were eager to file an application and wanted the nurse's help in filling it out. Several days later, Mrs. L. phoned to say that Mrs. F. had been taken to the hospital by ambulance, and had had a baby girl by caesarean section. Mrs. F.'s condition was good and she was expected home in a few days.

Later The school nurse telephoned that the F. children had been absent for several days and wanted to know if they were ill. The nurse explained that Mrs. F. was in the hospital for delivery and thought it was possible Mr. F. had kept them at home. She planned a visit soon and would let the school nurse know if the children were ill.

The nurse learned that a summer "head start" program would begin soon at the school and that Maria would be eligible and also that there were plans to offer English classes for the foreign-born at the school building in the evenings during the summer.

Visit 3 When the nurse and Mrs. L. called they found the children had returned to school. Mr. F. had kept them at home during Mrs. F.'s hospitalization because he was lonely and afraid. With the help of their minister, they had filled out Carlos' application for River Falls, and mailed it, and were waiting to hear from the institution. The nurse explained the "head start" program for Maria and the English classes for the parents and older children. Mrs. F.'s condition appeared good. She was obviously trying hard to follow the doctor's orders and the prescribed diet. Panchita appeared to be a normal, healthy baby.

Visit 4 A few days later, as the nurse was in the neighborhood, she stopped to see Mrs. F. and check on her clinic appointments. When Maria saw the nurse, she ran out the door and soon returned with Mrs. L. Mrs.

F. showed the nurse a letter from River Falls to the effect that Carlos was on the waiting list, and that there would be a place for him in about a month. Mrs. L. and Mrs. F. had a conversation in rapid Spanish. Then Mrs. L. explained that Mr. and Mrs. F. felt that they should not have any more children, and could the nurse tell them of a clinic where they could go for help. The nurse explained about the planned parenthood clinic and gave Mrs. F. a card to the clinic. The nurse arranged for a call about a month later.

Visit 5 Mr. and Mrs. F. were home when the nurse called. Mr. F. had found work as a fisherman and thought it would be permanent. He had arranged for time off so that he could be home when the nurse called. Manuel and Tito had summer jobs, thanks to Mrs. L.'s help and that of their minister. Carlos had been admitted to River Falls. A neighbor had taken them to visit him, and they were happy with the care he was receiving. They and the older children were attending the evening classes and Maria was enrolled in the "head start" program. The parents had attended the planned parenthood clinic. Mr. F. hoped they would be able to go off welfare the following month. The nurse urged Mrs. F. to take the preschool children to the children's clinic for immunizations. It appeared to the nurse that this family had achieved a certain amount of independence and could probably handle future health problems. She left her card and asked the family to call the nursing service if a need arose.

Later The nurse reported to the social worker and the school nurse that she had closed the case, as Mr. and Mrs. F. now seemed able to manage their own situation. Case closed.

DISCUSSION

1 What resources did this family appear to have within itself?
2 What emotional problems might you expect this family to have as a result of their experiences since leaving Cuba?
3 Should the nurse have closed the case when she did? Why?

Infant Health Supervision

Mr. H., age twenty-six, laundry driver
Mrs. H., age twenty-three, housewife.
Tommie, age four months.

A student nurse made the visit described here. She wished to do a self-evaluation of her call, and wrote it up on a process recording basis.

Purpose of visit   On my previous visit I had suggested that Mrs. H. attend the well-baby clinic with Tommie, which she did. On this visit I planned to discuss the clinic experience and any problems that Mrs. H. might have in caring for her baby.

Introduction   Mr. and Mrs. H. are high school graduates and have been married for two years. They are buying their home, which is in an old part of the city, in a middle-class neighborhood and close to a college where Mr. H. attends night school. He hopes to be a certified public accountant some day. Prior to her marriage, Mrs. H. worked for the telephone company. She is an intelligent young woman, eager to learn to care for her first child.

The visit   Mrs. H. greeted me warmly at the door, but then her facial expression became one of grave concern. After we were seated, Mrs. H. opened the conversation.

Mother-Nurse Verbal and Nonverbal Exchange and Interaction

Nurse Comments and Analysis

Mrs. H.: Last week at the well-child clinic, the doctor took my baby's diaper and handed it to the nurse. He told her to do a PKU test. At the time I didn't think to ask him what that meant, but I have been wondering: does this mean he thinks something is wrong with my baby?

Mrs. H. was obviously quite anxious about this test and the baby's health. I wondered if the test were the real cause of her anxiety or if she had some other reason for inquiring. I needed more information before answering her question.

Nurse: You're concerned about your baby's health?

This interpretation would allow Mrs. H. to expand upon the problem further, and allow me to evaluate it.

Mrs. H.: Yes, I am [Silence, but she seemed to want to say more.]

I nodded, telling her nonverbally to go on.

Mrs. H.: You see I've been leaving the window open in the bedroom at night because the baby's been perspiring so much. My husband keeps telling me the baby is going to get sick sleeping in that draft, and I knew deep down he was right. When I went to the clinic I was afraid the doctor would find something wrong with him.

It seems Mrs. H. may feel guilty that she might have caused an illness in her baby. Before clarifying her first question I wanted information about the general condition of her baby in order to relieve her fears.

Nurse: I see.

This was said in an understanding tone to let her know that I understood her explanation.

Nurse: What did the doctor say about Tommie's health?

I wanted to ascertain if the baby had a cold or other symptoms that could be related to the draft.

Mrs. H.: Oh, he said the baby was in absolutely perfect health and gaining weight.

The mother smiled for the first time—she seemed very pleased.

Nurse: That's fine, Mrs. H.

I shared in her delight and showed my approval.

Mrs. H. (her face clouded): I was so happy until I came home and remembered that PKU test. What does it mean?

She still may have connected the test with the draft in the bedroom, and now was the time to clarify this misunderstanding of her initial question.

Nurse: Do you remember, Mrs. H., when you had your chest x-ray at the health department?

I knew she had had an x-ray for tuberculosis.

Mrs. H. (puzzled): Yes, but that was a routine check for TB. My baby doesn't have TB, does he?

I was going to use this to correlate it with her baby's test, and I accepted her momentary puzzlement.

Nurse: No, but you see, just as you had a routine x-ray to check for tuberculosis, so the PKU test is a routine check for a disease in children called phenylketonuria.

I was going from the known (her own x-ray) to the unknown, the PKU test, so that she could understand better.

Mrs. H.: What does that mean?

Mother wants more explanation.

Nurse: Well, remember when we talked about the importance of protein, fats, and sugar foods in the diet?

Again, I attempted to enable the mother to recall what she knew in order to help her understand this condition.

Mrs. H.: Yes, I understand that.

She was eager for me to go on and I now knew she was following and understanding my explanation so far.

Nurse: This disease is concerned with proteins. Before they can be used to build strong bodies they have to be broken down to smaller parts, and to do this there is a substance called an enzyme. Do you understand so far?

Mrs. H.: Yes, I think I do. What you're saying is that a substance breaks proteins down in order to give my baby a strong body.

This feedback from Mrs. H. was evidence that she understood and was able to relate her learning to incident concerning the baby.

Nurse (smiling): That's right. In the disease phenylketonuria this substance, or enzyme, that breaks down a particular part of the protein isn't there and can't be used by the body. Therefore this part of the protein keeps building up in the body and can cause brain damage. Some of it comes out in the baby's urine, too, and that's one way to know if the baby has the disease. Do you understand so far?

I wanted to show my approval.

I was explaining it in lay terms, but before proceeding I asked for indication of her understanding.

Mrs. H.: I see, then this is what the nurse was testing for?

Again, feedback from Mrs. H. showed she understood.

Nurse: That's right.

I smiled to show my approval.

Mrs. H.: Can the nurse do the test there, or did she take something off the diaper and send it somewhere?

It seemed she was worried that she might be informed later about the test, and was concerned about whether her baby had the condition.

Nurse: No, they do the test right away at the clinic. Do you remember when your mother stayed with you after she was told she had diabetes and you did her urinalysis for her—and how the urine changed color after you dropped the tablet into the tube?

Again going from the known to the unknown and using my knowledge of family history.

Mrs. H. (with interest): Yes.

Using correlation in explanation.

Nurse: They tested the baby's urine like that. They drop a testing solution on a small spot on a wet diaper, and if the spot turns green, they know the baby has the disease. That is, they are pretty sure of it.

Mrs. H.: Then my baby doesn't have it, because the nurse brought the diaper back, smiled at me, and didn't say anything. Come to think of it, it was after the nurse talked to the doctor that he came back and said Tommie was in perfect health. Oh! I feel so much better now that I understand it wasn't the draft that had anything to do with this.

Evidence she understood the test; she seemed happy—perhaps in knowing that the draft had caused no harm.

There was marked relief in her voice. I nodded.

My suspicions were confirmed, and this was the opportunity to deal with the draft problem, which I did.

Summary   Although Mrs. H. was concerned about the test for PKU, her concern stemmed from her guilt feelings about the draft. By allowing the mother to talk further about her feelings and not answering the question directly at the beginning of the visit, I found a problem that could be dealt with. After answering Mrs. H.'s questions about the test, I focused on the draft problem. It was discovered that Mrs. H. had kept the four wool blankets she had used during the winter months on Tommie's bed. She had not removed any of the blankets with the approaching spring weather, and this was the reason for the baby's perspiration. Hence the open window, which was creating a draft, would not be necessary if some of the blankets were removed. This action served two purposes: first, alleviating the draft on the baby, and second, alleviating the guilt feeling of Mrs. H. that she might cause the baby illness. Mrs. H. was pleased and happy at the end of the visit and appeared relieved. From the course of the discussion, Mrs. H. now also understood something about PKU. I planned to discuss it further with her next time so that she would be a well-informed mother regarding this current problem.

DISCUSSION

1 What purposes did this visit serve?
2 What principles of learning did this nurse utilize?
3 What concomitant learning is it reasonable to hope took place?
4 How does the process recording method help in self-evaluation?
5 Should or should not the nurse have completed the discussion of PKU (e.g., incidence, symptoms, treatment, and problems) on this visit? Why?

Getting Acquainted with a New Community

You are a seventy-year-old widow who is hardy, curious (nosy), and full of energy. You want to volunteer your services wherever there seems to be a need. You can do just about anything that a nonprofessional person does (cook meals, serve coffee, visit lonely people, babysit with handicapped persons, etc.).

You want to visit community facilities that may be interested in your volunteer services, i.e., senior service centers, handicapped children's facilities, nursing homes, free clinics etc. Or perhaps you want to get an idea about what elderly people do in this community for health, recreation, social outlets, or constructive activities?

Activity assignment   Find a variety of community facilities that may be responsive to receiving volunteer services from an able geriatric citizen. Visit these places and get a "feel" of the environment. Be prepared to report about these places in writing and verbally.

DISCUSSION

1   Describe briefly the community facilities that were visited.
2   Is the local community responsive to the needs of the elderly?
3   In general, how were your inquiries received in the local community?

Getting Acquainted with a New Community

You are a seventeen-year-old girl who has lived all aspects of the alternative life-style—meaning drugs, alcohol, sex, poverty, etc. You have a vaginal discharge that is getting worse, and you do not know where to go for medical help (or health care). You are considering going off drugs since you are fed up with the life you have been living. The guy you have been living with does not want you around anymore—he has a new girlfriend. If you go straight, who will help you?

Activity assignment   Visit a variety of community facilities that may be of assistance to you, i.e., free women's clinics, drug and alcohol information centers, health department, etc. Find out if these places are actually helpful for young women in distress. Be prepared to write a written report and/or describe your findings verbally.

DISCUSSION

1 Describe briefly the community facilities that were visited.
2 Is the local community responsive to the needs of youth?
3 In general, how were your inquiries received in the local community?

Getting Acquainted with a New Community

You are a young wife and mother who recently arrived in this community. Your husband is out of work but is making the rounds regarding job possibilities. Your child is sixteen-months-old, is developing normally, but tends to have too many bouts of U.R.I. You wonder if you are feeding the child on an adequate diet. You are in the second trimester of pregnancy and beginning to think about supplies needed for the new baby. You have just visited the office of social and health services (welfare) and received a check of ——. —— (the monthly allotment for a man, wife, and one child). You wish to rent an apartment or home and want to find one today. According to the welfare worker, you can pay up to —— a month for a place. The remaining —— should be enough for food since you can buy food stamps.

Activity assignment   Look for a place to live today that will not cost over ——. Look for a place that you think will satisfy your needs. Is there a grocery store nearby? How about a physician's office? Since your husband uses the car daily, are you able to walk to your destinations? Is there a play area outside that is satisfactory for your child? Do you like the looks of the neighborhood? Be prepared to report your findings in writing or verbally.

DISCUSSION

1 Describe briefly the activities undertaken in finding a place to live.
2 Was a suitable place found? If so, what criteria were used in making the selection?
3 Is the local community concerned about the needs of low-income families?

Index